The COVID-19 Pandemic an
East Asia

Using "risk" as a conceptual lens, this book analyzes how communities across East Asia responded to the disruption unleashed by the COVID-19 pandemic.

The contributors to this book look at how governments, societies, and individuals have perceived, experienced, dealt with, and interpreted the pandemic and the transformations it has brought across countries like Japan, South Korea, Taiwan, Vietnam, and the Philippines. They examine pressing concerns such as infodemic, digital health literacy, media cynicism, telework, and digital inequalities in conjunction with issues such as public trust, identity formation, nationalism, and social fragmentation. They look at a wide range of questions relating to communication, mediation, and reactions to the challenges of the pandemic.

An insightful resource for scholars of risk studies and of East Asian societies, the book is also a valuable reference for students and researchers of media and communication studies and sociology.

Nobuto Yamamoto is Professor at the Department of Politics, Keio University, Japan. His areas of research include politics and history of Southeast Asia, in particular Indonesia. He is the author of *Censorship in Colonial Indonesia, 1901–1942* (2019) and editor of many books in Japanese.

COVID-19 in Asia

COVID-19, Business, and Economy in Malaysia
Retrospective and Prospective Perspectives
Edited by Weng Marc Lim, Surinderpal Kaur and Chong Huey Fen

COVID-19, Education, and Literacy in Malaysia
Social Contexts of Teaching and Learning
Edited by Ambigapathy Pandian, Surinderpal Kaur and Chong Huey Fen

COVID-19, Psychology, and Social Behaviour in Malaysia
Psychosocial Effects, Coping and Wellbeing Strategies
Edited by D. Gerard Joseph Louis, Surinderpal Kaur and Huey Fen Cheong

The COVID-19 Pandemic and Risks in East Asia
Media, Social Reactions, and Theories
Edited by Nobuto Yamamoto

Covid-19 in South, West, and Southeast Asia
Risk and Response in the Early Phase
Edited by Mohd Mizan Aslam and Rohan Gunaratna

The COVID-19 Pandemic and Risks in East Asia

Media, Social Reactions, and Theories

Edited by Nobuto Yamamoto

Routledge
Taylor & Francis Group

LONDON AND NEW YORK

First published 2023
by Routledge
4 Park Square, Milton Park, Abingdon, Oxon OX14 4RN

and by Routledge
605 Third Avenue, New York, NY 10158

Routledge is an imprint of the Taylor & Francis Group, an informa business

© 2023 selection and editorial matter, Nobuto Yamamoto; individual
chapters, the contributors

The right of Nobuto Yamamoto to be identified as the author of the editorial
material, and of the authors for their individual chapters, has been asserted in
accordance with sections 77 and 78 of the Copyright, Designs and Patents
Act 1988.

British Library Cataloguing-in-Publication Data
A catalogue record for this book is available from the British Library

ISBN: 978-1-032-26137-9 (hbk)
ISBN: 978-1-032-26138-6 (pbk)
ISBN: 978-1-003-28668-4 (ebk)

DOI: 10.4324/9781003286684

Typeset in Galliard
by Deanta Global Publishing Services, Chennai, India

Contents

vi *Contents*

Figures

Tables

Contributors

Pauline Gidget Estella is Assistant Professor at the University of the Philippines and a PhD candidate at Technische Universität Ilmenau in Germany. Her research interests lie in the areas of journalism education, Global South studies, digital mis- and disinformation, and crisis communication. Ms. Estella has published academic articles on global journalism competence and digital populism, as well as expert analyses on the state of the Philippine media. She has served as a consultant for research in international organizations, like the European Journalism Centre, and a consultant for workplace communication training in government and private agencies in the Philippines.

Leticia Nien-Hsuan Fang is Associate Professor of Journalism at the National Chengchi University, where she teaches in-depth news reports, discourse analysis, and communication and culture. Her interests are in the field of mediatization, gender, and technology, and her recent works are about relations between digital sexual violence and misogyny. Her research into misogyny online and digital violence appears in several edited collections. More recently, she has been studying the overall prevalence rate of online gender violence in Taiwan and how the misogyny that takes place online is woven into the full fabric of daily communication.

Chiung-wen Hsu is Professor and Chair at the Department of Radio and Television, National Chengchi University, Taiwan. Research interests focus on the interdisciplinary study of disaster risk reduction and communication, media coverage of disaster and trauma, TV journalism, and Internet communication. She has published in the fields of disaster management, media studies, and Internet communication. In addition to her scholarly work, Professor Hsu has collaborated with the newsrooms, non-government organizations, and government agencies on a wide range of applied research and educational projects.

Samantha P. Javier is Lecturer at the Department of Communication in Ateneo de Manila University and De La Salle University, the Philippines. She also serves as a communication consultant to international development and private organizations. A paper that was based on her Master's Thesis bagged the

Best Paper Award at the 9th National Social Science Congress. It was recently published by the Philippine Social Science Council as a chapter in the book *Resilience in Our Times*. Her other academic publications cover media and information literacy and disaster literacy.

Jinah Lee is Professor at the Institute for Journalism, Media & Communication Studies, Keio University, Japan. Her areas of interest are advertising, consumer psychology, political communication, gender, and diaspora. She is the author of *The Content and Reception of Political Advertising* (Shinyosha, 2011, in Japanese) and a book chapter of *Routledge Handbook of Political Advertising* (2017). She has published journal articles and book chapters on media psychology research, focusing on Japan and Korea.

Kwangho Lee is Professor at the Department of Humanities and Social Science, Keio University, Japan. His research interests include media psychology of news and entertainment, news diffusion, and homeland media use of diaspora. He is the author of *Media as a "Territory"* (Keio University Press, 2016, in Japanese) and the co-editor of *Social Psychology of Media Audience* (Shinyosha, 2017, in Japanese). Recently, he has published journal articles and book chapters on the causes and consequences of media cynicism.

Chang-De Liu is Professor in the Department of Journalism at National Chengchi University, Taiwan. His research interests include (but not limited to) media and sports, globalization of sports, political economy of communication, and media policy. He has been the Chairman of the Board in the Reporter, a not-for-profit online media focusing on investigative journalism in Taiwan, and the Chairman of the Board in the Campaign for Media Reform, an advocacy group formed mainly by communication scholars.

Martin Löffelholz is Professor of Media Studies, Head of the International Crisis Communication Research Group at the Ilmenau University of Technology, Germany, and former President of the Swiss German University in Jakarta, Indonesia. Since June 2021, he has been a spokesperson for the DECIPHER research consortium, which analyzes the communication strategies of governments and healthcare institutions in Europe and the US on COVID-19. His research focuses on crisis communication, journalism, organizational communication, and international communication. He is the author or (co-)editor of more than 300 scholarly publications, including *The Palgrave Handbook of Cross-Border Journalism* (co-edited with Liane Rothenberger and David Weaver, forthcoming).

Fumie Mitani is Associate Professor at the Department of Journalism, College of Law, Nihon University, Japan. Her research fields are political communication, mass communication, and journalism studies. She is the author of the book *Media and Politics on History Issue in Japan* (Keiso, 2021, in Japanese) and has contributed chapters to the edited books, including *Routledge International Handbook on Electoral Debates* (Routledge, 2020) and *Media and Nuclear Energy in the Post-War Japan* (Minerva Shobo, 2017, in Japanese).

Tsung-Jen Shih is Associate Professor of the International Master's Program in International Communication Studies at National Chengchi University, Taiwan. His research scholarship centers around the communication of science, technology, health, and risks. His research topics range from cyberbullying to climate change. Recently, he has expanded his research program to COVID-19, with a specific focus on how misinformation shapes public reactions to the disease. Dr. Shih serves as an associate editor for *Environmental Communication* and the *Journal of Information Society*. From 2021 to 2022, he was a Fulbright visiting scholar at the Fairbank Center for Chinese Studies, Harvard University, the US.

Yun-Chung Tang is a PhD candidate at the College of Communication, National Chengchi University, Taiwan. His research interests include Internet community and behavior, Internet meme and troll, media literacy, genre film, and virtue ethics.

Violet B. Valdez is Associate Professor at the Department of Communication and Director of Ateneo Center for Asian Studies at the Ateneo de Manila University. She was the founding director of the Konrad Adenauer Asian Center for Journalism at the Ateneo. Recently she edited and co-wrote a reference on media and information literacy. Presently her research focuses on the digital divide and on journalism education in Myanmar and Indonesia. Dr. Valdez is a member of the editorial board of *Journalism and Mass Communication Educator* (JMCE), as well as other journals in communication and Asian studies.

Vu Le Thao Chi is Assistant Professor at the Faculty of Policy Management, Keio University, Japan. Her primary research areas include the study of risk and choice-making behaviors in everyday life, human security, policy analysis in poverty, public health, disabilities, among others. She is active in Vietnam, Japan, and other Southeast Asian countries. Her recent publications include *Agent Orange and Rural Development in Post-war Vietnam* (Routledge, 2020).

Yi Xu is a PhD candidate at the Institute of Media and Communication Science, Technische Universität Ilmenau, Germany. She is working as a research associate in the DECIPHER project funded by the German Research Foundation (DFG), which aims at comparing government communication, media discourses, and citizens' responses to COVID-19 in Europe and the US. Her research interests include journalism studies, visual communication, risk and crisis communication, and public diplomacy. She has published articles in leading journals with regard to multimodal news frames of national images, textual-visual frames in German news, China's digital diplomacy, as well as cultural and media diversity.

Shuzo Yamakoshi is Professor at the Department of Politics, Keio University, Japan. His research fields are journalism studies, political communication, and critical media studies. He is the author of *The Political Sociology of News* (Keiso Shobo, 2022, in Japanese), journal articles, and book chapters on media and journalism studies.

Nobuto Yamamoto is Professor at the Department of Politics, Keio University, Japan. His primary areas of research include the political history of Indonesia, nationalism in Southeast Asia, the Chinese diaspora in Southeast Asia, and international relations in Southeast Asia. He is the author of *Censorship in Colonial Indonesia, 1901–1942* (Brill, 2019), numerous journal articles, and book chapters on Indonesia and Southeast Asia, as well as editor of many books on the Southeast Asian region and beyond.

1 Introduction

Risk Society and the COVID-19 Pandemic in East Asia

Nobuto Yamamoto

Introduction

In his 1998 book *World Risk Society*, the German sociologist Ulrich Beck contends that we live in a global risk society (Beck, 1998). A viral outbreak in 2020, nearly a quarter-century later, appears to confirm Beck's assessment. The outbreak was brought by a highly infectious new coronavirus, officially named SARS-CoV-2, which caused a severe respiratory disease. As the disease was discovered in 2019, the World Health Organization (WHO) named it COVID-19, and as of March 2020, the outbreak was officially declared a global pandemic. By April 2022, when this introduction is written, the novel coronavirus has spawned many new variants, and its spread has not subsided. It marks a watershed in all our lives in the twenty-first century.

History shows that pandemics have affected society in many ways. In the past, humans have experienced a variety of pandemics, such as the bubonic plague, influenza, and malaria (Harper, 2021). In 2015, the International Risk Governance Council recognized pandemics as an emerging risk but not as a major risk then (IRGC, 2015). We have experienced two epidemics in the twenty-first century—the original severe acute respiratory syndrome (SARS) in 2004 and Middle East respiratory syndrome (MERS) in 2018, but they did not develop into a global pandemic. There was a more recent pandemic, the 2009 swine flu caused by the H1N1 influenza virus, which curiously is rarely brought up in the context of the COVID-19 pandemic. Instead, mainstream media tend to look back to the 1918 Spanish influenza pandemic as the most appropriate comparison to the devastation presently unleashed upon the world by a contagion (Honigsbaum, 2020). This comparison seems to underscore the scale of impact and severity of the COVID-19 pandemic, in that in terms of global and historical consequences, it is a public health crisis that only happens once in a hundred years.

By the time the present volume reaches the public, COVID-19 might have become less consequential and its grip on our daily lives relaxed. But we lose an important opportunity to learn if we let the pandemic goes by without reflecting on the way our society, though connected through by globalization, nevertheless responded to the crisis within the national frameworks. This volume reexamines the concept of risk society in connection with the COVID-19 pandemic. It

DOI: 10.4324/9781003286684-1

investigates how citizens and governments in five East Asian countries—namely Japan, South Korea, Taiwan, the Philippines, and Vietnam—received, perceived, and communicated the COVID-19 pandemic, which thus informed and shaped their responses to it.

Risk Society Reconsidered

In 1986, Beck coined the term "risk society" to describe modern globalized societies and the inherent risks they hold. He defines risk society as "a systematic way of dealing with hazards and insecurities induced and introduced by modernisation itself" (Beck, 1992, p. 21). Incidentally, it was in 1986 when the Chernobyl nuclear power plant accident unfolded to a stunned world. Its impact on the environment and public health became an immediate concern. In the past four decades, risk society has become a key term to describe the emergence of a new type of risk that is difficult to predict or anticipate how the risk itself evolves. As globalization progressed, Beck subsequently developed the idea of a risk society in the context of globalization (Beck, 1998; 2008). When the new coronavirus disease rapidly spread across the globe, many scholars, in particular sociologists, picked up this term to refer to the uncertainties brought by a full-blown global pandemic (e.g., Arias-Maldonado, 2020; Chernilo, 2021; Belayeth Hussain, 2022). Indeed, the concept of risk society seems convenient and suitable to the situation, but it is important to remind ourselves of the specific context in which Beck formulated this concept.

Beck's original intention with this concept was to question the historical process of modernity. Since the nineteenth century, modernity has increased predictability and certainty through scientific and technological progress and the accumulation of knowledge. The knowledge invented by social science was institutionalized for the purpose of public policy (Wallerstein, 1991). This historical process of modernization, Beck argues, has now reversed itself, and the expansion of science, technology, and knowledge has been bringing about new uncertainties. In his view, the modernization process was based on the idea that one could benefit from anticipating, diversifying, and controlling risk. In contrast, he argues that in modern times the nature of risk has been fundamentally transformed, and as a result, risk has unexpected and comprehensive consequences on a scale that involves the entire world. Beck notes that it is extremely difficult to predict and control the consequences of risk in advance. Herein lies the historical irony. As Anthony Giddens argues, risks are "manufactured uncertainty" by human beings (Giddens, 1994, p. 97); the new risks are risks created by human knowledge and technology. As the world becomes more complex and interconnected economically and politically, risks have become global, engulfing, and expanding the entire globe.

In the age of globalization, conventional administrative controls have been proven inadequate, if not ineffective, once risks become global. Theoretically and historically, in the traditional approach to control, social problems that impede the smooth operation of society are identified as potential risks. Their causes are investigated through statistical surveys. For the sake of public policy, targeted measures are formulated and then implemented. The effectiveness of the measures is later evaluated, and problems that need to be eliminated are identified. This cycle of administrative practice derives from a statistical picture of the world in which a large number of events can be observed, and the probability of occurrence of such events can be determined (Hacking, 1990). These administrative controls have helped create the welfare state in nineteenth-century Europe, which provides social security as a form of insurance policy. The welfare state functions as a hedge against social risks based on the statistical picture.

However, as a risk society entails uncertainty, the welfare state has not had the intended effect, because it fails to fulfill its role as the risk manager of society. Both the experts who serve as advisors of traditional administrative control and the administrative officers who function as the enforcers of policy are no longer the sole risk managers today, as we explain below (Beck, 1998, pp. 72–90).

Risk society compels both individual lifestyles and public decisions to change, and it may change how politics work in a country (Beck, 1998). The authority for risk perception, risk management, its evaluation, and decision-making will be taken away from experts and government officials, while a wide range of stakeholders, including citizens and NGOs, will be involved. A risk society, Beck argues, recreates politics through the revitalization of various forms of participation, which he calls subpolitics (Beck, 1998, pp. 91–108). By raising questions about existing institutional power, the idea of subpolitics suggests a radical reimagining of liberal democracy. Subpolitics does not take for granted statistical data about individual preferences or majority-based decision-making. Rather, it assumes that open information will reach individuals and that individuals will make decisions about social risks based on that information. It enables individuals to act both as risk managers and as risk-takers. Activating subpolitics may shed light on the development of risk societies.

Beck's argument about risk society and subpolitics leaves some questions unanswered. The way public and individual decision-making interact remains unclear. It is impossible to deny that individual decisions do not always match public decisions. In such a case, subpolitics itself could pose a new risk for society. However, Beck projects a possible democratic turn in subpolitics in confronting risks. Since subpolitics operates within national borders, he implies that risks should be managed at national and community levels. It is at this point that an individual has a political role to play. The concept of risk society raises the question of how individuals perceive and understand risks. As we learn from two classic novels below, individuals rely on the information they gather from neighbors and the authorities when they are confronted with unexpected dangers. When they lose trust in the government or doubt its ability to manage risks, they will turn to rumors and misinformation. This creates a new risk in society. It implies how risk is socially constructed in terms of reality.

We also need to remember that risk society has a national dimension—even when risks have become global. Each country has its own government, its own particular history, particular political and social culture, particular social infrastructures and systems, and particular citizenry. Information about a particular risk may circulate, but people may interpret it differently. People may have different attitudes toward it, depending on how they receive and comprehend related information and how they communicate in their community. Risk may exacerbate social division if a society is structurally and systematically divided before the risk occurs. As we learned during the COVID-19 pandemic, the social division triggered by it normally reveals the character of the society, as well as its preexisting risks.

COVID-19 Revisited

What is the COVID-19 pandemic, and what kind of risks are associated with it? In sum, it is the kind of pandemic whose magnitude in terms of consequences is measured centennially, thus the frequent comparison with the 1918 Spanish flu pandemic. COVID-19 has changed the way people live in fundamental ways. It spread rapidly and globally within a few months due to the mobility and interconnectedness afforded by globalization. There was little knowledge of the new virus or how to contain it, so in the first few months of its detection, COVID-19 not only cost many lives, it felt exceptionally threatening. On January 30, 2020, the WHO declared the outbreak a Public Health Emergency of International Concern but took more than a month to officially declare it a pandemic. The delay indicated, if not added, much of the uncertainty regarding the new disease. As COVID-19 spread to various parts of the globe, toward the end of 2020 major mutations of the new coronavirus became the cause for concern. In late 2020, the Alpha variant took over the original one in some parts of the world, while in 2021 the Delta variant became dominant, only to be upstaged months later by the Omicron variant. As of April 1, 2022, there have been more than 486 million cases of COVID-19, including more than six million deaths (WHO, 2022).

The COVID-19 pandemic reflected the way states and societies perceived risks. To tackle it, almost all governments introduced a series of lockdowns internally and closed or heavily restricted national borders—measures which all but halted ordinary economic activities and local and transnational mobility. People were compelled to wear masks when they were out in public spaces and to maintain a physical distance from others. From early 2021, COVID-19 vaccines became available, and there was hope that it was the best and quickest way out of the crisis before effective medicines could be produced. But even after more than 11 billion vaccine doses were administered by the end of March 2022 (WHO, 2022), the pandemic has not subsided. Along the way, the so-called "vaccine nationalism," which led wealthy countries to prioritize their population and therefore monopolize early batches of the vaccines, has hampered the global battle against COVID-19. As a consequence, developing nations were lagging in terms of vaccination rates. In the face of a highly infectious disease that has made national borders meaningless, each country in effect has adopted policies and measures to contain it in ways that are only applicable or beneficial nationally. Only after studies and data showed that the Omicron variant that had replaced the Delta was milder in terms of effects that the situation appeared to change; from February 2022, a number of countries in Asia and the West began to relax restrictions and attempted to get back to "normal" life, even as the Omicron sub-variant (BA.2) proved to be even more infectious than its predecessor.

In the era of the COVID-19 pandemic, we have gone through the "new normal." Some of the changes are so profound that it is simply not possible to expect a return to pre-pandemic form. Under the new circumstances, societies have adapted in various ways. Many of the measures taken to mitigate the spread of infection such as lockdown, distancing, and masking were effective to a certain extent. But the more people adapt to living with the threat of COVID-19, the more they become resistant to measures that disrupt their day-to-day activities and personal comfort. This has put a growing number of citizenries in opposition to their governments, which remain obliged to change, even tighten, the policies to contain the pandemic whenever new variants emerge. The shifting policies, as governments are compelled to adapt to the latest data on COVID-19, have contributed to the anxiety and distrust among citizens toward the authorities. The pandemic has demonstrated that scientific information is difficult to revise once circulated, while distrust breeds misinformation that is rampant on social and alternative media. Rifts in society have materialized, among others between a segment of the population who takes COVID-19 to be a matter of life or death, and another who makes light of its effects on health even doubts its existence. While COVID-19 might be an all-encompassing affair in the last two years, people's reactions to it and their perceptions of risk related to it have been proved to be vastly varied.

Fiction Revived

The magnitude of the COVID-19 pandemic not only inspired comparison with a hundred-year-old plague, journalists and scholars from Europe to Asia reached into the past and to the realm of fiction for clues of how societies have emerged from the dark days of deadly plagues. In the early stages of the pandemic, when the end was far from sight, references to fiction—from science fiction to classic novels—featuring a plague in the storyline were frequent in publications as well as on social media chatter. Hoping to find answers, to comprehend the confounding situation, and ultimately to get a sense that, as in fiction, this plague too would eventually pass, many turned to novels and films on plagues.

Among the classics often invoked in connection with the COVID-19 pandemic, two novels stood out. One is Albert Camus' *The Plague* (*Le Peste*, 1947), and the other is Daniel Defoe's *A Journal of the Plague Year* (1722). *The Plague* especially has regained popularity during the pandemic. It certainly helps that Camus was a Nobel Prize winner in literature, and the straightforward title announces its relevancy to our plague-ridden time.

In *The Plague*, the epidemic takes place in the city of Oran. Oranians are utterly unprepared for it and have doubts concerning pestilences. Dr. Rieux in the novel fears that a "mysterious fever" is spreading in the city, compounded by a rising number of deaths. Convinced that this mysterious fever is a plague, he appeals to the authorities to take urgent measures. However, since the law and the government value formal words more than reality, instead of responding to the plague, they spend time discussing how to define the word "plague" and what impact it would have on social activities if the current fever were to be recognized as a plague. This prevents them from taking action to contain the plague. They fail to acknowledge the contagion as a plague, and the number of deaths in Oran swells before any effective countermeasures are put in place. The plague is finally recognized when a telegram arrives from the governor, who has been avoiding responsibility; the telegram orders the colonial governor to declare a plague situation and close the city, which is essential to seal off the entire city and quarantine it as a plague district—what we in today's parlance call a lockdown.

The bureaucratic blunder described in *The Plague* reminds us of the situation in 2020, at the height of uncertainties regarding COVID-19 (e.g., Banerjee, Sathyanarayana Rao, Kallivayalil, & Javed, 2020; Kabel, & Phillipson, 2021). The health and bureaucratic authorities in many countries were slow to recognize the seriousness of the disease. Many governments mishandled the situation, and very few received satisfactory marks from their citizens. The popularity of the 1947 classic and its translations was revitalized during the pandemic due to the parallels it offers. In Japan since February 2020, printing presses rushed to produce 360,000 copies of *The Plague* in Japanese translation, while in South Korea it became a top seller. The sudden popularity of *The Plague* is also witnessed in the United Kingdom (UK), Italy, and France (Saeki, 2020). In November 2021, the American publisher Knopf published the latest version of the English translation by Laura Marris (Camus, 2021).

Meanwhile, Defoe's *A Journal of the Plague Year*, published over two centuries before *The Plague*, drew less media attention overall (University of Nottingham, 2019; Yousif, Razzyq, & Nsaif, 2021), but Japan's public service broadcaster, NHK, featured it in four series in September 2020. The director of NHK believed that the novel was relevant to thinking and understanding what happened to people and society when the COVID-19 pandemic hit (NHK, 2020).

A Journal of the Plague Year is a novel featuring the great plague in London in 1665. It begins thus:

> It was about the beginning of September, 1664, that I, among the rest of my neighbours, heard in ordinary discourse that the plague was returned again in Holland; for it had been very violent there, and particularly at Amsterdam and Rotterdam, in the year 1663, whither, they say, it was brought, some said from Italy, others from the Levant, among some goods which were brought home by their Turkey fleet; others said it was brought from Candia; others from Cyprus. It mattered not from whence it came; but all agreed it was come into Holland again.

In writing fiction using a journalistic style, Defoe pioneered the modern novelistic technique of realism. His concern was to give a detailed picture of the turmoil in London under the grip of the plague. The story portrays the devastation of London from the standpoint of a single chronicler, the merchant H.F., who reports as the contagion unfolds. The originality of Defoe's description lies in the way he recreates what happens when a plague strikes a large city. The city dwellers become an uncontrollable horde of delusional people, who turn to phony astrologers and swindlers peddling questionable cures. The plague has in effect destroyed the social system that facilitates the flow of reliable information, and made people irrational. Defoe juxtaposes the arrival of the plague and the collapse of trust. Calling it social suicide, he criticizes the self-destructive responses of the panicked population, judging them worse than the horror of the plague itself.

In reading *A Journal of the Plague Year*, one sees a mirror of our contemporary society when it comes to irrational behavior in the face of a full-blown pandemic. We see Defoe's city dwellers in our neighbors and fellow citizens, terrified people who confronted COVID-19 by relying on their personal judgment rather than on the existing social trust system and expert advice. Some cast doubt on the advice of government officials and medical experts and chose to follow dubious information found on social media regarding how to cure COVID-19. Many acted in a self-centered manner rather than as responsible members of a community. These attitudes in themselves constitute a new risk in society.

Another thing we learn from the two classics is that in a time of uncertainty and great stress, information is difficult to control. In *The Plague*, the city authorities of Oran attempted to control information regarding the plague but ultimately fail, while in *A Journal of the Plague Year* the residents of London tend to rely on rumors and false information. In both stories, the technology of information is far less sophisticated compared to ours, and the scopes of information circulation are much smaller, i.e., French Algeria and the City of London. It is thus imperative to reflect on the potential consequences of our current digital communication technology and global information circulation, which is what our present volume will attempt to address in subsequent pages.

Organization of the Book

The COVID-19 Pandemic and Risks in East Asia: Media, Social Reactions, and Theories offers comparative and theoretical perspectives of the risks related to the COVID-19 crisis in East Asia. As a versatile concept, "risk" captures the way diverse communities (from national to urban and rural) perceive and respond to disruptive events, such as a pandemic. Owing to its versatility, the concept of "risk" is utilized to highlight often divisive responses to disruptive events. The key to perceiving and understanding risk is also communication. Risk and danger can be distinguished conceptually, according to Niklas Luhmann (Luhmann, 1993, pp. 1–31). Risk arises because a certain decision has been made, while danger can occur regardless of the decision. This book takes the pandemic as a risk that includes the concept of danger. As COVID-19 spreads through human contact, information about the potential risks associated with the disease is not shared equally and accurately. Information or misinformation influences perceptions of risk. Risk perception may in turn create additional risks for society. We believe that the book's strength lies in its emphasis on media as a vector of risk, as well as in its focus on East Asia.

Because of the emerging risk conditioned by the COVID-19 pandemic, since late 2020 studies in the fields of social sciences, in addition to medical and natural sciences, featuring the COVID-19 pandemic and the risk associated with it have begun to appear in English. Most of them draw cases from Western countries (e.g., Goyal & Gupta, 2020; Linkov, Keenan, & Trump, 2021; Mabille, 2021), while few pay attention to those in East Asia (e.g., Jing, Han, & Ogawa, 2021; Seneviratne & Muppidi, 2021), albeit the latter's comparative success in confronting COVID-19. This volume spotlights East Asian nations in the early phase of the pandemic. This phase matters because this was the time when neither the WHO nor the national governments had a clear picture of what exactly the COVID-19 contagion would bring about. During the initial phase, precisely due to the lack of authoritative sources of information concerning COVID-19, people were especially anxious and confused. The initial phase shaped much of the government, the media, and the public's perception of COVID-19. Despite early praises for their comparative success in containing COVID-19 in the first half of 2020—a stark contrast with Italy, the United States (US), or the UK—East Asian nations actually responded to COVID-19 in dissimilar ways and they each had their share of challenges.

The COVID-19 Pandemic and Risks in East Asia holds that risks must be understood as complex constructions of materiality, experience, embodiment, and practice. Five nations from East Asia are studied in this volume—Japan, South Korea, Taiwan, the Philippines, and Vietnam—with three paired comparisons. It examines how government, society, and individuals perceived, processed, and interpreted the pandemic through diverse forms of communication, which resulted in divergent perceptions and interpretations.

The volume consists of eleven chapters in which different approaches are used to address national issues related to COVID-19 in East Asian countries. Pandemic-related risks are discussed in some chapters from the perspective of communication studies and in others from a sociological standpoint. Each chapter employs empirical research methods, including interviews, surveys, and data analysis. Analyses and data illustrate the way government regulations responded to the pandemic, and how the public perceived and reacted to COVID-19 and related regulations. Based on their original data, some chapters have revealed that the conventional wisdom of communication studies does not stand.

The subsequent chapter by Martin Löffelholz, Pauline Gidget Estella, and Yi Xu introduces a comprehensive research mapping in the field of risk and crisis communication. Research on risk and crisis communication has evolved along with the rapid transformation of media environment over the decades. This chapter provides a comparative and global overview of the history of risk and crisis communication research to gain a better understanding of the role communications play in global and national risk societies. By addressing major works in the field, Chapter 2 illustrates key differences between mainstream "West" and Asia in terms of norms and perspectives. It demonstrates that many empirical studies in Asian countries have contributed to alternative and expanding perspectives in the field of study. The chapter also addresses critical issues, such as misinformation and disinformation, arising from today's increasingly sophisticated communication technologies.

East Asian countries fared comparatively well in the initial phase of the pandemic, but Taiwan received the most praise for its digital administrative measures. Chapter 3 showcases a successful case of risk management using digital technology. Chiung-wen Hsu and Yun-Chung Tang examine the Taiwanese government's strategy in dealing with the novel coronavirus and in particular the torrent of information it unleashed. With the spread of COVID-19 in early 2020, the term infodemic became a buzzword. It combines "information" and "epidemic" to refer to the rapid spread of accurate and inaccurate information about the disease, which inundated mainstream media outlets and social media from early on. The authorities in Taiwan however succeeded in controlling information by diligently refuting misinformation, even turning infodemic into political propaganda about the government's success in containing COVID-19. The nation's previous experiences with SARS in 2004 and MERS in 2018 have helped the government to swiftly install preventative measures. The chapter demonstrates how the Taiwanese government made use of the information technology and surveillance systems installed over the years.

In the digital age when information circulates globally, it is easy to overlook the fact that infodemic primarily takes shape within national boundaries. As in other countries, infodemic in Taiwan flourished on social networking sites. In Chapter 4, Tsung-Jen Shih details how social networking sites influenced the circulation and delivery of information about COVID-19. During the time of crisis, uncivil online messages, which Shih calls "noise," were abound on such sites in Taiwan, nevertheless did not develop into a social panic. In fact, Shih's data find that such "noise" indicated a heightened risk perception and public support for government policies and strategies in containing the pandemic.

The extent of public trust in the government is conditioned in part by history, as Vu Le Thao Chi demonstrates in Chapter 5. Vu makes a comparative analysis between Vietnam and Japan, whose governments adopted opposite approaches to tackle COVID-19; Vietnam imposed strict measures on people's activities, whereas Japan introduced only moderate restrictions. From Vu's interviews, we learn that citizens in the two countries perceived the COVID-19 threats differently, each shaped by their nation's history. The Vietnamese, who have a more recent memory of war, used combat terminologies when talking about the contagion. Their government also resorted to wartime rhetoric to garner people's support for its policies. In Japan, the Edo-derived custom of public courtesy helped secure public compliance with mitigating measures. Vu's study illustrates how the sense of the public can attenuate the development of risk in society.

COVID-19-related regulations have been in place for approximately two years, but social reactions to them vary from country to country. The varying responses have to do with the level of risk people perceive with regard to the contagion and with a country's past experiences with epidemics. In Chapter 6, Jinah Lee compares Koreans and Japanese in terms of digital health literacy and highlights the differences between the two populations in responding to information related to COVID-19. Her survey shows that Koreans' recent experience with MERS in 2018 has made them more cautious and respond more swiftly to the new contagion. Koreans in general were also more eager to search for information concerning COVID-19, while information avoidance was more noticeable among the Japanese. Japanese were also more likely to express fatigue and feeling overwhelmed by infodemic. Lee's findings underscore the importance of psychological factors and digital health literacy in a risky society.

While citizens in Korea and Japan responded differently to COVID-19 information, there is a similar tendency in the way people perceived the messengers. In Chapter 7, Kwangho Lee utilizes the concept of media cynicism to illustrate how citizens in Japan and Korea responded to mainstream media's coverage of COVID-19. In the conventional wisdom of media cynicism, the global decline in press credibility has contributed to the widespread rejection of mainstream media in favor of alternative media. During the pandemic, citizens turn instead to social media to obtain information, which thus affects their risk perception. Lee's surveys in Japan and Korea in 2021, however, do not support these assumptions. He remains cautious of the disruptive effects of media cynicism, which hinders the reception of appropriate risk information, especially in the era of pandemics.

The question of media alerts us to the fact that in the present media environments, our experiences are essentially mediated, and what we perceive to be "reality" is a construct of our media experience. This is what Shuzo Yakamoshi and Fumie Mitani explore in Chapter 8 by highlighting today's hybrid media system and its conditions, which thus shape the way people experience the pandemic. To understand mediated experience, they look at the role of emotions during the first wave of COVID-19 in Japan. In their study, they find that a sense of moral panic emerged among the audience of a popular TV information show that regularly featured COVID-19 and related government policies. Anxiety, fear, and anger were among the emotions that in turn shaped a collective identity among its audience. The effects of COVID-19 on identity formation are not limited to Japan as one recalls the phenomenon in the US where mask wearers tend to be Democrats, while the resistors tend to be Republicans (Leonhardt, 2022). Unlike in the US, however, pandemic-related emotions in Japan did not develop into social risks or social divisions.

In Taiwan, too, the COVID-19 pandemic had occasioned the opportunity for identity confirmation with the emergence of pandemic-related discourses of nationalism. In Chapter 9, Chang-de Liu discusses the Taiwan professional baseball, which reopened its 2020 season in April and became the only professional baseball event held at that time. Baseball is a popular sport in Taiwan, and the return of the professional season amid the pandemic was regarded as a national triumph over the viral threat. It is undeniable that Taiwan's geopolitical position in East Asia contributes to such nationalistic feeling. While the pandemic has exposed fissures in many societies, including problems such as racism and xenophobia, Liu reads the attendant nationalist discourses as symptoms of desire in the Taiwanese society for sovereignty and recognition in an increasingly globalized world.

While Liu's chapter focuses on the more constructive effect of the pandemic in terms of national cohesion in Taiwan, the study by Nien Hsuan Fang exposes a potential rift in society regarding sexual minorities. This has become a visible social risk that the pandemic divulged. In Chapter 10 Fang examines pandemic-related reports in Taiwan news media, in particular a newly coined term "special social cluster" to signify the chain of COVID-19 transmission among homosexuals. The special designation, adopted by local governments as well, has in effect revived the stigmatization of gay people in the first Asian country to legalize same-sex marriage. Fang's chapter offers in-depth interviews with gay people and their account of this turn of events.

Digital technology has quite often made the world seem like a flat, unvarying plain. The concluding chapter by Violet B. Valdez and Samantha P. Javier is a good reminder of the great digital divide that was acutely felt during the pandemic when many activities—from schooling to religious worship—moved online. In Chapter 11, Valdez and Javier present their study of women dwellers in a slum area of Manila who had to rely on the Internet for coping and survival, despite obvious limitations and challenges. Using mostly smartphones and tablets, they were able to provide their children with the necessary device to attend online classes, connect with their families, and enact their spirituality, among others. As we battle through the first great pandemic of the digital age, this chapter draws much-needed attention to the worsening digital inequalities and the risks they entail.

As we conclude our interrogation of the risks that the COVID-19 pandemic has brought to East Asian nations, we are acutely aware of the absence of China among the countries studied. There is no doubt that the book would have benefitted from studies of cases in China. We accept this shortcoming as a motivation to do further research on the topic that covers more regions of the globe. Our research has revealed unique social realities and reactions to the unprecedented risk of the COVID-19 pandemic in East Asia. Further explorations of other countries and other regions would only enrich our understanding of the diverse realities and reactions to risk.

Acknowledgments

This volume includes papers first presented online at the international conference "Risk Society and the Media in an Uncertain Age" on February 23, 2021, organized by Keio University Global Research Institute (KGRI) and co-sponsored by the formerly Japan Society in Journalism and Mass Communication. Since the volume focuses on the ongoing COVID-19 pandemic, all papers have been significantly revised and updated to reflect the most current situation. At the same time, fresh names have joined the book project to make the research and analyses more cohesive thematically. The 2021 conference was the final phase of the three-year-long international collaborative project "Risk Society and the Media" (2018–2021), which was a continuation of the "Crisis Reporting Project" (2015–2018) at KGRI. I would like to thank KGRI for their generous funding and support. The institutional collaborators for the two projects were the Department of Communication at Ateneo de Manila University (The Philippines), the College of Communication at National Chengchi University (Taiwan), (then) the Centre for Policy Research on Science and Technology at Simon Fraser University (Canada), the Department of Communication at Yonsei University (South Korea), the Faculty of Law and Politics at Keio University (Japan), and the Institute for Journalism, Media & Communication Studies at Keio University. I would like to extend my sincere gratitude for their collaborations and engagements over the years and, most obviously, to all the contributors in this volume.

References

Aris-Maldonado, M. (2020). COVID-19 as a global risk: Confronting the ambivalences of a socionatural threat. *Societies*, *10*(4), 92. https://doi.org/10.3390/soc10040092

Banerjee, D., Sathyanarayana Rao, T. S., Kallivayalil, R. A., & Javed, A. (2020). Revisiting '*The Plague*' by Camus: Shaping the 'social aburdity' of the COVID-19 Pandemic. *Asian Journal of Psychiatry*, *54*. https://doi.org/10.1016/j.ajp.2020.102291.

Beck, U. (1992/1986). *Risk Society: Towards a New Modernity*. Sage.

Beck, U. (1998). *World Risk Society*. Polity Press.

Beck, U. (2008/2007). *World at Risk*. Polity Press.

Belayeth Hussain, A. H. M. (2022). Social distancing in risk society: A cross-national analysis of policy responses to the COVID-19 pandemic. *International Review of Sociology*, *32*: 40–62. DOI: 10.1080/03906701.2022.2051981

Camus, A. (2021/1947). *The Plague*. Knopf.

Chernilo, D. (2021). One globalisation or many?: Risk society in the age of the Anthropocene. *Journal of Sociology*, *57*(5), 144078332199756. DOI:10.1177/1440783321997563.

Defoe, D. (1990/1722). *A Journal of the Plague Year*. Oxford University Press.

Giddens, A. (1994). *Beyond Left and Right: The Future of Radical Politics*. Stanford University Press.

Goyal, M. K., & Gupta, A. K. (Eds.) (2020). *Integrated Risk of Pandemic: Covid-19 Impacts, Resilience and Recommendations*. Springer.

Hacking, I. (1990). *The Taming of Chance*. Cambridge University Press.

Harper, K. (2021). *Plagues Upon the Earth: Disease and the Course of Human History*. Princeton University Press.

Honigsbaum, M. (2020). *A History of Global Contagion from the Spanish Flu to Covid-19*. Penguin.

IRGC. (2015). *IRGC Guidelines for Emerging Risk Governance: Guidance for the Governance of Unfamiliar Risks*. International Risk Governance Council.

Jing, Y., Han, J-S., & Ogawa, K. (Eds.) (2021). *Risk Management in East Asia: Systems and Frontier Issues*. Routledge.

Kabel, A., & Phillipson, R. (2021). Structural violence and hope in catastrophic times: From Camus' The Plague to COVID-19. *Race & Class*, *62*(4), 3–18.

Leonhardt, D. (2022, January 25). Two covid Americas. *The New York Times*. https://www.nytimes.com/2022/01/25/briefing/covid-behavior-vaccinated -unvaccinated.html

Linkov, I., Keenan, J. M., & Trump, B. D. (Eds.) (2021). *COVID-19: Systemic Risk and Resilience*. Springer.

Luhmann, N. (1993/1991). *Risk: A Sociological Theory*. Walter de Gruyter.

Mabille, F. (Ed.) (2021). *Covid 19: Toward a World Risk Society*. Editions L'Harmattan.

NHK. (2020). Producer A no Omowaku: 9 gatsu no meicho: Pest no kioku (Producer A's Speculation: September's best book, Memories of the Plague). https://www.nhk.or.jp/meicho/famousbook/101_defoe/index.html#:~ :text=患者を出したため、行政,滑稽な行動などなど

Saeki, K. (2020, July 12). A book beyond borders: Why the world is reading Albert Camus' "The Plague." *NHK World-Japan*. https://www3.nhk.or.jp/nhkworld/ en/news/backstories/1188/

Seneviratne, K., & Muppidi, S. R. (Eds.) (2021). *COVID-19, Racism and Politicization: Media in the Midst of a Pandemic*. Cambridge Scholar Publishing.

University of Nottingham. (2019). 'Yet I Alive!': COVID-19 and the future of the novel. https://www.nottingham.ac.uk/vision/vision-future-of-the-novel

Wallerstein, I. (1991). *Unthinking Social Science: The Limits of Nineteenth Century Paradigms*. Polity.

World Health Organization (WHO). (2022). WHO coronavirus (COVID-19) dashboard. https://covid19.who.int. (Accessed on 1 April 2022).

Yousif, M. K., Razzyq, W. K., & Nsaif, Q. K. (2021). Epidemic manifestation in Daniel Defoe's *A Journal of the Plague Year* and Covid 19: A comparative study. *Turkish Journal of Computer and Mathematics Education*, *12*(7), 628–633.

2 COVID-19 as a Catalyst of Global Risk Society

Institutionalization, De-Westernization, and Datafication of Crisis Communication Research

Martin Löffelholz, Pauline Gidget Estella, and Yi Xu

Introduction

The world has been upended by the COVID-19 pandemic, a global health emergency that also unfolded as economic, political, organizational, and even personal crises. For many global institutions, the coronavirus crisis was unprecedented (e.g., Guterres, 2020; World Bank, 2020) and has shown how even many developed countries were ill-prepared for a crisis of this magnitude (John & Frater, 2020; Wilensky, 2021). Already in its third year, the pandemic continues to force shifts in life routines as countries struggle to cope with new waves, variants, and "trade-off" dilemmas (i.e., to what extent can economic losses due to restrictions be justified?). The current pandemic is a "systemic event" (Kunelius, 2020, p. 1) juxtaposed with another "systemic crisis": the climate emergency, to which countries worldwide are vulnerable. These "overlapping" (Kunelius, 2020, p. 1) systemic events are global in nature and ultimately require global perspectives and solutions, despite the persistence of nation-centric approaches.

Therefore, in historicizing and mapping risk and crisis communication research, a truly global perspective is needed, one that goes beyond the reality and history of risk and crisis communication scholarship in affluent Western societies, which was already described in much of the literature in the past decades (e.g., Löffelholz, 2022; Schwarz et al., 2016). In an increasingly globalized world, marked by shifts in geopolitics, the rise of transnational economic flows, and the hybridization of public spheres, it is imperative to discuss how risk and crisis communication are studied beyond the so-called "West" (primarily Western Europe and North America). This chapter will deal with the development of risk and crisis communication research across the world, the core themes and findings, and emerging trends, with attention given to how the respective scholarship particularly in Asia fared in comparison with that in Europe and the US, leading to a discussion on both the de-Westernization of the discourse and future research trajectories.

DOI: 10.4324/9781003286684-2

Chernobyl and the Emergence of Crisis Communication Research

The history of risk and crisis communication research is laden with events that either triggered waves of new studies or led to paradigm shifts in scholarship. More than any event before, the Chernobyl reactor accident on April 26, 1986, marked a turning point, especially in the mainstream of "Western" research activities. It signaled "the end of the nineteenth century, the end of classical industrial society" (Beck, 1986, p. 10; authors' translation) and its often-naïve belief in modernization. The nuclear catastrophe in the former Soviet Union attests to the reflexivity of techno-economic progress, whose unintended consequences have no regard for national boundaries and affect the modernization process itself. In this other form of modernity, termed "risk society" by the German sociologist Ulrich Beck (1986), the production of risks increasingly overshadows the production of wealth. As a result, the promise of security gains in importance, but this promise "must be constantly reaffirmed against a vigilant and critical public by symbolic or real interventions in techno-economic development" (Beck, 1986, p. 26; authors' translation).

Shortly before the events in Chernobyl, Beck completed the manuscript for his seminal study on risk society. When the Chernobyl incident occurred, he added a second preface in May 1986, arguing that his conceptual unfolding of the risk society had acquired a "bitter taste of truth" (Beck, 1986, p. 10). This conclusion was in line with the zeitgeist of the time, as protests against the civilian use of nuclear energy grew in many countries in the 1970s, especially after the (albeit localized) nuclear accident in Harrisburg ("Three Mile Island") in the US in 1979. Against this background, in this first phase of risk and crisis communication research in the 1970s, governments, the nuclear industry, and (affiliated) research institutions were primarily concerned with analyzing the "perception and acceptance of technical risks" (Renn, 1981; authors' translation), assuming that a better understanding of risk communication could contribute to the acceptance of risky technologies (Peters, 1991).

However, both risk and crisis communication "grew organically out of a variety of perspectives and initiatives, whether they are community-based activism, government response or industry initiated" (Palenchar, 2009, pp. 31–32). Other starting points for risk and crisis communication research emerged in disaster sociology, which in its early stages "focused on two communication issues: disaster warning systems and evacuations processes and behaviors" (Seeger et al., 2016, p. 424). For example, Miletti and Beck (1975) explained "evacuation symbolically" as early as in the mid-1970s by being one of the first scholars to explicitly invoke the notion of "communication in crisis." Disaster research centers, especially in the US, were established even earlier, e.g., at Ohio State University in 1963. In 1985, this disaster research center moved to the University of Delaware (www .drc.udel.edu).

In other regions of the world, such research centers were established much later than in the US. In Germany, for example, the first disaster research center was founded in 1987 at the University of Kiel. Here, sociologists analyzed disasters as behavior-changing events, e.g., based on the "Chernobyl syndrome" (Dombrovsky, 1987), explicitly introducing the concept of crisis communication (Dombrovsky, 1991). During these years, communication scholars, not least in Europe, still focused on media coverage examining, for example, how "Chernobyl in the media" (Teichert, 1987) or "nuclear energy in the press" (Kepplinger, 1988) was portrayed.

In many parts of Asia, the 1970s–1980s were not bereft of critical incidents that could be subjects of analysis in risk and crisis communication research, but the nature of these incidents was quite different from that of the Chernobyl or Harrisburg incidents. These decades saw protracted political crises, social unrest, and the beginnings of independent governance in many Asian countries, e.g., the power struggle in China, a coup in South Korea, the fall of a dictatorship in the Philippines, and the early years of Singapore as an independent republic. However, risk and crisis communication studies during this period were few and far in between. A notable example would be Liao's (1980) analysis of the "reactive behavior" of the Chinese mass media during the 1962 India–China border conflict. Remarkably, the study already used the term "crisis communication," at around the same time Western scholars introduced the concept of "communication in crisis."

We assume that the dearth of studies at this time in Asian countries results from the fact that many educational institutions were either in transition or in their formative years, primarily due to the turbulent political circumstances during this period. As indicated by the lack of submissions to established journals in the field, the fundamental concepts of crisis communication have yet to be fleshed out in research, similar to the case of Western scholarship at this time. Risk and crisis communication research in Asia started to expand in the early 2000s, as evidenced by the number of studies published around this period, which will be discussed later in this chapter.

Triggered by studies of both media at war and public relations, however, the analytical perspective of communication studies broadened and differentiated in the early 1990s, especially in Europe and North America. Scholars increasingly used the term "crisis communication" (Benoit, 1997; Coombs, 1999; Fearn-Banks, 1996; Löffelholz, 1993a; Marra, 1998; Sellnow, 1993), ushering in the second phase of risk and crisis communication research.

Internationalization and the Intra-Asian Research Gap

In the first decades of risk and crisis communication research, the analytical frame of reference was predominantly the nation-state, and accordingly, scholars regarded the respective media system or the population of a particular nation-state as material objects. Transnational and comparative research, as well as international academic networking among risk and crisis communication researchers, picked up speed in the 2000s, thus forming the third phase of risk and crisis communication research. An important trigger of internationalization was the activity of the International Research Group on Crisis Communication (IRGoCC), founded in 2002 at the Technische Universität Ilmenau, Germany. In 2009, the research group organized the first international conference dedicated exclusively to risk and crisis communication research, which has since been held every two years at various locations in Europe (Löffelholz, 2022). Similar goals, but more focused on the US context, are pursued by the International Crisis and Risk Communication Conference, which the University of Central Florida has been organizing since 2011. Both conference series have sustainably promoted networking in risk and crisis communication research and set the framework for greater institutionalization.

Research in East Asia also started to internationalize in the early 2000s, and at this point, one can already see the gap between East Asia and other Asian countries when it comes to research development, a gap that only widened in the next decades, and which poses an argument against generalizing Asian scholarship as a singular tradition. For example, in the early 2000s, works dealing with risk and crisis communication in China were steadily increasing in number, peaking in 2009, and are already somewhat diverse in terms of themes and approaches, although still far less than the number of studies published in the next decade. With the internationalization came further differentiation of crisis types in research. There were already some studies on governmental crisis communication (e.g., Chen, 2008; Chen, 2009; Lee, 2009), often with recommendations regarding best practices, as some propose conceptual frameworks for information systems and message strategies (e.g., Shi & Yu, 2008; Wang & Xi, 2009), while others look at how Chinese media report on crises (e.g., Fu et al., 2009; Wang et al., 2009). In as early as the 2000–2010 decade, some Chinese scholars in the field of computer science or web intelligence were also starting to create automated tools to aid crisis communication (e.g., Goh et al., 2006). It must be noted, however, that this is different from the use of machine learning or automated tools for risk and crisis communication research, which was gaining steam in the next decade. Works regarding South Korean risk and crisis communication research, meanwhile, were already looking at stakeholders' crisis perception (e.g., Jeong, 2009), media framing of crises (e.g., Wertz & Kim, 2010), and corporate crisis communication (e.g., Hwang & Cameron, 2009).

The critical incidents that affected much of Asia in the early 2000s also served as the impetus for risk and crisis communication research, in particular as case studies, such as the SARS and swine flu pandemics (e.g., Lee, 2009; Xia, 2007) or the 2008 Sichuan earthquake in China (e.g., Chen, 2009; Fang et al., 2009; Fu et al., 2009). Indeed, the character of scholarship is largely shaped by the political, economic, and other systemic contexts of the time.

On the other side, risk and crisis communication research in developing regions of Asia was still struggling to gain footing in the early 2000s, when scholarship in developed East Asian countries was starting to internationalize and scholars in these countries were proposing their own frameworks or models for research (e.g., Shi & Yu, 2008). In fact, even now, our literature search shows that in areas like South and Southeast Asia, risk and crisis communication research remains fragmented, with systematic empirical research scant and wanting. For example, much of the literature in many Southeast Asian countries consists of descriptive case studies and still needs proper conceptualization of fundamental ideas, key variables, and analytical frameworks, all of which are crucial in developing empirical studies. This could be explained by the poor research infrastructure in many developing countries, an issue that begs to be addressed in light of the reality that these regions are most vulnerable to disasters, political crises, or mis- and disinformation.

Institutionalization and the Growth of Systematic Research

The next decade, 2010 onwards, has seen further institutionalization of risk and crisis communication research and an exponential increase in the number of studies even in developing Asian countries. An important step for the institutionalization of research, which can be interpreted as the fourth phase in the development of the field, was the establishment of a temporary working group on crisis communication of the European Communication Research and Education Association (ECREA) in 2011. In view of the great interest, the group was elevated to the status of a division shortly afterward. Another contribution to the institutionalization of the field is *The Handbook of International Crisis Communication Research* (Schwarz et al., 2016). The basic idea of which goes back to a proposal to merge analyses of war communication and studies of corporate crisis communication developed in the early 1990s (Löffelholz, 1993b). In the handbook, scholars from across the world describe the state of the art in risk and crisis communication research in a multidisciplinary manner and thus— in conjunction with other seminal works (Sellnow & Seeger, 2013; Heath & O'Hair, 2009)—contribute to its canonization. The handbook, in its attempt to have a truly global perspective on the state of research, included literature reviews for environments beyond the Western mainstream, such as Asian countries like China (Huang et al., 2016), India (Dhanesh & Srimamesh, 2016), and South Korea (Kim, 2016). Also contributing to the institutionalization of the field is *The Journal of International Crisis and Risk Communication Research* (JICRCR), which was founded in 2018 and is the first scholarly journal dedicated to human and mediated communication issues associated with crises, risks, and emergencies around the world (Seeger, 2018).

The decade has also seen significant growth in systematic crisis communication research, particularly in terms of case studies and quantitative approaches, especially in East Asia, and partly in some Asian developing countries. Research on risk and crisis communication related to disasters—volcanic eruptions, typhoons, to name a few—are quite common in developing (and also developed) Asian countries and are often discussed in relation to disaster preparedness, policy, development communication, and government accountability. For instance, several studies investigated crisis communication during the time of super typhoon Haiyan in 2013 (e.g., Hugelius et al., 2016; Tandoc & Takahashi, 2017), described to be one of the strongest cyclones in history, which barreled across the Philippines and other parts of Southeast Asia. Others looked into the post-crisis communication in the aftermath of the 2015 Nepal earthquake (e.g., Ketter, 2016; Subba & Bui, 2017).

At this point, the differentiation by crisis types even in developing Asian countries also becomes clearer, as some studies have examined crisis communication in natural disasters, organizational crises, and conflicts. Furthermore, theory-driven research, as well as studies that test established theories and frameworks in risk and crisis communication, e.g., the Situational Crisis Communication Theory (SCCT) or the Image Repair Theory, appear to be on the rise in these countries (e.g., Kriyantono & McKenna, 2019; Purworini et al., 2019). This indicates that while research advances in developing Asia might be lagging (due in large part to the persistent systemic dilemmas of these societies, such as high levels of education deprivation and intergenerational poverty), scholarship is becoming more competitive. This is driven partly by increased global academic exchange, i.e., more opportunities to participate in international conferences, more collaborations with colleagues abroad, and more scholars studying overseas. However, in the de-Westernization perspective, one must be wary of the European–North American bias pervading global academic exchange, which will be further discussed in the following section.

Social media research has also become much more common in the recent decade, even in the developing regions of Asia (e.g., Malasig & Quinto, 2016; Tandoc & Takahashi, 2017). Scholars in (and from) developed countries of Asia, in particular China and South Korea, published large-sample analyses of crisis communication and crisis perception in social media (e.g., Cho et al., 2013; Zhang et al., 2020). The popularity of social media research should not come as a surprise given the sharp increase in social media use especially in developing countries, but systematic research on risk and crisis communication in social media is far less common in these areas compared with East Asian countries.

The rapid rise of risk and crisis communication research in East Asia coincided with what Wu et al. (2016) described as "ultrafast economic development," a "mixed blessing" that led to "an increasing proportion of crises, including financial, environmental, and food-safety crises" (Wu et al., 2016, p. 1). This encouraged some scholars to describe some Asian countries as risk societies as early as the 2000s (Wishnick, 2005; Yuan, 2021), including global tourist areas like Bali, Indonesia (e.g., Connor & Vickers, 2003). Overall, risk and crisis communication research has developed in four partially overlapping phases (Löffelholz, 2022), which, however, gained different momentum in the world regions:

- *Risk orientation*: In the first phase starting in the 1980s, research focused on the perception of technologically induced risks by different stakeholders, but the dearth of risk and crisis communication studies in Asia at this time makes it difficult to determine how this phase took shape in the continent. This might have something to do with the political climate of many Asian countries at the time, as some countries had just started governing themselves independently from colonial rule, while others are still reeling from political crises, with their social institutions and research infrastructure far from their current state.

- *Differentiation*: In the second phase from the beginning of the 1990s (Europe and the US) and from the early 2000s (Asia), the term "crisis communication" was used more often, and associated with it, different types of crises came into focus. The differentiation and internationalization phases coincided especially in East Asia, which could perhaps be explained by the rapid economic development—driving and partially driven by globalization—in these societies.
- *Internationalization*: In the third phase from the early 2000s, risk and crisis communication research became interconnected, initially with a strong European–North American bias.
- *Institutionalization*: In the fourth phase, beginning in the early 2010s, an ECREA section and the publication of the first handbooks solidified risk and crisis communication research.

While mostly the material objects differ, methodologically there are a number of commonalities of research across the globe. Most analyses still focus primarily on country-specific case studies, while cross-border or international comparative studies are scarce. The research focus is mainly on those crises that trigger great media attention in the respective country. In the US, for example, the nuclear accident in Harrisburg (1979), the terrorist attacks on September 11, 2001, or the flood disaster in New Orleans (2005) led to a large number of studies (Seeger et al., 2016). In Sweden, which was directly affected by the nuclear disaster in Chernobyl due to radioactive fallout, the accident led to more attention on crisis communication, similar to other European countries (Frandsen & Johansen, 2016). In Colombia, the "drug crisis" or the bloody fight against the FARC (Fuerzas Armadas Revolucionarias de Colombia) rebels was a recurrent theme in the research agenda (Arroyave & Erazo-Coronado, 2016). In many parts of Asia, disasters were common subjects of analysis, such as those related to super typhoon Haiyan (e.g., Tandoc & Takahashi, 2017) or the 2015 Nepal earthquake (e.g., Subba & Bui, 2017).

While there are similarities, there are also differences in the national and regional development of risk and crisis communication research. In the Global South as well as in some authoritarian-controlled political systems, crisis-related research developed more hesitantly than in democratically constituted industrial societies, which underscores the relevance of political, socioeconomic, and cultural contexts for understanding risk and crisis communication (Schwarz, 2016). In the former Soviet Union, concepts such as "risk" and "crisis" were considered outgrowths of a Western social order and were used in the context of anti-capitalist propaganda, but not to describe problematic situations at home (Samoilenko, 2016). Research in and about China turns less often to crisis communication in companies, but focuses more on state actors. Since the government often assumes "the role of the patriarch, like a father who rewards, disciplines, and protects his children" (Huang et al., 2016, p. 274), the executive branch often becomes the main actor in crises and is, therefore, more frequently the subject of academic research.

Theorizing and the Pandemic as a "Wicked Problem"

Impulses for theory-building, especially with regard to corporate risk and crisis communication research, came initially primarily from the US (Sellnow & Seeger, 2013). However, a constructionist understanding of crisis formed a central theoretical starting point of crisis communication research in Germany already in the early 1990s (Löffelholz, 1993a, 2022). Accordingly, whether an event or a process is understood as a crisis depends on the perception and interpretation of the respective observers. As a result,

> situations threatening the existence of a company are not objective phenomena that can be found empirically [...]. The assessment of a [...] crisis therefore depends on which sections of reality the observer considers relevant [...]. Management philosophy, value system, and attitudes act here as perception filters. In this respect, the identification of a crisis situation is the result of individual or collective processes of perception and consciousness formation.
>
> (Staehle et al., 1999, p. 903; authors' translation)

In this respect, how nuclear accidents, flood disasters, or mismanagement are perceived is contingent on collective or social consciousness. "Only when corporate actors, media, or government officials agree to label a problem a 'crisis,' for example, do they respond to it as such" (Hearit & Courtright, 2004, p. 206).

Although theory-building began earlier in Europe and North America, scholars in East Asia, particularly in China, have also proposed models or frameworks for crisis communication (e.g., Shi & Yu, 2008). Wu et al. (2016) even created the "Chinese model of crisis communication" based on a review of literature from Chinese societies (Mainland China, Hongkong, and Taiwan), while Huang et al. (2016) identified the features of Chinese crisis communication through the same method. However, this is also indicative of the abovementioned gap between East Asia and other Asian regions in terms of research development: We have yet to see reflections on the state of the art (which in the first place would be difficult for countries with little to no research) and works on theory-building in the developing regions in and beyond Asia.

By the 2020s, however, the scientific analysis of risk and crisis communication presents itself as an internationally well-connected and productive field of research, in which diverse empirical findings as well as an increasingly sophisticated theoretical debate have created a good basis for guiding professional practice and educational work (Ha & Boynton, 2014). The growing body of crisis communication research increasingly helps explain relevant problems and advances the professionalization of the field. However, with the radical connectivity of people through mobile and social media, the automation of communication, and the growing relevance of artificial intelligence, new challenges are emerging that require a reorientation of risk and crisis communication research.

As if the range of issues to be explored has not widened enough as an outcome of digitalization, the COVID-19 pandemic has acted as a catalyst for global risk and crisis communication research, accelerating it enormously, as a crisis unlike anything before begged to be examined in so many aspects. At the same time, however, the pandemic is a "wicked problem," because "all possible actions have uncertain effects, and because they are intertwined with other problems in complex and, to a large extent, unmanageable systems" (Schiefloe, 2021, p. 5). For instance, the pandemic response in each country cannot be fully understood without a familiarity with political systems, which can be described by variables like "regime type," "formal political institutions," and autonomy of concerned government institutions (Greer et al., 2020, p. 1413).

Indeed, the pandemic "embodies a perfect storm of modern risk society"—a result of a "man-made ecological disturbance" and rapidly spreading "along the modern infrastructures of transportation and migration" (Yuan, 2021, p. 2). The pandemic and its multiple crises, which started in early 2020 and continue to burden citizens and governments as of the time of writing, triggered an "explosion" in risk and crisis communication research across the globe. For China and the US, for example, the number of studies in this field of research published in 2020–2021 was almost thrice the number of studies in the past years, and most of these are related to the pandemic. Moreover, because the pandemic is a global dilemma, comparative studies become all the more necessary especially in terms of evaluating risk and crisis communication, the crucial question being "which worked in what context, and why?" One notable example of comparative projects is the DECIPHER (Deciphering the Pandemic Sphere) consortium, based in Technische Universität Ilmenau in Germany, which aims to compare the risk and crisis communication of governments, health institutions, and the media in Europe and the US during the coronavirus pandemic (www.tu-ilmenau.de/decipher).

"Western" Mainstreaming and the Need for a Truly Global Perspective

Since the early 1990s, the IRGoCC at Technische Universität Ilmenau has been reviewing theoretical approaches and empirical findings in risk and crisis communication research, primarily published in Europe and North America (Löffelholz, 1993b, 2004, 2022; Löffelholz & Schwarz, 2008; Schwarz, 2015, 2016; Schwarz & Löffelholz, 2014, 2022). Based on our most recent literature reviews (Löffelholz, 2022; Schwarz & Löffelholz, 2022), risk and crisis communication can be understood as a process that proceeds in four phases: (1) prevention, (2) preparation, (3) management, and (4) evaluation (cf. Coombs, 2019). For each of these phases, influencing factors and measures can be identified that shape the management of crisis communication institutionally (i.e., roles, organizational culture), instrumentally (i.e., press releases, crisis plans), and symbolic relationally (i.e., messages, stakeholder relationships) (Löffelholz & Schwarz, 2008).

In terms of crisis prevention, issues management, reputation management, and risk communication can reduce the likelihood of a crisis outbreak or at least create better conditions for more effective crisis management (Coombs, 2019). Issues monitoring helps to identify crisis signals earlier (Wiedemann & Riess, 2014), while long-term reputation management can delay the onset of crises, thus creating time and scope for decision-making (Einwiller, 2014) and helping to avoid premature blame or early scandalization (Coombs & Holladay, 2006). Risk communication, in turn, anticipates possible crisis scenarios and raises awareness among relevant stakeholders (Renn, 2009). Approaches such as the Extended Parallel Processing Model (Roberto et al., 2009) or the IDEA model (Sellnow et al., 2017) describe how to apply certain risk communication strategies.

With regard to institutional factors influencing the prevention of crises, research is primarily concerned with the question of to which extent the organizational culture and specific organizational structures can reduce susceptibility to crises. Pauchchant and Mitroff (2006) conclude that "unhealthy" organizational cultures tend to suppress crisis signals and operate with a simplistic good–evil dichotomy according to which, for example, media are considered hostile. In contrast to these defensive organizational cultures, proactive and cooperative organizational cultures support the success of crisis communication (Marra, 1998). In addition, the embedding of the public relations function in the top management of an organization and the greater decision-making autonomy that comes with it are among the key success factors of crisis communication. Public relations' access to resources and the support of organizational management form important prerequisites for being able to react quickly and appropriately in crises (Schwarz & Büker, 2018; Cloudman & Hallahan, 2006). However, various studies show that crisis prevention continues to be neglected in many organizations (Schwarz et al., 2017; Schulz, 2001).

With regard to crisis preparation, crisis plans, crisis management teams, and crisis training are analyzed in particular to enable faster and more effective action in corresponding situations. Crisis plans bundle relevant information, assign responsibilities, and prepare courses of action (Coombs, 2019); in some cases, however, their importance is overestimated (Marra, 1998). Only about one-third of the German organizations surveyed, but as many as three-quarters of US organizations, are equipped with crisis plans (Lee et al., 2007; Schwarz & Pforr, 2011). Other crisis preparation tools include training and simulations in which crisis teams are prepared for an emergency (Coombs, 2019). Although relatively many organizations have appropriate staffing, some operate sub-optimally in crises because they have not been adequately trained (Cloudman & Hallahan, 2006; Schulz, 2001). Intranet- and Internet-based tools, such as dark sites, social bots, or geo-mapping, can also contribute to effective crisis preparation.

During acute crisis management, the main aspects to consider are symbolic relational aspects, i.e., selecting appropriate rhetorical communication strategies, assessing the impact of these strategies, and considering the relationships between organizations and their stakeholders. In crises, organizations should communicate quickly, consistently, transparently, and openly to journalists in order to influence the public interpretation of a crisis (Coombs, 2019). In terms of content, behavioral instructions and information on how to process a crisis must be provided in the acute phase in order to protect those affected from harm and to support them in coping with the crisis (Sturges, 1994). Furthermore, in order to protect the reputation of organizations in crises, a research tradition has been established in which rhetorical crisis communication strategies are studied (Benoit, 1995; Coombs, 2010b). In this context, Coombs and Holladay (2004) have presented the most significant approach to explaining the relationship between crises, the selection of crisis communication strategies, and organizational reputation. According to the Situational Crisis Communication Theory, attributions of responsibility depend on the type of crisis, the crisis history, and an organization's relationships with its stakeholders (Coombs & Holladay, 2004; Coombs, 2019).

Other aspects that support crisis management relate to organizations' relationships with their stakeholders, specifically the relationship between public relations and journalism and the role of emotions. This is because both company spokespersons and their stakeholders tend to react emotionally in crises (Claeys & Schwarz, 2016). Thus, in the case of crises caused by organizations, spokespersons should show a mix of anger and hope; in contrast, in the case of crises in which organizations themselves are among the victims, angry reactions are more effective than mixed (anger and hope) or non-emotional reactions (Xiao et al., 2018). Regarding stakeholder relationships, it appears that positive relationships established before a crisis have positive effects during crises, based on a study on an oil spill incident in South Korea (Jeong, 2009). Pre-established relationships between press offices and newsrooms also prove useful in crises. At the same time, however, journalists in such situations increase their own research, incorporate more evaluations, and cut input material more than in routine reporting (Barth & Donsbach, 1992).

The analysis of the fourth phase of the process of managing crisis communication has been largely neglected in research to date, although crisis-related learning processes can make a decisive contribution to crisis prevention and avoidance (Ulmer et al., 2007). However, organizations can draw on concepts and instruments of general PR evaluation (Besson, 2008) and incorporate findings from research on the prevention and early detection of crises. In addition to the previously mentioned aspects, it is important to break down barriers that prevent early warning signals from being perceived in time and learning processes from being initiated in a pre-crisis phase. To this end, what must be created is an organizational culture that not only emphasizes past successes but also promotes a learning culture that makes it possible to identify and address trouble spots (Veil, 2011).

This brief overview shows how dynamically crisis communication research has developed over the past decades. Although relatively few scholars across the world regularly work on the subject area, crisis communication has become the "dominant topic in public relations research. It could soon be the case where the tail (crisis communication) wags the dog (public relations)" (Coombs, 2010a, p. 61). Even if one may not entirely follow this optimistic assessment, it is certainly true that a productive and further growing scholarly community has emerged that is aware of both the successes and desiderata of crisis communication research as well as further challenges. In the future, we can therefore expect to see more studies on the description and explanation of communication under crisis conditions that take a decidedly theory-based approach, focus more on communication within organizations (Johansen et al., 2012) and transnational crises (Schwarz, 2016), and examine the consequences of technological disruptions in greater detail. However, a more global perspective is particularly important, as we would like to illustrate with the example of the increasing importance of risk and crisis communication research in Asia. In this context, the main question is to what extent concepts originating from the European–North American mainstream are applicable to settings beyond the "West," or more generally, what does it mean to de-Westernize risk and crisis communication research?

De-Westernization and the "Contextual Perspective" in Asia

Communication studies have long been influenced by traditions and perspectives coming from Europe and North America (Waisbord & Mellado, 2014, p. 361), in particular the Western liberal democracies, which have systems and realities different from the Global South or high-income nations with tightly controlled political systems. The Western-centric scholarship could be described as a consequence of a long colonial past and the cultural mindset that it created and that continues to persist, the North–South gap in terms of resources and soundness of welfare institutions, and geopolitics in the past decades. Waisbord and Mellado argue that because internationalization of scholarship occurred earlier in the West (as we also observed in our review of the development of risk and crisis communication literature), Western theories, perspectives, and subjects of study, in particular those from the US, gained "ascendancy" as the measure or gold standard of research (Waisbord & Mellado, 2014, p. 362).

This "academic Eurocentrism" was deemed "inadequate" in explaining the realities or circumstances of many environments beyond the West (Waisbord & Mellado, 2014, p. 362). The argument becomes more of a cause for concern when juxtaposed with the findings of Diers-Lawson (2017): Based on a review of risk and crisis communication literature in English published from 1953 to 2015, it is clear that the field is "shockingly American-centric and fails to reflect the needs and global reality of crisis communication today" (Diers-Lawson, 2017, p. 1). Moreover, the interest in Asian studies is declining in Western academia, at a time when Asia's "geo-political footprint grows" (Lau, 2021). In the United Kingdom, for example, the number of Asian studies degrees conferred has declined in the past years (Lau, 2021).

Using approaches originating from the West without the necessary critique (or at the very least retrofitting) may result in "ontological and analytical distortions" that usually come with merely transferring "foreign categories and perspectives" (Waisbord & Mellado, 2014, p. 362). For instance, some categories, dimensions, variables, or typologies may not capture the intricacies of Global South systems, or some normative definitions from the West cannot be used as the yardstick for such environments. To de-Westernize communication studies is not only to avoid such distortions (or as a form of backlash against centuries of colonization), it is also to take into account geopolitical shifts and the rise of new powers (Waisbord & Mellado, 2014, p. 362).

In de-Westernizing communication studies, Waisbord and Mellado (2014) proposed four key dimensions: (1) the subject of study, (2) the body of evidence, (3) analytical frameworks, and (4) academic cultures. The subject of study reflects the realities and horizon of societal and academic imagination in certain societies, and so there are issues or circumstances that are alien to the West and therefore understudied. The idea, then, is to bring such issues or circumstances into focus. De-westernizing the body of evidence, meanwhile, means avoiding "universalistic pretensions based on a narrow slice of context-specific cases," and "evidence from the rest of the world" has to be duly considered (Waisbord & Mellado, 2014, p. 365).

To illustrate how the first two dimensions can be used as tools for analysis, we can use Wu et al.'s (2016) review of risk and crisis communication research in Mainland China, Hong Kong, and Taiwan across a period of 16 years. In Asian risk and crisis communication research, it is crucial to consider a "contextual perspective," or "broader factors" such as political and media systems (Wu et al., 2016, p. 2) in trying to understand the subject of the study, e.g., the concept of the crisis, crisis communication goals, or communication habits of institutions. Wu et al. (2016) analyzed the applicability of established Western theories in the context of each country and described stark differences between Western theoretical ideals and those of Chinese risk and crisis communication. For example, the authors found that

> with regards to the hierarchical authoritarianism and relation-centered values derived from Confucianism, Chinese crisis managers would probably attach more salience to the maintenance of a courteous image than to the analysis of the four major variables for crisis management posited by Western theories.
>
> (Wu et al., 2016, p. 16)

These variables include crisis type, stakeholder, crisis system, and crisis phase based primarily on Pearson and Mitroff's (1993) work on crisis management. In addition, they posited that the "separation of powers and juristic and media autonomy are conditional features of Western theories' predictions" (Wu et al., 2016, p. 12), and therefore should be less applicable in authoritarian systems like Mainland China. Huang et al. (2016) also observed that the "current theories of crisis communication are predominately applied to democratic societies, especially the US-American society, where corporations, interest groups, and policymakers reach the public and influence their opinions by building mass media agendas" (Huang et al., 2016, p. 203).

Some features of crisis communication in Chinese societies, like the preference for "ambiguous communicative strategies such as diversion and avoidance for the purpose of face-saving" (Wu et al., 2016, p. 2) or the avoidance of direct or extreme communication strategies (Huang et al., 2016, p. 203) might seem strange to those who are not familiar with the cultural context. Pang and Hu (2018) also found "inconsistencies with Western frameworks" (p. 118) in their analysis of corporate crisis response in China: for example, contrary to the recommendations of the SCCT framework, organizations tend to use denial and corrective action together, even if the circumstances call for only the denial strategy based on the theory (Pang & Hu, 2018, p. 122). The same goes for South Korean research. Citing the studies of Lee and Lee (2006) and Kim et al. (2008), Kim (2016, p. 409) observed that South Koreans prefer "accommodative crisis response strategies, regardless of crisis type," issuing an apology in all types of crises, contrary to the recommendations of the SCCT framework. Therefore, in consolidating global research, identifying the best practices and most salient frameworks should be based on the body of evidence that includes settings previously underrepresented or misrepresented.

To de-Westernize research is also to direct "attention to issues that might be absent in the analytical radar of Western scholars, but are important in the non-Western world" (Waisbord & Mellado, 2014, p. 361). "Intellectuals in the periphery" are likely to look into perennial conditions of poverty, corruption, digital divide, and other types of systemic dilemmas (Waisbord & Mellado, 2014, p. 361), contextual realities that strongly influence risk and crisis communication practice. The de-Westernization project also calls for the creation of "analytical frameworks" anchored on empirical research and an emphasis on "theoretical perspectives original to the global South" (Waisbord & Mellado, 2014, p. 365) that are absent or omitted in the state of research. This can be in the form of indigenous frameworks grounded on local conditions but are still based on a dialogue with Western perspectives, such as the Chinese model of crisis communication created by Wu et al. (2016). Scholars can also criticize and test known frameworks as what Wu et al. (2016), Kim (2016), and Pang and Hu (2018) did in their works. Apart from proposing and analyzing conceptual frameworks, the de-Westernization project will also benefit from theories that are truly global in terms of perspective, taking account of the particularities of regions, their differences, as well as universalities or trends that run across continents and cultures.

The fourth dimension of de-Westernizing scholarship is "academic cultures," defined as "the network of interrelated and explicit beliefs about the practice of teaching and research, and the social significance of these practices" (Ringer, 1992, cited by Waisbord and Mellado, 2014, p. 369). As of the time of writing this chapter, there is still no empirical study on academic cultures specifically for risk and crisis communication research. Citing Averbeck's (2008) study on European academic cultures, Waisbord and Mellado (2014, p. 370) argued that, despite the opportunities for internationalization and the rise of international collaboration, the "values of specific academic cultures have become dominant." This is where the North–South dialogue and negotiation of positions in risk and crisis communication research come in: Self-reflexiveness and critique of established research traditions (is there another way of looking at the problem apart from the established approach?) is a prerequisite for global theory-building. Differences and commonalities of academic cultures in risk and crisis communication scholarship could also be examined through empirical designs in future research. Furthermore, a truly global perspective is required due to the increasing hybridization, datafication, and algorithmization of risk and crisis communication.

Hybridization and the Dissemination of "Topical Disinformation"

With the emergence of "hybrid media systems" (Chadwick, 2017), characterized by the interdependence of traditional and Internet-based media and the destabilization of an elite-driven public sphere, research has increasingly turned to online communication in crisis contexts. The hybridization of media is leading organizations to tap into additional communication channels to reach stakeholders directly (Schultz et al., 2011). Messages can thus be more easily tailored to specific crises and different stakeholder groups. At the same time, the importance of new public actors such as bloggers, YouTubers, or social media influences is growing. Organizations must therefore operate more and more in multidirectional communication processes and can lose trust in the process (Johansson & Odén, 2018), because in the new communication spaces created by the Internet, not least, crises can also arise or be dynamized (Ettl-Huber et al., 2013). Other problems with the use of Internet-based media relate to the lack of confidentiality of information about people affected, the danger that unverified or incorrect information can reach millions of people in a very short time, and the risk of panic if too much information is disseminated at a very early stage of a crisis (Valentini & Kruckeberg, 2016).

With the increased relevance of Internet-based platforms such as Facebook, YouTube, Twitter, or Instagram, a large number of studies emerged in the last two decades, focusing on "crisis PR on the internet" (Köhler, 2006) and increasingly on the growing importance of social media in crises (Valentini & Kruckeberg, 2016; Liu et al., 2011). Through a systematic review of literature on risk and crisis communication research in social media, Rasmussen and Ihlen (2017) found a rising interest in the topic, as seen in the increasing number of studies since 2009, which should be expected given the rapid rise in social media use for different life transactions worldwide. Aspects analyzed include, for example, the use of chat apps, video platforms, and social networks to identify and monitor crisis signals, the possibilities of dialogic communication with stakeholders, or the effectiveness of social media in disseminating crisis-related behavioral instructions (Schwarz & Löffelholz, 2022). Findings show that the choice of communication medium (social versus traditional media) indeed has an impact on reputation, emotions, and follow-up communication. In some cases, the choice of communication medium proved to be more significant than the respective content message (Schultz et al., 2011). It is therefore not surprising that governments and other institutions are using crisis communication via the Internet or social media more and more strategically (Rasmussen & Ihlen, 2017).

The state of research in social-mediated or digital risk and crisis communication also justifies the call for de-Westernization. Rasmussen and Ihlen (2017) looked into the geographical spread of social media users studied in the extant literature and observed that research mostly focused on the US, Europe, and East Asia. The authors believe that this inadequacy has to be addressed; otherwise, this field will become "too particularistic and Western-centred without even demonstrating an awareness of these limitations" (Rasmussen and Ihlen, 2017, p. 12), a disservice at the time of global or transboundary risks and crises.

Admittedly, a systematic, empirically saturated conceptualization of the influence of social media in crises is not yet available (Zhao et al., 2018). However, with the Social-Mediated Crisis Communication (SMCC) model, there is at least an attempt to theorize the crisis communication of organizations and their stakeholders mediated via social media (Jin et al., 2014). According to this, organizations represent a central source of crisis information that is confronted by different types of public actors. Most relevant target groups are those who actively participate in social media-based communication about crises as bloggers, YouTubers, or Instagrammers some of whom have a large number of followers and should therefore be reached by organizations at an early stage. This is distinguished from those who are not creatively active themselves, but who share information online or offline and are thus involved in the dissemination of information in crises. Finally, the inactive, who neither actively nor reactively use social media, but at best obtain information about crises indirectly, i.e., mediated via traditional mass media, must be taken into account (Austin & Jin, 2017). With the SMCC model, the analysis of stakeholder groups and new public actors is moving more into the focus of scientific attention alongside the previously dominant organization-related crisis communication research. This is because only a few studies to date have dealt with the question of how individuals or groups use social media to share ideas and experiences for coping with crises with others (Valentini & Kruckeberg, 2016).

However, the hybridization of media systems, the associated simplification of access to media-mediated public spaces, and the radicalization of connectivity through powerful stationary and mobile communication devices do not only have positive consequences for communication in crises. Under the conditions of an increasingly fluid public sphere, false information can be spread deliberately, which can prolong, intensify, or even trigger crises (Ettl-Huber et al., 2013). However, to what extent and in what way the dissemination of "topical disinformation" (Zimmermann & Kohring, 2018) via social media, which is not satisfactorily captured by the buzzword "fake news" (Tandoc et al., 2018), contributing to the initiation or aggravation of crises (Coombs & Holladay, 2012) has hardly been empirically investigated so far. The destabilization of the previously strongly elite-dominated public sphere of democratic societies due to the de-oligopolization of the media system is obvious (Chadwick, 2017). Consequently, as the findings of the European Communication Monitor suggest, it is becoming increasingly difficult to build or maintain stakeholder trust in organizations (Zerfaß et al., 2019). This situation appears to be more pronounced in developing regions: In Pakistan, for example, social media users "ascribe more legitimacy to user-generated content" compared to Western social media users (Rasmussen & Ihlen, 2017, p. 8), which, in turn, can make it more problematic to manage organizational crises unless appropriate countermeasures are taken.

Datafication and the Reflexivity of Innovations

In addition to the interdependence of traditional and participatory media, risk and crisis communication research is challenged by the rapidly growing interconnectedness of a wide variety of objects. The ubiquity of mobile devices and constantly available sensors in smartphones, sports wristbands, entertainment technologies, industrial machinery, and many others is gradually leading to the comprehensive "datafication" (Mayer-Schönberger & Cukier, 2013, p. 73) of all areas of life. The term refers to the generation of a wide variety of information, "including what we never used to think of as information, such as a person's location, the vibration of an engine, or the load on a bridge" and its transformation "into a data format in order to quantify it" (Mayer-Schönberger & Cukier, 2013, p. 15). With datafication, public as well as private communication is changing seriously, for example, through the possibility of automated tracking of human (purchase) decisions in real time or new forms of advertising, marketing, and public relations based on (predictive) analytics of extremely large data sets ("big data"), for example, generated from social media. For public communication, and thus also for the early detection, management, and evaluation of crises, datafication represents both an opportunity and a threat (Holtzhausen, 2016; Weiner & Kochhar, 2016).

In the fast-developing societies of East Asia, particularly South Korea and China, "the responsive socio-technological webs of a wide range of actors and resources" are a strong part of the "governance in risk society" (Yuan, 2021, p. 1). In the pandemic response of South Korea and China, "technological solutions to the pandemic operated as actor-networks embedded in the complex cross-boundary interactions among different social sectors and close collaboration among various government agencies" (Yuan, 2021, p. 11). At the same time, however, the pervasiveness of technological applications can be a cause for worry because of the possibility of using surveillance and big data technologies as a threat to civil rights (Yuan, 2021, p. 10). Large amounts of data also enable the software-supported automation of activities that were previously the preserve of human actors. This algorithmization of communication began as early as the 1970s with the introduction of digital word processing in newsrooms (Weischenberg, 1982). Today, the search, selection, and publication algorithms of huge tech companies such as Google, Facebook, or Twitter shape public and private communication worldwide. In addition, a vast number of special software helps newsrooms to automatically generate journalistic texts, companies to decide on the optimal marketing mix, or agencies to monitor social media for early detection of potential crises. However, as the theory of a reflexive modernization of society suggested (Beck, 1986), automated systems can become the cause of crises, as the scandal surrounding the company Cambridge Analytica in 2018 (González et al., 2019), or the case of Microsoft chatbot Tay showed. Based on a deep learning-based analysis of messages from human actors on Twitter and other platforms, Tay posted racist, sexist, and conspiracy-theory content after a short time and was soon after taken offline (Neff & Nagy, 2016).

Datafication, algorithmization, and automation of communication are among the most important challenges facing risk and crisis communication management and research in the 2020s. However, the findings of a survey of communication managers from more than 40 countries point to a still large gap between the presumed great importance and the actually not too advanced use of automated systems in organizational communication (Wiesenberg et al., 2017). For risk and crisis communication research, however, it is in any case a very relevant topic, as illustrated by studies on the use of autonomous agents in political propaganda (Woolley & Howard, 2016) or of social bots during the Manchester bombing in May 2017 (Brachten et al., 2018), for example. Furthermore, advances in artificial intelligence should be included in the context, as the use of which can accelerate crisis responses and tailor them more precisely to target groups and communication channels. In this respect, risk and crisis communication research is at the beginning of a new phase of development. Driven by the need to under-stand and elaborate hybrid, algorithmic, and automated crisis communication, it is necessary to closely link communication and computational theories and methods. Appropriate conceptual and methodological tools are being developed in many countries within the framework of computational crisis communication.

With the increasing availability of digital data, the importance of computational data analysis requiring algorithmic solutions is growing (Domahidi et al., 2019), but has limited application in risk and crisis communication research (Stieglitz et al., 2018). Computational analyses facilitate cross-national analyses of public communication in social media and a more effective study of temporal aspects of government communication, media coverage, and citizen responses. In relation to the current pandemic, for example, computational analysis allows researchers to examine the impact of government response on changes in infection rates (Abd-Alrazaq et al., 2020) and explore sources of conspiracy allegations (Singh et al., 2020; Del Pilar Zaras-Sarate, et al. 2017) or echo chambers (Eady et al., 2019). Computational approaches to analyzing risk and crisis communication could even support data-driven policies as well as corporate decision-making. The reflexivity of these innovations, as conceptually described by Beck (1986) almost 40 years ago, is already casting its shadows, as a look at authoritarian states shows.

It is clear that risk and crisis communication research has developed into a far richer field of study compared to its beginnings in the early 1980s. However, it is also clear that misbalances in research development and perspectives remain unaddressed, despite the rise of globalized academic settings and exchanges. The deficiency in research especially in the Global South is a function of systemic circumstances that have long hindered research development in these regions, and to de-Westernize risk and crisis communication research primarily requires understanding these contextual realities. It is therefore necessary for communities working in the field of risk and crisis communication to engage more intensively with the project of de-Westernization, not least in light of the rise of transnational crises such as the current pandemic.

References

Abd-Alrazaq, A., Alhuwail, D., Househ, M., Hamdi, M., & Shah, Z. (2020). Top concerns of tweeters during the COVID-19 pandemic: Infoveillance Study. *Journal of Medical Internet Research, 22*(4), e19016. doi: 10.2196/19016.

Arroyave, J., & Erazo-Conado, A. M. (2016). Crisis and risk communication research in Colombia. In Schwarz, A., Seeger, M. & Auer, C. (Eds.). *Handbook of international crisis communication research* (pp. 411–421). Wiley Blackwell.

Austin, L., & Jin, Y. (2017). Social media and crisis communication. Explicating the social-mediated crisis communication model. In Dudo, A. & Kahlor, L. (Eds.). *Strategic communication: New agendas in communication* (pp. 163–186). Routledge.

Averbeck, S. (2008). Comparative history of communication studies: France and Germany. *The Open Communication Journal, 2*(1), 1–13.

Barth, H., & Donsbach, W. (1992). Aktivität und Passivität von Journalisten gegenüber Public Relations. Fallstudie am Beispiel von Pressekonferenzen zu Umweltthemen. *Publizistik, 37*(2), 151–165.

Beck, U. (1986). *Risikogesellschaft: Auf dem Weg in eine andere Moderne.* Suhrkamp.

Benoit, W. L. (1995). *Accounts, excuses, apologies: A theory of image restoration strategies.* State University of New York Press.

Benoit, W. L. (1997). Image repair discourse and crisis communication. *Public Relations Review, 23*, 177–186.

Besson, N. A. (2008). *Strategische PR-Evaluation. Erfassung, Bewertung und Kontrolle von Öffentlichkeitsarbeit.* VS.

Brachten, F., Mirbabaie, M., Stieglitz, S., Berger, O., Bludau, S., & Schrickel, K. (2018). *Threat or opportunity? Examining social bots in social media crisis communication.* Australasian Conference on Information Systems.

Chadwick, A. (2017). *The hybrid media system. Politics and power.* 2nd. ed., Oxford University Press.

Chen, L. (2008). Open information system and crisis communication in China. *Chinese Journal of Communication, 1*(1), 38–54.

Chen, N. (2009). Institutionalizing public relations: A case study of Chinese government crisis communication on the 2008 Sichuan earthquake. *Public Relations Review, 35*(3), 187–198.

Cho, S., Jung, K., & Park, W. (2013). Social media use during Japan's 2011 earthquake: How twitter transforms the locus of crisis communication. *Media International Australia, 149*(1), 28–40.

Claeys, A.-S., & Schwarz, A. (2016). Domestic and international audiences of organizational crisis communication: State of the art and implications for cross-cultural crisis communication. In Schwarz, A., Seeger, M. W. & Auer, C. (Eds.). *Handbook of international crisis communication research* (pp. 224–235). Wiley-Blackwell.

Cloudman, R., & Hallahan, K. (2006). Crisis communications preparedness among U.S. organizations: Activities and assessments by public relations practitioners. *Public Relations Review, 32*(4), 367–376.

Connor, L., & Vickers, A. (2003). Crisis, citizenship, and cosmopolitanism: Living in a local and global risk society in Bali. *Indonesia, 25*(April 2003), 153–180.

Coombs, W. T. (1999). *Ongoing crisis communication: Planning, managing, and responding.* Sage.

Coombs, W. T. (2010a). Crisis communication and its allied fields. In Coombs, W. T. & Holladay, S. J. (Eds.). *The handbook of crisis communication* (pp. 54–64). Wiley-Blackwell.

Coombs, W. T. (2010b). Parameters for crisis communication. In Coombs, W. T. & Holladay, S. J. (Eds.). *The handbook of crisis communication* (pp. 17–53). Wiley-Blackwell.

Coombs, W. T. (2019). *Ongoing crisis communication: Planning, managing, and responding,* 5th ed., Sage.

Coombs, W. T., & Holladay, S. J. (2004). Reasoned action in crisis communication: An attribution theory-based approach to crisis management. In Millar, D. P. & Heath, R. (Eds.). *Responding to crisis: A rhetorical approach to crisis communication* (pp. 95–115). Lawrence Erlbaum.

Coombs, W. T., & Holladay, S. J. (2006). Unpacking the halo effect: Reputation and crisis management. *Journal of Communication Management, 10*(2), 123–137.

Coombs, W. T., & Holladay, S. J. (2012). The paracrisis: The challenges created by publicly managing crisis prevention. *Public Relations Review, 38*(3), 408–415.

Del Pilar Salas-Zárate, M., Medina-Moreira, J., Lagos-Ortiz, K., Luna-Aveiga, H., Rodríguez-García, M. Á., & Valencia-García, R. (2017). Sentiment analysis on tweets about diabetes: An aspect-level approach. *Computational and Mathematical Methods in Medicine, 2017*(5), 1–9. https://doi.org/10.1155/2017/5140631.

Dhanesh, G. S., & Sriramesh, K. (2016). Risk and crisis communication research in India. In Schwarz, A., Seeger, M. & Auer, C. (Eds.). *Handbook of international crisis communication research* (pp. 302–312). Wiley Blackwell.

Diers-Lawson, A. (2017). A state of emergency in crisis communication: An intercultural crisis communication research agenda. *International Journal of Intercultural Communication Research, 46*(1), 1–54. doi:10.1080/17475759.2016.1262891.

Domahidi, E., Yang, J., Niemann-Lenz, J., & Reinecke, L. (2019). Computational communication science. Outlining the way ahead in computational communication science: An introduction to the IJoC special section on "Computational Methods for Communication Science: Toward a Strategic Roadmap." *International Journal of Communication, 13*, 3876–3884.

Dombrovsky, W. R. (1987). *Das Tschernobyl-Syndrom: Katastrophen als verhaltensändernde Ereignisse.* Westdeutscher Verlag.

Dombrovsky, W. R. (1991). *Krisenkommunikation. Problemstand, Fallstudien und Empfehlungen.* Kernforschungsanlage.

Eady, G., Nagler, J., Guess, A., Zilinsky, J., & Tucker, J. (2019). How many people live in political bubbles on social media? Evidence from linked survey and Twitter data. *Social Media and Politics*, *9*(1). https://journals.sagepub.com/doi/full/10.1177/2158244019832705)

Einwiller, S. (2014). Reputation und Image: Grundlagen, Einflussmöglichkeiten, Management. In Zerfaß, A. & Piwinger, M. (Eds.), *Handbuch Unternehmenskommunikation* (2nd ed., pp. 371–391). Springer Gabler.

Ettl-Huber, S., Nowak, R., Reiter, B. & Roither, M. (Eds.) (2013). *Social media in der Organisationskommunikation: Empirische Befunde und Branchenanalysen.* Springer VS.

Fang, J., Li, X., & Li, Y. (2009). The breakthrough and revelation of Government crisis communication in "5.12" Wenchuan Earthquake. In Proceedings of 2009 International Conference on Public Administration (5th) (Vol III, pp. 486–490). Chengdu, PRC.

Fearn-Banks, K. (1996). *Crisis communications: A casebook approach.* Mahwah. Lawrence Erlbaum Associates.

Frandsen, F., & Johansen, W. (2016). Crisis communication research in Northern Europe. In Schwarz, A.; Seeger, M. & Auer, C. (Eds.). *Handbook of international crisis communication research* (pp. 373–383). Wiley Blackwell.

Fu, K., Zhou, L., & Chan, Y. (2009). 21 of 26 analyzing media coverage on government's disaster management practices after Wenchuan earthquake: A preliminary result. In Proceedings of International Disaster and Risk Conference Chengdu 2009 (pp. 55–58). Chengdu, PRC.

González, F., Yu, Y., Figueroa, A., López, C., & Aragon, C. (2019). Global reactions to the Cambridge Analytica scandal: An inter-language social media study. In International World Wide Web Conference Committee, May 13–17, 2019. https://doi.org/10.1145/3308560.3316456.

Goh, O., Fung, C., Wong, K., & Depickere, A. (2006). An embodied conversational agent for intelligent web interaction on pandemic crisis communication. In 2006 IEEE/WIC/ACM International Conference on Web Intelligence and Intelligent Agent Technology, Workshops Proceedings. Hongkong, PRC. doi: 10.1109/WI-IATW.2006.37.

Greer, S. L., King, E. J., da Fonseca, E. M., & Peralta-Santos, A. (2020). The comparative politics of COVID-19: The need to understand government responses. *Global Public Health*, *15*(9), 1413–1416.

Guterres, A. (2020, April 8). Now is the time for unity. Retrieved from United Nations: https://www.un.org/en/un-coronavirus-communications-team/%E2%80%9Cnow-time-unity%E2%80%9D

Ha, J. H., & Boynton, L. (2014). Has crisis communication been studied using an interdisciplinary approach? A 20-year content analysis of communication journals. *International Journal of Strategic Communication*, *8*(1), 29–44.

Hearit, K. M., & Courtright, J. L. (2004). A symbolic approach to crisis management: Sears defense of its auto repair policies. In Heath, R. L. & Millar, D. P. (Eds.). *Responding to crisis. A rhetorical approach to crisis communication* (pp. 201–212). Lawrence Erlbaum Associates.

Heath, R. L., & O'Hair, H. D. (Eds.) (2009). *Handbook of risk and crisis communication.* Routledge.

Holtzhausen, D. R. (2016). Datafication: Threat or opportunity for communication in the public sphere? *Journal of Communication Management*, *20*(1), 21–36.

Huang, Y. C., Wu, F., Cheng, Y., & Lyu, J. C. (2016). Crisis communication research in the Chinese Mainland. In Schwarz, A., Seeger, M. & Auer, C. (Eds.).

Handbook of international crisis communication research (pp. 269–282). Wiley Blackwell.

Huang, Y., Wu, F., & Cheng, Y. (2016). Crisis communication in context: Cultural and political influences underpinning Chinese public relations practice. *Public Relations Review, 42*(2016), 201–213.

Hugelius, K., Gifford, M., Örtenwall, P., & Adolfsson, A. (2016). Disaster radio for communication of vital messages and health-related information: Experiences from the Haiyan Typhoon, the Philippines. *Disaster Medicine and Public Health Preparedness, 10*(4), 591–597. doi: doi:10.1017/dmp.2015.188.

Hwang, S., & Cameron, G. (2009). The estimation of a corporate crisis communication. *Public Relations Review, 35*(2), 35–38.

Jeong, S. (2009). Public's responses to an oil spill accident: A test of the attribution theory and situational crisis communication theory. *Public Relations Review, 35*(3), 307–309.

Jin, Y., Liu, B. F., & Austin, L. L. (2014). Examining the role of social media in effective crisis management: The effects of crisis origin, information form, and source on publics' crisis responses. *Communication Research, 41*, 74–94.

Johansen, W., Aggerholm, H. K., & Frandsen, F. (2012). Entering new territory: A study of internal crisis management and crisis communication in organizations. *Public Relations Review, 38*(2), 270–279.

Johansson, B., & Odén, T. (2018). Struggling for the upper hand. News sources and crisis communication in a digital media environment. *Journalism Studies, 19*(10), 1489–1506.

John, T., & Frater, J. (2020, March 6). Why isn't Europe better prepared for the coronavirus outbreak? Retrieved from CNN: https://edition.cnn.com/2020/03/06/europe/europe-coronavirus-covid-19-intl/index.html

Kepplinger, H. M. (1988). Die Kernenergie in der Presse. Zum Einfluss subjektiver Faktoren auf die Konstruktion der Realität. *Kölner Zeitschrift für Soziologie und Sozialpsychologie, 40*, 659–683.

Ketter, E. (2016). Destination image restoration on facebook: The case study of Nepal's Gurkha Earthquake. *Journal of Hospitality and Tourism Management, 28*(September 2016), 66–72.

Kim, S. (2016). Crisis communication research in South Korea. In A. Schwarz, C. Auer, & M. Seeger (Eds.), *The handbook of international crisis communication research* (pp. 404–409). Wiley.

Kim, Y., Cha, H. & Kim, J. R. (2008). Developing a crisis management index: Applications in South Korea. *Journal of Public Relations Research, 20*(3), 328–355. doi:10.1080/10627260801962962

Kriyantono, R., & McKenna, B. (2019). Crisis response vs crisis cluster: A test of situational crisis communication theory on crisis with two crisis clusters in Indonesian public relations. *Jurnal Komunikasi: Malaysian Journal of Communication, 35*(1), 222–236.

Köhler, T. (2006). *Krisen-PR im Internet: Nutzungsmöglichkeiten, Einflussfaktoren und Problemfelder*. VS.

Kunelius, R. (2020). On the overlap of systemic events: Covid-19, climate, and journalism. *Social Media + Society, 6*(3), 1–4.

Lau, J. (2021, September 30). Is Western academia keeping up with Asia's rise? Retrieved from The World University Rankings: https://www.timeshighereducation.com/features/western-academia-keeping-asias-rise

Lee, J., Woeste, J. H., & Heath, R. L. (2007). Getting ready for crises: Strategic excellence. *Public Relations Review, 33*(3), 334–336.

Lee, K. (2009). How the Hong Kong government lost the public trust in SARS: Insights for government communication in a health crisis. *Public Relations Review, 35*(1), 74–76.

Lee, S., & Lee, M. (2006). 기업위기에서 기업이미지가 사과의 수용, 책임귀인, 반복성 판단에 미치는 영향: 삼성 현대 자동차 CEO위기를 중심으로 [The effect of positive corporate image on publics' acceptance of corporate apology: Focusing on CEO crises of Samsung and Hyundai]. 홍보학연구. *Journal of Public Relations Research, 10*(2), 197–231.

Liao, K. (1980). Mass media and crisis communication in China: Chinese press reactions in the 1962 Sino-Indian border conflict. *Communication Research, 7*(1), 69–94.

Liu, B. F., Austin, L., & Jin, Y. (2011). How publics respond to crisis communication strategies: The interplay of information form and source. *Public Relations Review, 37*(4), 345–353.

Löffelholz, M. (Ed.) (1993a). *Krieg als Medienereignis. Grundlagen und Perspektiven der Krisenkommunikation*. Westdeutscher Verlag.

Löffelholz, M. (1993b). Krisenkommunikation. Probleme, Konzepte, Perspektiven. In Löffelholz, M. (Ed.). *Krieg als Medienereignis. Grundlagen und Perspektiven der Krisenkommunikation* (pp. 11–32). Westdeutscher Verlag.

Löffelholz, M. (2004). Krisen- und Kriegskommunikation als Forschungsfeld. Trends, Themen und Theorien eines hoch relevanten, aber gering systematisierten Teilgebiets der Kommunikationswissenschaft. In Löffelholz, M. (Ed.). *Krieg als Medienereignis II. Krisenkommunikation im 21. Jahrhundert* (pp.13–55). VS.

Löffelholz, M., & Schwarz, A. (2008). Die Krisenkommunikation von Organisationen: Ansätze, Ergebnisse und Perspektiven der Forschung. In Nolting, T. & Thießen, A. (Eds.). *Krisenmanagement in der Mediengesellschaft: Potenziale und Perspektiven in der Krisenkommunikation* (pp.21–35). VS.

Löffelholz, M. (2022). Von Tschernobyl zur Corona-Infodemie. Entwicklung, Ergebnisse und Herausforderungen der Risiko- und Krisenkommunikations-forschung. In Beuthner, M., Bomnüter, U., & Kantara, J. A. (Eds.). *Risiken, Krisen, Konflikte. Herausforderungen und Perspektiven medialer Vermittlungen* (pp. 27–48). Springer.

Malasig, B., & Quinto, E. (2016). Functions of and communication behavior on twitter after the 2015 Nepal earthquake. *Jurnal Komunikasi: Malaysian Journal of Communication, 32*(1), 87–102.

Marra, F. J. (1998). Crisis communication plans: Poor predictors of excellent crisis public relations. *Public Relations Review, 24*(4), 461–474.

Mayer-Schonberger, V., & Cukier, K. (2013). *Big data: A revolution that will transform how we live, work and think*. John Murray.

Miletti, D. S., & Beck, E.M. (1975). Communication in crisis: Explaining evacuation symbolically. *Communication Research, 2*, 24–49.

Neff, G., & Nagy, P. (2016). Talking to bots: Symbiotic agency and the case of tay. *International Journal of Communication, 10*, 4915–4931.

Palenchar, M. J. (2009). Historical trends of risk and crisis communication. In Heath, R. L. & O'Hair, H. D. (Eds.). *Handbook of risk and crisis communication* (pp. 31–53). Routledge.

Pang, A., & Hu, Y. (2018). The indigenization of crisis response strategies in the context of China. *Chinese Journal of Communication, 11*(1), 105–128.

Pauchant, T. C., & Mitroff, I. I. (2006). Crisis prone versus crisis avoiding organizations: Is your company's culture its own worst enemy in creating crises? In Smith, D. & Elliott, D. (Eds.). *Key readings in crisis management. Systems and structures for prevention and recovery* (pp. 136–146). Routledge.

Pearson, C. M., & Mitroff, I. I. (1993). From crisis prone to crisis prepared: A framework for crisis management. *The Academy of Management Executive, 7*(1), 48–59.

Peters, H. P. (1991). Durch Risikokommunikation zur Technikakzeptanz? Die Konstruktion von Risiko„wirklichkeiten" durch Experten, Gegenexperten und Öffentlichkeit. In Krüger, J. & Ruß- Mohl, S. (Eds.). *Risikokommunikation. Technikakzeptanz, Medien und Kommunikationsrisiken* (pp 11–66). Sigma.

Purworini, D., Purnamasari, D., & Hartuti, D. (2019). Crisis communication in a natural disaster: A chaos theory approach. *Jurnal Komunikasi: Malaysian Journal of Communication, 35*(2), 35–48.

Rasmussen, J., & Ihlen, Ø. (2017). Risk, crisis, and social media: A systematic review of seven years' research. *Nordicom Review, 38*(2), 1–17. doi: 10.1515/nor-2017-0393.

Renn, O. (1981). *Wahrnehmung und Akzeptanz technischer Risiken. Spezielle Berichte der Kernforschungsanlage Jülich, 6 Bände.* Kernforschungsanlage Jülich. http://dx.doi.org/10.18419/opus-7503

Renn, O. (2009). Risk communication: Insights and requirements for designing successful communication programs on health and environmental hazards. In Heath, R. L. & O'Hair, H. D. (Eds.). *Handbook of risk and crisis communication* (pp.80–98). Routledge.

Ringer, F. (1992). *Fields of knowledge: French academic culture in comparative perspective, 1890-1920.* Cambridge University Press.

Roberto, A. J., Goodall, C. E., & Witte, K. (2009). Raising the alarm and calming fears: Perceived threat and efficacy during risk and crisis. In Heath, R. L. & O'Hair, H. D. (Eds.). *Handbook of risk and crisis communication* (pp. 285–301). Routledge.

Samoilenko, S. (2016). Crisis management and communication research in Russia. In Schwarz, A., Seeger, M., & Auer, C. (Eds.). *Handbook of international crisis communication research* (pp. 397–410). Wiley Blackwell.

Schiefloe, P. M. (2021). The Corona crisis: A wicked problem. *Scandinavian Journal of Public Health, 49*(1), 5–8. doi: 10.1177/1403494820970767.

Schultz, F., Utz, S., & Göritz, A. (2011). Is the medium the message? Perceptions of and reactions to crisis communication via twitter, blogs and traditional media. *Public Relations Review, 37*(1), 20–27.

Schulz, J. (2001). Issues management im Rahmen der Risiko- und Krisenkommunikation. Anspruch und Wirklichkeit in Unternehmen. In Röttger, U. (Ed.). *Issues Management. Theoretische Konzepte und praktische Umsetzung. Eine Bestandsaufnahme* (pp. 217–234). Westdeutscher Verlag.

Schwarz, A. (2015). Strategische Krisenkommunikation von Organisationen. In Bentele, G., Fröhlich, R., & Szyszka, P. (Eds.). *Handbuch der Public Relations. 3. Auflage* (pp. 1001–1016). Springer VS.

Schwarz, A. (2016). Crisis communication research in Germany. In Schwarz, A., Seeger, M., & Auer, C. (Eds.). *The Handbook of international crisis communication research* (pp. 357–372). Wiley Blackwell.

Schwarz, A., Seeger, M., & Auer, C. (2016). Significance and structure of international risk and crisis communication research: Toward an integrative approach. In Schwarz, A., Seeger, M., & Auer, C. (Eds.), *The Handbook of international crisis communication research* (pp. 1-10). Wiley Blackwell.

Schwarz, A., & Büker, J. (2018). Die Krisenkommunikation von Hochschulen. In Fähnrich, B., Metag, J., Post, S. & Schäfer, M. S. (Eds.). *Forschungsfeld Hochschulkommunikation* (pp. 271–295). Springer VS.

Schwarz, A., & Löffelholz, M. (2014). Krisenkommunikation: Vorbereitung, Umsetzung, Erfolgsfaktoren. In Zerfass, A. & Piwinger, M. (Eds.). *Handbuch Unternehmenskommunikation: Strategie – Management – Wertschöpfung. 2. Auflage* (pp. 1303–1319). Springer Gabler.

Schwarz, A., & Löffelholz, M. (2022). Krisenkommunikation: Vorbereitung, Umsetzung, Erfolgsfaktoren. In Zerfass, A., Piwinger, M. & Röttger, U. (Eds.). *Handbuch Unternehmenskommunikation. 3. Auflage* (pp. 963–979). Springer Gabler.

Schwarz, A., & Pforr, F. (2011). The crisis communication preparedness of nonprofit organizations: The case of German interest groups. *Public Relations Review, 37*(1), 68–70.

Schwarz, A., Schleicher, K., Srugies, A., & Rothenberger, L. (2017). *Die Krisenkommunikation von Jugendämtern in Deutschland: Befunde zur Medienberichterstattung und strategischen Kommunikation insbesondere im Kontext schwerer Fälle von Kindeswohlgefährdung.* Universitätsverlag.

Seeger, M. W. (2018). Answering the call for scholarship: The Journal of International crisis and risk communication research. *Journal of International Crisis and Risk Communication Research, 1*(1), 7–10.

Seeger, M. W., Sloan, A. G., & Sellnow, T. (2016). Crisis communication research in the United States. In Schwarz, A., Seeger, M. & Auer, C. (Eds.). *Handbook of international crisis communication research* (pp. 422–433). Wiley Blackwell.

Sellnow, T. L. (1993). Scientific argument in organizational crisis communication. The case of Exxon. *Argumentation and Advocacy, 30*, 28–42.

Sellnow, D. D., Lane, D. R., Sellnow, T. L., & Littlefield, R. S. (2017). The IDEA model as a best practice for effective instructional risk and crisis communication. *Communication Studies, 68*(5), 552–567.

Sellnow, T. L., & Seeger, M. W. (2013). *Theorizing crisis communication.* Wiley.

Shi, J., & Yu, M. (2008). Crisis response: The message strategies and media coverage model. In 2008 IEEM International Conference on Industrial Engineering and Engineering Management (Vols 1–3, pp. 585–589). doi: 10.1109/IEEM.2008.4737936.

Singh, L., Bansal, S., Bode, L., Budak, C., Chi, G., Kawintiranon, K., Padden, C., Vanarsdall, R., Vraga, E., & Wang, Y. (2020). A first look at COVID-19 information and misinformation sharing on Twitter. http:// arxiv.org/abs/2003.13907

Staehle, W. H., Conrad, P., & Sydow, J. (1999). *Management: Eine verhaltenswissenschaftliche Perspektive* (8th ed.). Vahlen.

Stieglitz, S., Mirbabaie, M., Fromm, J., & Melzer, S. (2018). The adoption of social media analytics for crisis management: Challenges and opportunities. In Twenty-Sixth European Conference on Information Systems (ECIS2018), Portsmouth, UK. Retrieved from https://www.researchgate.net/publication/325416290_The_Adoption_of_Social_Media_Analytics_for_Crisis_Management_-_Challenges_and_Opportunities

Sturges, D. L. (1994). Communicating through crisis: A strategy for organizational survival. *Management Communication Quarterly, 7*(3), 297–316.

Subba, R., & Bui, T. (2017). Online convergence behavior, social media communications and crisis response: An empirical study of the 2015 Nepal earthquake police twitter project. In Proceedings of the 50th Annual Hawaii International Conference on System Sciences (pp. 284–293). Hawaii, USA.

Tandoc, E. C., & Takahashi, B. (2017). Log in if you survived: Collective coping on social media in the aftermath of Typhoon Haiyan in the Philippines. *New Media & Society, 19*(11): 1778–1793. https://doi.org/10.1177/1461444816642755

Tandoc, E. C., Lim, Z. W., & Ling, R. (2018). Defining 'fake news': A typology of scholarly definitions. *Digital Journalism, 6*, 137–153.

Teichert, W. (1987). Tschernobyl in den Medien. Ergebnisse und Hypothesen zur Tschernobyl- Berichterstattung. *Rundfunk und Fernsehen, 35*(2), 185–204.

Ulmer, R. R., Sellnow, T. L., & Seeger, M. W. (2007). *Effective crisis communication: Moving from crisis to opportunity*. Sage.

Valentini, C., & Kruckeberg, D. (2016). The future role of social media in international crisis communication. In Schwarz, A., Seeger, M. & Auer, C. (Eds.). *Handbook of international crisis communication research* (pp. 478–488). Wiley Blackwell.

Veil, S. R. (2011). Mindful learning in crisis management. *Journal of Business Communication, 48*(2), 116–147.

Waisbord, S., & Mellado, C. (2014). De-westernizing communication studies: A reassessment. *Communication Theory, 24*, 361–372.

Wang, S., Jin, S., & Shi, Y. (2009). Function study of media crisis communication-based on case analysis of China media coping with Wenchuan earthquake. In Proceedings of International Disaster and Risk Conference Chengdu 2009 (pp. 125–129). Chengdu, PRC.

Wang, Y., & Xi, B. (2009). Research on crisis information network of crisis communication: A case study of Songhua River Pollution in China. In Proceedings of 2009 International Conference On Public Administration (5th) (Vol II, pp. 349–354). Chengdu, PRC.

Weiner, M., & Kochhar, S. (2016). *Irreversible: The public relations big data revolution*. Institute for Public Relations.

Weischenberg, S. (1982). *Journalismus in der Computergesellschaft. Informatisierung, Medientechnik und die Rolle der Berufskommunikatoren*. Saur.

Wiedemann, P. M., & Riess, K. (2014). Issues monitoring und issues management in der Unternehmenskommunikation. In Zerfaß, A. & Piwinger, M. (Eds.). *Handbuch Unternehmenskommunikation, 2. Auflage* (pp. 493–512). Springer Gabler.

Wiesenberg, M., Zerfass, A., & Moreno, A. (2017). Big data and automation in strategic communication. *International Journal of Strategic Communication, 11*(2), 95–114.

Wertz, E., & Kim, S. (2010). Cultural issues in crisis communication: A comparative study of messages chosen by South Korean and US print media. *Journal of Communication Management, 14*(1), 81–94.

Wilensky, G. (2021). 2020 Revealed how poorly the US was prepared for COVID-19—and future pandemics. *JAMA, 325*(11), 1029–1030. doi:10.1001/jama.2021.1046.

Wishnick, E. (2005). *China as a risk society.* East-West Center. https://www
.eastwestcenter.org/system/tdf/private/PSwp012.pdf?file=1&type=node&id
=32086

Woolley, S. C., & Howard, P. N. (2016). Political communication, computational
propaganda, and autonomous agents. *International Journal of Communication,
10,* 4882–4890.

World Bank. (2020, April 17). Decisive action in an unprecedented crisis. Retrieved
from The World Bank: https://www.worldbank.org/en/news/feature/2020
/04/17/decisive-action-in-an-unprecedented-crisis

Wu, F., Huang, Y.-H., & Kao, L. (2016). East meets West: A new contextual
perspective for crisis communication theory. *Asian Journal of Communication,
26*(4), 350–370.

Xia, B. (2007). Risk communications: The performance of Chinese Government –
Research on the case of Avian Influenza. In ISCRAM CHINA 2007: Proceedings
of the Second International Workshop on Information Systems for Crisis Response
and Management. Harbin, PRC.

Xiao, Y., Hudders, L., Claeys, A.-S., & Cauberghe, V. (2018). The impact of
expressing mixed valence emotions in organizational crisis communication on
consumer's negative word-of-mouth intention. *Public Relations Review, 44*(5),
794–806.

Yuan, E. (2021). Governing risk society: the socio-technological experiences of China
and South Korea in the COVID-19 pandemic. *Asian Journal of Communication,
31*(5). doi: 10.1080/01292986.2021.1913620.

Zerfass, A., Verčič, D., Verhoeven, P., Moreno, Á., & Tench, R. (2019). *European
Communication Monitor 2019. Exploring trust in the profession, transparency,
artificial intelligence and new content strategies. Results of a survey in 46 countries.*
EUPRERA / EACD, Quadriga Media Berlin.

Zhang, X., Nekmat, E., & Chen, A. (2020). Crisis collective memory making on
social media: A case study of three Chinese crises on Weibo. *Public Relations
Review, 46*(4). doi: https://doi.org/10.1016/j.pubrev.2020.101960.

Zhao, X., Mengqi, Z., & Liu, B. F. (2018). Disentangling social media influence in
crises: Testing a four-factor model of social media influence with large data. *Public
Relations Review, 44*(4), 549–561.

Zimmermann, F., & Kohring, M. (2018). „Fake News" als aktuelle Desinformation.
Systematische Bestimmung eines heterogenen Begriffs. *Medien und
Kommunikationswissenschaft, 4,* 526–541.

3 Information Literacy or Political Propaganda

Analyzing the Taiwan Government's Responsive Strategies to COVID-19 Infodemic

Chiung-wen Hsu and Yun-Chung Tang

Introduction

Taiwan was predicted to be one of the countries most affected by COVID-19 due to its geographic proximity to China and frequent interactions between the two nations. Because of the painful lessons of the severe acute respiratory syndrome (SARS) in 2003, the Taiwan government and people had high alerts early on. In addition, the democratic mechanism ensures transparency and publicity, with which Taiwan has implemented prevention measures in fighting disease successfully. However, Taiwan cannot have a narrow escape from the infodemic and misinformation prevails.

The Taiwan government is concerned about the misinformation and mobilizes the relevant authorities to fight against it. The Taiwan Centers for Disease Control (CDC), Ministry of Health and Welfare (MOHW), is the uppermost infectious disease control authority in charge of disease prevention and control, and it is also responsible for providing real-time information regarding disease surveillance and notification of the relevant units in Taiwan. During the breaking time of unknown pneumonia in Wuhan, China, the CDC was aware of it. It launched "advanced deployment" (超前部署, chaoqian bushu) such as onboard quarantine of passengers on direct flights from Wuhan starting from December 31, 2019.

Following the international outbreak situation, the Executive Yuan approved the establishment of the COVID-19 Central Epidemic Command Center (CECC) by the CDC as a level 3 center on January 20, 2020, which was seen as a prompt response to the coronavirus in the early stage of the pandemic. Premier Tseng-chang Su upgraded it to a level 2 center on January 23 and to a level 1 center (the highest level) on February 27. The CECC relies on the support of the CDC both in the office area and in its affairs.

Several units have distributed the anti-misinformation messages via several channels. The Executive Yuan, MOHW, and CDC make relevant announcements through each website, Facebook account, or Line account. The Taiwan government took this strategy as a critical factor in controlling the pandemic. On

DOI: 10.4324/9781003286684-3

the Minister of Health and Welfare website, a banner named crucial policies for combating COVID-19.[1] The ministry provides the essential success factors for Taiwan to control the pandemic, including SARS experience, Central Epidemic Command Center, information transparency, good resources allocation, timely border control, smart community transmission prevention, advanced medical technology, and the good etiquette of citizens. The government is optimistic about its response to COVID-19. To provide immediate, transparent, and first-hand information to the media and to the public, the CECC hosts a daily press conference and publishes press releases every day. Unprecedently, the daily press conferences have been live streaming since January 22, 2020; a sign language interpreter has joined the press conferences since January 27 to ensure the rights of people with hearing impairments, and Hakka real-time oral interpretation done by Hakka TV has been included in the press conferences since June 7, 2021, to help Hakka people to get the information faster.

The CECC has produced self-protection materials and provided the materials through various media outlets to promote public health. The TV noncommercial ad serials are well known in Taiwan called protecting Taiwan through mutual support (防疫大作戰) with local dialect varieties and foreign language versions accessible to different kinds of residents in Taiwan, such as migrant workers and foreign nationals.

The hotline of 1922 for communicable disease reporting and consultation plays an essential role in giving away information and responding to the public's inquiries. Ideally, the calls should be directed to the related official departments to make sure any individual's situation is taken care of.

In addition to the offline media outlets, the above press conferences, self-protection materials, data on the outbreaks, contact tracing results, and new policies are provided on the website, Line, and Facebook accounts. Clarifications of misinformation, disinformation, and malinformation are essential during the pandemic. This study examines how the Taiwan government fights against the infodemic and the anti-misinformation messages made by the officials.

Study's Theoretical Framework

Since the early awareness of the outbreak of COVID-19, the Taiwan government adopted proper countermeasures to block the spread and prevent a tremendous number of casualties. However, it did not alleviate the dissemination of infodemic in Taiwan. Misinformation prevailed immediately at the start of the outbreak. According to the Taiwan FactCheck Center, in the first three months of 2020, there was a lot of misinformation regarding virus characteristics, remedies, cures, measures, then conspiracy mixed with scientific papers, and Taiwan's losing control.[2] The huge amount of misinformation, to some extent, could seriously jeopardize the hard work of the society of the whole citizens during the pandemic and turn the nation into a chaotic situation. It is vital and urgent to understand the infodemic in Taiwan and fight it. Due to the effort of many researchers, a fruitful finding is displayed in front of us.

Lin (2022) also accumulated 153 messages from Taiwan FactCheck Center from January 1, 2020, to June 30, 2020, and found that common themes of misinformation are COVID-19 cures, the characteristics and means of transmission of COVID-19, global and local pandemic governance, disinformation, pandemic in countries other than China and Taiwan, and others. She also found that some misinformation might be traceable to China's operations against Taiwan due to simplified Chinese characters and mainly focusing on Taiwan's out of control. The themes of misinformation mainly encompass COVID-19 and its measures, and the troll from China is considered a crucial transmitter. By understanding the themes of misinformation, it is important to come up with a better solution to refute the misinformation.

Besides the themes of misinformation, the types of information also draw people's attention and engagement, which should inform the public. Pulido and her colleagues' study (2020) found that false information is more tweeted. But tweets with science-based evidence or fact-checking were more retweeted. By definition, science-based evidence tweets comprise science-based information guaranteeing the content's reliability and fact-checking tweets contain reliable information to debunk false information. These two types of tweets captured more engagement, implying that the health authorities could publish such information to prompt anti-misinformation and health literacy information.

On top of the characteristics of misinformation, Kim (2020) thought that it is essential to investigate who believes the misinformation regarding COVID-19 and identify structural factors that determined belief in fake news to manage infodemic. In addition to the demographics, higher perceived risk and stigma toward the confirmed patients positively affect belief in fake news. People with higher perceived benefit of the consequences caused by COVID-19 and higher trust in the community negatively affect belief in fake news. Lastly, the amount of information and heuristic thinking without analyzing information logically have positive effects on belief in fake news, and the source credibility has a negative effect. The positive effects of stigma and heuristic thinking on belief in fake news especially show that people did not process information rationally and systematically. Thus, Kim (2020) further suggested when the government communicates with the public, it needs to use a communication strategy based on a more "humane and emotional approach" rather than a simple, mechanical, and fact-based approach. As for the perceived risk, health literacy should be addressed.

The consequences of the misinformation about COVID-19 are multilayered. It distorted people's risk perception, which is related to rejection of information, improper preventative public health behaviors, and the spread of the pandemic (Krause et al., 2020; Dryhurst et al., 2020). The countermeasures to control the infodemic are also multilayered. Health literacy is considered a determinant of health and debunks misinformation by the above research. van der Linden et al. (2020) also proposed that behavioral scientists should identify the scope of the negative influences on health-protective behaviors and adopt the theory of psychological inoculation to manage an effective response to control the spread of misinformation about COVID-19.

People in Taiwan also have faced fear and limited knowledge about this unknown disease, paralyzing their rational judgment and distorted risk perception. Given that health literacy played a vital role in stopping the misinformation and facilitating health behaviors, it is crucial to examine how the Taiwan government responded to the misinformation about COVID-19 to empower people's health literacy to influence their public health's behaviors and attitudes to survive from the pandemic.

Before COVID-19, there was little research focusing on health misinformation but more on health literacy of diseases or behaviors. Some research paid attention to patients and information-seeking users (Phlypo et al., 2020; Wingard, 2005), and some research focused on messages (Belogianni et al., 2019; Ezika, 2020). This study adopted the theoretical framework of the message quality of health literacy and examined the anti-misinformation messages from the Taiwan government accordingly.

Walsh and her team conducted the content analysis and heuristic evaluation of My Health Record (MyHR), the Australian government-announced health system, in 2016 and 2018 (Walsh et al., 2017, 2021). Their criteria to evaluate information quality, themes, target audiences, and usability provided this study to scrutinize the government messages. There was readability, currency, information source, presentation style, and links between resources included in the information quality criteria. Except for the website's usability requirements in the heuristic evaluation, this study followed the rest criteria. This study included the items to fit in the contexts of the Taiwan government's responding platforms and messages: describing the health behavior, positive tone, action steps, plain language, checking content for accuracy, using links effectively, disability accessibility, social media sharing options, and offering content in multiple languages.

In Walsh's studies, they found there was not much change in two years. There were some improvements in information quality, such as increases in resources from non-government organizations, video resources, translated resources, and resources with themes of privacy, security, and post-registration use. But there were gaps unresolved in information quality and usability which may hinder the usefulness of people with low health literacy, such as lack of plain English or low literacy resources, lack of resources in community languages, lack of diversity in presentation styles, and lack of targeted resources for the target audiences (older or people with health conditions).

Fan and his colleagues' work (2020) found similar arguments. They analyzed 321 English websites from 34 countries employing search engine results using 12 search terms. They claimed that the websites with higher quality provided multiple aspects of COVID-19 and used a variety of sources that facilitated a better understanding of the pandemic. However, most websites addressed COVID-19 prevention but neglected treatment issues that became the public's concerns reflected on search trends.

Things are slightly different when it comes to social media. Previous research (Martin & MacDonald, 2020) focusing on scientific communication suggested that interpersonal communication strategies are quite important and supportive for engagement. In social media, such as Facebook, Twitter, or Instagram, using selfies, non-scientific content, and first-person style communication are solid strategies to encourage engagement and discussion, which will increase the possibility of information transmission. The above research sheds light on the higher quality of literacy messages, offering a comprehensive perspective via science communication, health communication, communication strategy, content text, and literacy.

Based on the above literature review, the research questions are listed below:

1. What kind of misinformation does the government respond to more?
2. What channel does the government use more to respond to misinformation?
3. What strategy does the government use to respond to misinformation?
4. In terms of literacy, what does the government do in the messages?

Research Methods

This study adopts mixed methods to depict the message presentation and contexts of government information (GV) against misinformation about COVID-19. This research has two phrases (study I and study II). First, the content analysis of government information allocated on websites, Facebook, LINE, Twitter, and Instagram of the Executive Yuan, Ministry of Health and Welfare, Prime Minister Su, and Taiwan Center for Disease Control starting from December 31, 2019, to February 1, 2021 (Table 3.1).

To examine the characteristics of anti-misinformation messages, the two undergraduate students majoring in Communication were trained to analyze the origins of anti-misinformation messages (website, Facebook, Line, Twitter, and Instagram), the sources of misinformation, PNG images of misinformation, PNG images of anti-misinformation messages, content (regulations, penalty, fact-checking), language (Taiwanese dialect and English), and political figures (Premier Tseng-chang Su and President Ing-wen Tsai). The intercoder reliability is identical.

This study conducted an in-depth interview with the spokesman of Central Epidemic Command Center (CECC), Jen-hsiang Chuang, Taiwan Centers for Disease Control (CDC) Deputy Director-General, and another Deputy

Table 3.1 Online Channel for Relative Governmental Units

	Website	Facebook	LINE	Twitter	IG
Executive Yuan	+	+	–	–	–
Premier Tseng-chang Su	–	+	+	+	+
MOHW	+	+	+	+	–
CDC	+	+	+	+	+

Director-General, Yi-chun Lo, on February 25, 2021. And the in-depth interviews with the Chair of the Department of Public Relations of CDC, Kai-ling Tsao, were on February 25, 2021, and May 4, 2021. The participatory observation was executed twice in the same period.

On May 19, 2021, Taiwan faced the first outbreak after recording over 100 locally transmitted cases for several consecutive days and declared a nationwide level 3 COVID-19 alert. There was more misinformation circulation during the unprecedented explosion in Taiwan. The study further started the second phrase research. According to study I, the government information is cross-posting in several social media outlets. The CDC takes the lead in releasing anti-misinformation messages on its websites, Facebook, Line, Twitter, and Instagram.

The LINE official account of the CDC (@taiwancdc, 疾管家) is recognized as the primary protocol of government information after President Tsai Ing-wen's recommendation in her Facebook post.[3] The LINE official account of the CDC established in 2017 initially functions to prevent influenza, vaccination, and inquire about more than 90 kinds of epidemic information worldwide, with about 100,000 users. But with the outbreak of the epidemic, the number of users soared to 500,000 within a week during the 2020 Chinese New Year and then exceeded 2 million within a month and a half. As of the end of March 2020, 2.1 million people had followed. As of January 2022, there are 10,212,091 users.

Study II scrutinized the 198 messages posted on the LINE official account of the CDC employing text analysis. The in-depth interview with Chair Tsao was conducted online on January 22, 2022.

Results

Content Analysis

The research finding of study I suggests that the government responding message to misinformation during the pandemic in Taiwan features several strategies focused on multiple media channels and multiple formats, image spokespeople, humorous style, displaying the source of misinformation/rumor, and addressing the consequences of spreading misinformation. Besides responding to misinformation, government-created content is shared and distributed extensively via different social network services. The following paragraphs will demonstrate the features of responding strategies that the Taiwan government applied from three perspectives: media, content, and style. Afterward, the finding will further display its potential and ambition for sharing.

From the perspective of media, multiple media channels and formats were utilized for maximizing media coverage, both online and offline, new media, and traditional media. The CDC's daily press conference would spare time for responding to the misinformation out of routine pandemic information broadcasting. As for the online platform, the official website, Facebook, Twitter, Instagram, and Line were all frequently used to respond to misinformation. There

Table 3.2 The Online Media Platform Used for Responding to Misinformation

	Website	Facebook	LINE	Twitter	Instagram	Total
Executive Yuan	32	5				37
Premier		3		2	3	8
Tseng-chang Su						
MOHW	26	24	10	9		69
CDC	11	17	10	1		39
Total	69	49	20	12	3	153 (130 cross-posting)

were 151 collected pieces of responding information released from December 31, 2019, to February 1, 2021, from the Executive Yuan, Executive Dean, Ministry of Health and Welfare, and Taiwan Center of Disease Control.

The official websites play the role of the protocol of official documents and announcements, and the four relevant authorities posted more messages on the websites. Regarding public social network sites (hereafter, SNS) usage in Taiwan, Facebook and LINE are mainly used. Instagram and Twitter are usually for personal image display and international information and are less used (Table 3.2).

Besides the multiple platform use, almost every piece of information contained images for the image-oriented SNS feature and for the purpose of sharing. As mentioned above, the content was also shared and repeated from one media to another in both text and image formats. Specifically, 130 out of 153 pieces of responding information were cross-posting.

The most origins of anti-misinformation messages on SNS are from Facebook, Line, and Twitter in a descending order, which fits the current status quo of social media usage in Taiwan. The sources of misinformation mentioned in the text or PNG images are vague. The government authorities tend to respond more to online misinformation from Internet sources (63), communication apps (33), and SNS (21) and less to offline misinformation from press media (44) (Table 3.3).

Regarding the content, the result showed some features such as image orientation, displaying the source of misinformation/rumor, and consequences of spreading misinformation. The researcher discovered 56 responses indicating the origin of misinformation/rumor PNG images, and 110 responses were governmental created PNG images for helping clarification and information distribution. Some of them were memes to provide information humorously.

As for the political figures used in the anti-misinformation messages, unlike Premier Tseng-chang Su's frequently presented on the PNG images or text, President Ing-wen Tsai was mentioned only once inside the text about her policy of producing enough masks for the public distorted by one press media and there were no PNG images of her at all. Minister of MOHW and the commander of CECC, Shih-chung Chen, only appeared once on the anti-misinformation

Table 3.3 The Characteristics of Anti-Misinformation Messages

Items		Counts
Origins of anti-misinformation messages	Website	69
	Facebook	49
	LINE	20
	Twitter	12
	Instagram	3
Sources of misinformation	Press media	44
	Communication apps	33
	SNS	21
	Internet sources	63
PNG images of misinformation		56
PNG images of anti-misinformation messages		110
Political figures	Premier Tseng-chang Su	10
	President Ing-wen Tsai	1
	Minister Shih-chung Chen	1
Content	Regulations	114
	Penalty	74
	Fact-checking	30
Language	Taiwanese dialect	16
	English	1

message with PNG image regarding the intimidation about circulating misinformation. Although there are ten posts regarding Premier Tseng-chang Su, the significant impacts lead to the following government responses.

The first confirmed case of COVID-19 in Taiwan was imported from Wuhan, China, on January 22, 2020. Due to the well-organized advanced deployment, the case was found in the airport, and the strict border policy showed the effectiveness to stop spreading. Taiwan was safer than its neighborhood counterparts as a close country near China. The PNG images, especially those with Premier Tseng-chang Su, were designed more like memes.

The first meme against COVID-19 misinformation from Premier Tseng-chang Su makes fun of the imaginary enemy, China (Figure 3.1). The meme showed part of the fake epidemics text regarding one frog farmer in Pingtung County who incidentally found that Pingtung Gymnasium was locked down to build the portable cabin hospital and figured out that more than 700 confirmed cases in the south part of Taiwan. The visual center was Su's big teasing smile and words with funny wording: "lol~ What is the purpose of sending the frog to the temporary hospital?" There were two hashtags, #with the government (#有政府) and #please reset assured (#請安心), becoming a series of memes. The illustration mentioned that the fake information is exaggerated and unreasonable, and the

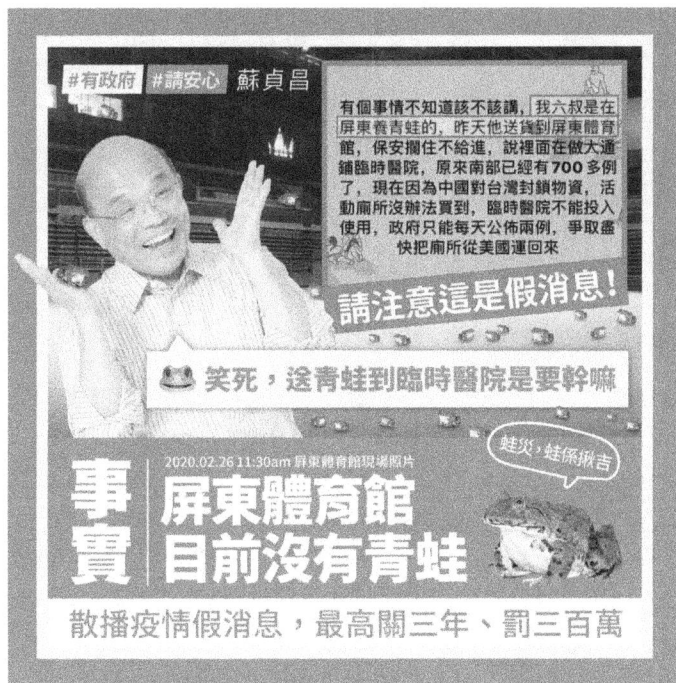

Figure 3.1 Premier Tseng-chang Su's meme against COVID-19 misinformation on February 26, 2020

wording and grammar are not Taiwanese. This humorous and funny expression prevails at the beginning of the pandemic.

The prevailing meme style was initiated by MOHW and started from the dog, CEO Shina, owned by the SNS team member and became the "spokesperson." The first post with CEO Shiba was published on February 3 to promote hygiene during the pandemic (Figure 3.2(a)). After that, CEO Shiba became a celebrity. There were more CEO Shiba's PNG images, and the style of the image reflected the commons in people's daily life, such as mimicking the popular Line PNG that senior people love to forward, which is easy to circulate in SNS (Figure 3.2(b)).

The first anti-misinformation message of MOHW was posted on February 15 to refute the outbreak in Taiwan and clarify that there were three doctors quarantined because of close contact with the confirmed cases, not because of being infected as media coverage (Figure 3.2). The CEO Shiba in the PNG images was in an angry face and with the "angry" word next to it, which showed that the CEO Shiba was mad with the fake news.

CEO Shiba and Premier's memes went viral during the pandemic, responding to the misinformation and making clarification in a less intimidating way. Besides the image spokespeople used, the text displayed a high sense of humor.

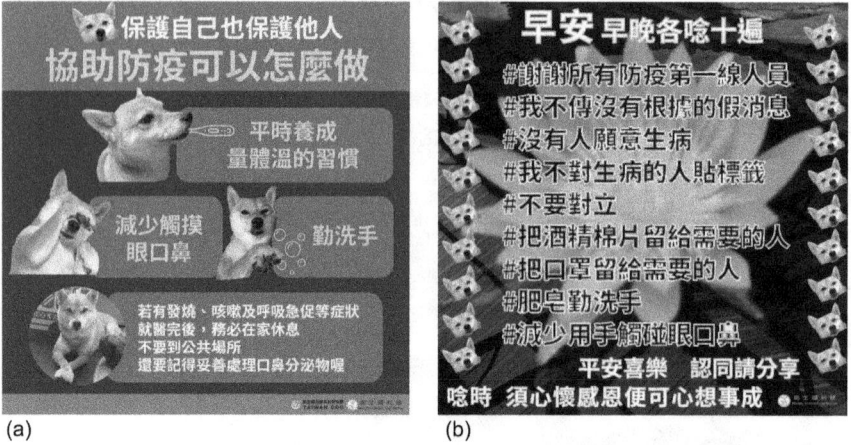

Figure 3.2 The meme-like PNG images with CEO Shiba of MOHW. (a) The first CEO Shiba PNG image regarding the pandemic on February 3, 2020. (b) The mimic style of popular LINE PNG image for seniors on February 14, 2020

Sixteen pieces use Taiwanese (language) slang or speaking for entertainment purposes. The researchers believe that using a humorous style aimed to ease the fear appeal and raise confidence in the government policy and the intention of sharing. But considering the foreigners' information access, only one message is made in English, let alone other languages.

A high percentage of responses also included the consequences of spreading misinformation. Related law statements were solemnly displayed, such as Article 14 of "Special Act for Prevention, Relief and Revitalization Measures for Severe Pneumonia with Novel Pathogens" (76), Social Order Maintenance Act (83), and other norms and laws (9), including Communicable Disease Control Act, and Article 313 of the Criminal Law. Besides the exact law statement, the amount of penalty was also mentioned in 74 responses. With the legal intimidation primarily, the responses addressed less how to do the fact-checking, the need and necessity for stopping the spread of misinformation to avoid panic, supply shortage, health issues, and policies misunderstanding. In other words, the Taiwan government tried to use fun, fear, and reasoning as communication appeals but provided little literacy of fact-checking and knowledge of COVID-19 at the same time.

Overall, the Taiwan government's responsive strategy toward misinformation demonstrated several features, and it all connected to the purpose of using one versatile material for all possible media platforms. The media perspective of responsive strategies suggested that the hyperlink, cross-media platform, and multiple formats lead to a fluid and interchangeable potential for sharing information. The numerous cross-posting within the government website and SNS is evidential for its interchangeability. The content and style perspectives show the government's intention to earn the public's confidence in the government's COVID-19 countermeasures, intimidation about circulating misinformation and encourage the public to disseminate the information via humorous style and meme-like content. However, information literacy was not an issue for the Taiwan government. Since the government's responsive strategy created numerous versatile materials waiting for modification and transmission, it is crucial to look at its responding information in detail.

Text Analysis and In-Depth Interview

In this section, the most crucial anti-misinformation platform, the Line official account of CDC, will be examined, focusing on the clarification zone, the specific anti-misinformation message hub. The CDC started to put the relevant information on the Line account on January 25, 2020. On top of the text analysis, the researchers conducted in-depth interviews online and offline twice to provide the contexts of the government's responsive strategies.

1) The confident and aggressive attitude toward Wuhan pneumonia and China

Taiwan had the first confirmed case on January 21, 2020, the first domestic confirmed case on January 28, and the first death on February 15. It aroused people's attention and care about COVID-19. The CDC launched several prevention plans and had the epidemic in control in January and February 2020. The government was confident, and the attitude toward China was aggressive. The officers mentioned the coronavirus disease as Wuhan pneumonia in the oral speeches and government documents even after the World Health Organization (WHO) has announced the official name, COVID-19, on March 12.

According to the Taiwan FactCheck Center, in the first three months of 2020, there was a lot of misinformation regarding virus characteristics, remedies, cures, measures, then conspiracy mixed with scientific papers, and Taiwan's losing control. The CDC's first anti-misinformation message posted on January 2, 2020, aimed at a picture of medical staff on board the fake information that there were confirmed cases on the airplane and entered Taiwan categorized as Taiwan's losing control. The CDC claimed that no confirmed cases entered Taiwan and mentioned that medical staff uniforms were not Taiwan authorities. In addition, the PNG image showed the above information and stated the Social Order Maintenance Act and the penalty (Figure 3.3).

Although the CDC didn't make explicit reasons for selecting the misinformation to clarify, the anti-misinformation messages from the CDC were mainly referred to those that originated from China and gave the impression that the misinformation was a type of information war of China. For example, the CDC's first anti-misinformation message against the Wuhan pneumonia entering Taiwan posted on January 2, 2020, only mentioned that the picture of the medical staff on the plane shown in the misinformation was not from Taiwan, judging from the uniforms. None of

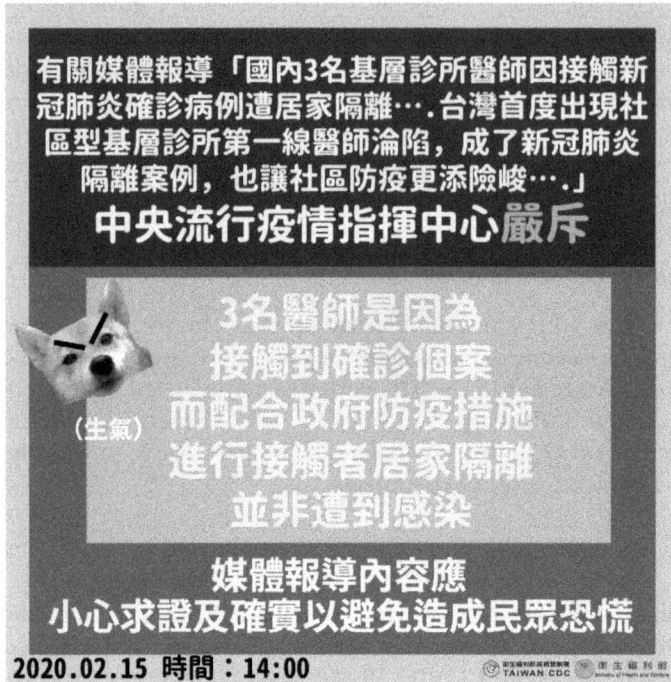

有關媒體報導「國內3名基層診所醫師因接觸新冠肺炎確診病例遭居家隔離….台灣首度出現社區型基層診所第一線醫師淪陷，成了新冠肺炎隔離案例，也讓社區防疫更添險峻….」

中央流行疫情指揮中心嚴斥

（生氣）

3名醫師是因為
接觸到確診個案
而配合政府防疫措施
進行接觸者居家隔離
並非遭到感染

媒體報導內容應
小心求證及確實以避免造成民眾恐慌

2020.02.15 時間：14:00

Figure 3.3 The first anti-misinformation message with CEO Shiba of MOHW was posted on February 15, 2020

the information mentioned about China (Figure 3.4). The LINE official account of CDC (@taiwancdc) released the assumption that the misinformation would be part of the information war of China. In the 198 posts on the clarification zone (澄清專區) from January 25, 2020, to July 10, 2021, the CDC claimed that 21 cases of misinformation as part of the information war were directly from China and implied that some cases might be the intended behaviors of Internet users from China.

2) The politics of government's responses in the first three months of the pandemic

The more increasing confirmed cases, the more misinformation messages. But it seems not always the case. When the pandemic started at the beginning of 2020, people were unfamiliar with the disease and had no experience. Under this circumstance, people tend to believe the information and circulate it. The CDC announced many anti-misinformation messages on the Line official account. Besides, when the confirmed cases burst suddenly, people were in panic. When the cases were over 100 on March 18, over 200 on March 24, and over 300 on March 30, 2020, the CDC also made great efforts to fight against misinformation. The amounts of anti-misinformation messages are 41 pieces in January and

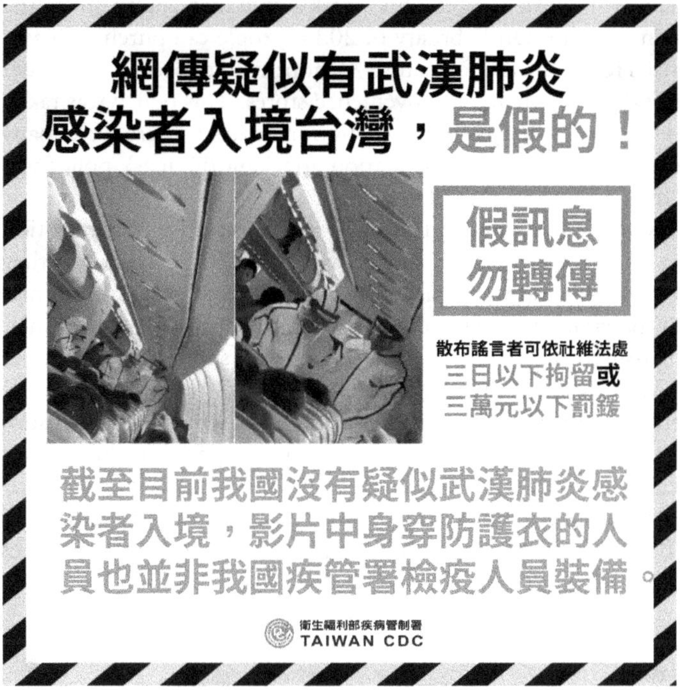

Figure 3.4 The CDC's first anti-misinformation message posted on January 2, 2020

February 2020 and 51 pieces in March, which are more than 17 pieces in the first risk period of community spread. This first risk period started around April 14 till the following two weeks because of the confirmed crew members of Panshi Fast Combat Support Ships traveling around Taiwan without quarantine when offboard.

Unlike the effort of the Taiwan FactCheck Center, the CDC fought against the misinformation in the first three months of 2020 mainly were Taiwan's losing control and epidemic prevention resources, such as medical masks and toilet papers. The government authorities, not only the CDC but also the Criminal Investigation Bureau of the National Police Agency and the Ministry of Justice Investigation Bureau, worked together to investigate the misinformation and stop further transmissions. The government had less tolerance for the misinformation regarding increasing confirmed cases, lockdown areas, and hot zones, doubting the government's ability to respond to the pandemic, especially the misinformation that might come from China. Nearly 90% of 90 pieces of anti-misinformation messages were to refute Taiwan's losing control and reinforce the correctness of the government countermeasures.

The lack of livelihood supplies and medical masks was also an important issue in Taiwan. The government coordinated with the private sector to set up new face mask production lines to stop panic. Digital Minister Audrey Tang teamed up with the engineers who developed the first mask search map app to create the name-based rationing system. On February 6, 2020, people can purchase masks with their National Health Insurance cards. A month later, people can order face masks online and collect them at convenience stores. This policy was taken as national pride in several government promotion materials.[4] There were many coverages by foreign media. The misinformation attacking the mask policy was also the target of the CDC.

In addition, Taiwan went through a toilet paper crisis because of speculation of imminent increases. The supermarket shelves were wiped clean as soon as they were refilled. The panic buying was believed to have triggered the misinformation that paper raw materials were being diverted to make surgical masks. Premier Tseng-chang Su reassured the public that the nation had sufficient toilet paper supplies with a meme-like PNG image on February 7, 2020 (Figure 3.5). The misinformation that threatened the government's commitment to sufficient supplies was not accepted. Nine out of ninety messages were related to the medical mask and toilet paper.

The government's political consideration in selecting misinformation to refute was apparent in the following case. A man living in Taoyuan posted pictures

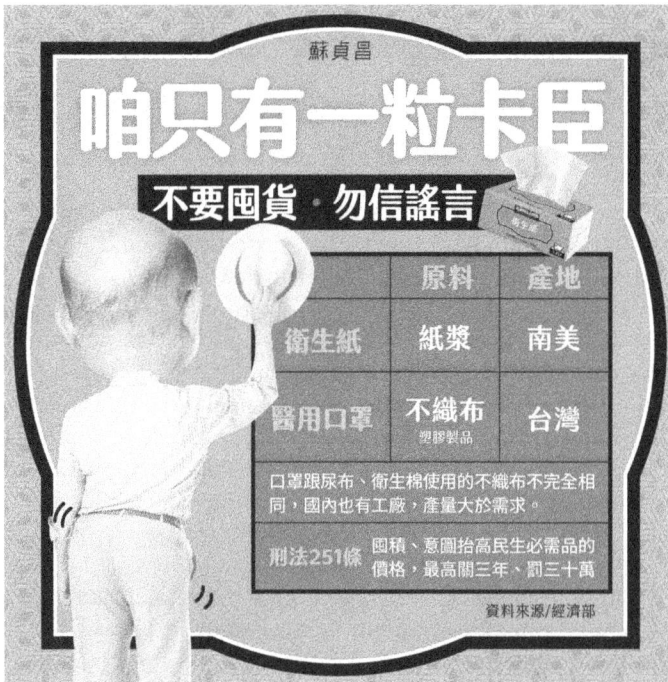

Figure 3.5 Premier Tseng-chang Su's meme to call for calm and refute the misinformation on February 7, 2020

of giving masks free in Vietnam and praised the policy of the Vietnam government being superior to Taiwan's long queues for purchasing medical masks on Facebook. The Criminal Investigation Bureau of the National Police Agency investigated the case and brought it to justice in accordance with Article 63 of the Social Order Maintenance Act. The anti-misinformation against Vietnam's free mask on the street was publicized in CDC's clarification zone on March 20, 2020. This case was not critical compared to the misinformation about virus characteristics, remedies, and cures that might endanger people's lives. It was likely chosen because it threatened the government's prestige in dealing with the pandemic. As for the anti-misinformation which might harm people's health, there were only four out of 90 cases in the first three months of the COVID-19 pandemic. The worse is that there were only four in the total 198 cases in the clarification zone of the Line official account of CDC throughout study II.

3) The government responses in the different surge periods

After the risk of community spread of Panshi Fast Combat Support Ships ended in late April 2020, there were fewer confirmed cases. By June 7, Taiwan had not reported domestic confirmed cases for 56 days (over four incubation periods). As a result, Taiwan lifted pandemic-related restrictions and held press conferences weekly[5] instead of daily. On October 29, Taiwan reached the milestone of 253[6] days without locally confirmed cases. Although there were some cases in the following year of 2020, a contact of a New Zealand pilot working for EVA Air was diagnosed with COVID-19 on December 22, marking the first local transmission since April. There were only eight pieces of anti-misinformation messages from May to September.

At the beginning of 2021, a domestic infection cluster was identified at Taoyuan General Hospital. The first case of the cluster was confirmed on January 11, and the cluster had been successfully capped at 21 cases and one death on February 15. There were only two pieces of anti-misinformation messages in January. These two cases of possible community spread were from the aviation and medical professions, which were relatively uncomplicated and controllable. A few people were impacted. Therefore, the government seemed not to respond to the misinformation.

Another peak of the government's anti-misinformation came with level 3 nationwide restrictions in the four-tier alert system started on May 19 and ended on July 26, due to the local transmissions starting from China Airline's cluster and moving to Novotel Taipei Taoyuan International Airport, Wanhua district, Huanan Market, overseas workers clusters, and more. There are 43 pieces of CDC anti-misinformation messages in May, 32 in June, and only 5 in July.

The number of cases between May and June were a little less than the unknown turmoil and rapidly confirmed-case increasing period in March 2020. In the same way, most of the cases in this surge were Taiwan's losing control. It is worth mentioning that 22 out of 80 messages were related to rapid tests, vaccines, the conspiracy of vaccine selection, and distribution. It showed that the public was worried about the quality of vaccines and the government's vaccine policy, and the consequences of being vaccinated. However, the anti-misinformation messages did not provide health information and further resources for fact-checking and only offered the official refutation and warned of the possible penalty of circulating the misinformation.

After the alert level was decreased to level 2, the pandemic slowed down a bit, and there was no more surge till the end of 2021. The latest messages were posted on July 10, 2021.

4) The government's fast response policy

This study conducted in-depth interviews with the spokesman of Central Epidemic Command Center (CECC), Jen-hsiang Chuang, Centers for Disease Control (CDC) Deputy Director-General, another Deputy Director-General, Yi-chun Lo, and the Chair of the Department of Public Relations of CDC, Kai-ling Tsao regarding the CDC anti-misinformation policy and practices.

These unprecedented challenges make the CECC and CDC learn to fight against misinformation. If the journalists brought up misinformation and asked for clarification in the live press conferences, the CECC needed to reply immediately. Therefore, they had to study the widespread misinformation circulated in SNS and the press and prepare the answers for the commander or the spokesman.

There were the so-called 222 guidelines for handling misinformation online. Except for vaccine-related misinformation, which the legal affairs team takes, the CDC PR office responded to the rest misinformation. It included posting messages in two hours with two PNG images and a 200-word text. The guideline makes sure that the widespread misinformation would be clarified immediately, the two PNG images for the convenience of SNS forwarding and the visual reading trend, and short text of around 200 words for readability.

Along with the immediateness of answering the misinformation, the government officers felt another difficulty in fighting misinformation, the proper manner to refute the misinformation in public, whether online or offline. Some misinformation was disguised as the correct information by providing partial truths and absolute photos. Without elaboration, the simple clarification would cause more misunderstanding. Thus, the refuting should be concise. Direct denouncement and waring of circulation were rules of thumb. Finally, as Digital Minister Audrey Tang suggested, the officers tried to respond to the misinformation humorously. Still, they recognized they were not good at it because they were not trained this way in their career of being government officers.

Parallel to the content analysis and text analysis findings, the anti-misinformation messages were short and lacked health literacy. The receivers know the message was incorrect but do not know why, which does not facilitate their judgment when facing misinformation again. Besides, the warning of violating laws and receiving penalties was in every piece that did not do any good for health literacy.

5) The government's passive attitude toward anti-misinformation after the meme controversial

The last anti-misinformation post on the LINE official account of CDC was on July 7, 2021, which clarified the policy of conditional reopens on July 13. The misinformation pointed out that the strict policy was for the family members but not for outside connections. Even though there was severe surge in January and February 2022, there were no more anti-misinformation messages from the CDC until this chapter was written.

Due to the first surge in 2022, the Department of Public Relations of CECC answered the study questions through Line chats and emails. It claimed that the clarification zone of the CDC website and the LINE official account of the CDC are updated simultaneously in terms of content and timing. The CECC will actively clarify some notorious and serious misinformation and make announcements. The Department of Public Relations of CECC didn't answer why the information stopped on July 7, 2021. Further, the PR of CECC mentions that they cooperate with the third-party fact-check centers to provide anti-misinformation messages. In addition, the CECC offers links to fact-check institutes for the public on the CDC website.

However, the website and LINE links of four major fact-check institutes are not easy to look upon the CDC website, including Taiwan FactCheck Center, Line fact-check, Rumor of Truth, and MyGoPen (Figure 3.6). The authors cannot find the leaf labels and inquire about the CDC again to obtain the website map routes. The links were posted and updated on May 25, 2021, after the government-imposed level 3 pandemic restrictions. The attitude to fight against COVID-19 misinformation turned inactive and passive suddenly.

Discussion

Before level 3 restrictions were issued on May 19, 2021, Taiwan had demonstrated its capacity to keep COVID-19 at bay; there were some controllable surges, though. The record of 253 days with no local confirmed cases and the #TaiwanCanHelp campaign launched by Ing-wen Tsai's government marked the national pride. To quell the COVID-19 rampancy, the government urged the public to follow the epidemic prevention measures. The successful control of outbreaks had built people's trust in the CECC and the government as a whole. Those who disagreed with the government measures were called anti-Shih-chung. The pronunciation of anti-Shih-chung sounds similar to "counterclockwise" in Chinese, which implied violating the CECC commander's orders and the government led by President Ing-wen Tsai and Premier Tseng-chang Su. The atmosphere prevailed and gave the government more power and confidence to make people comply with the COVID-19 policy.

The big government phenomenon was also reflected in the government's anti-misinformation policy. Similar to the policy of the Democratic Progressive Party (DPP), taking China as an enemy and COVID-19 as a war made the DPP-ruled government concentrate on comparing China's measures and proving the malice of China. The anti-misinformation messages do not show the consideration of people's benefits but more like the arena to fight against China and show the

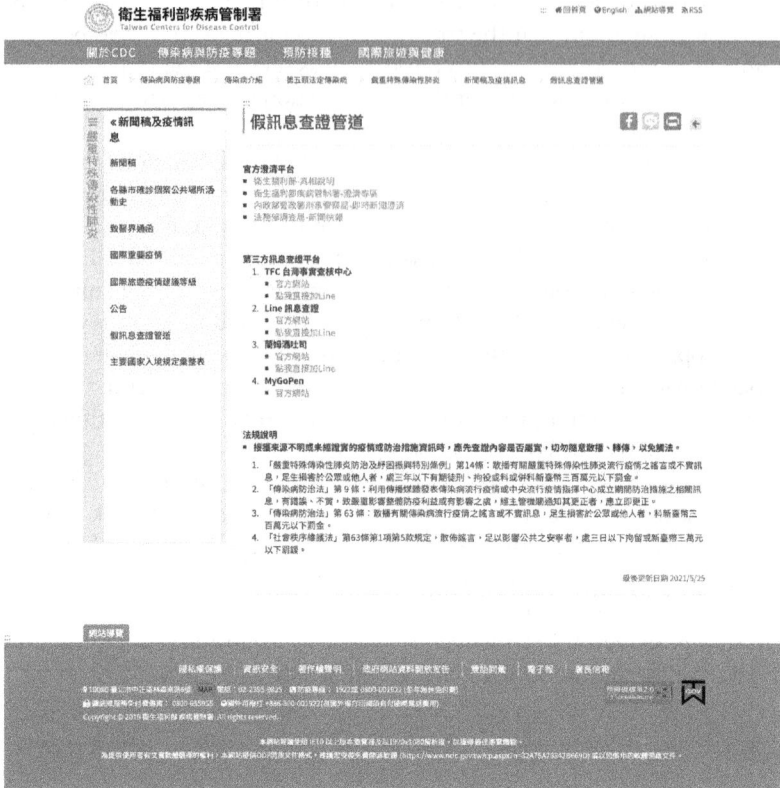

Figure 3.6 The links of four major fact-check institutes on the CDC website

efficacy and power of the government. Although the texts might not indicate the hidden purposes, the chosen misinformation and the PNG images disclosed the intentions of political propaganda.

Information literacy has been proved essential to facilitate comprehension and making mundane and critical decisions regarding health issues and diseases, also to mitigating COVID-19 infodemic by increasing critical verification practices before sharing on SNS (Melki et al., 2021; Rudd & Baur, 2020). As the leading public health authority, CDC should be familiar with the guideline and research. However, under the central theme of government policy and the unfamiliar info-demic situation, the CDC faced difficulties refuting the misinformation humor-ously and adequately.

The situation got even worse, after the controversy of the government's memes team, the cooperation between LINE and Taiwan government, 222 dis-cipline was abandoned. The government further let go of the fighting against COVID-19 misinformation and rendered the duty to the third-party fact-check centers. Fact-check is only one part of information literacy. There is so much that the government authority, research, and other actors have to contribute, such as language minorities. This study suggests a second thought to deal with misinformation. Instead of fighting against it, take it as a mirror of what the government has not done well. For example, in this study, the information about foreigners is rare, but the researchers did find that the misinformation tends to use oversea workers or immigrants, unfamiliar groups for local Taiwan people, as the subjects. As Lee et al. (2022) suggests, the attitudes toward outsiders in Taiwan were involved in the controversy as racial capitalism claimed. The authority also has the responsibility to manage it with information literacy.

The Taiwan government learned the lesson from SARS, including amending the Communicable Disease Control Act to facilitate the coordination among government agencies and private organizations, establishing the National Health Command Center to complete the epidemic prevention system, recognizing the lack of sources in the prevention network. The Taiwan government took the lessons to control the COVID-19 pandemic.

In this COVID-19, the government should learn another lesson regarding information distribution, including establishing the process of command, designing the accessible, readable, correct information content and channels, and, most importantly, cultivating the citizens' health literacy to stop the infodemic.

Notes

1 https://covid19.mohw.gov.tw/en/mp-206.html.
2 https://tfc-taiwan.org.tw/articles/3546.
3 https://www.facebook.com/tsaiingwen/posts/10157477092971065.
4 https://www.mofa.gov.tw/Upload/RelFile/2890/172267/20200517_1-4%20Public%20-private%20partnerships.pdf.
5 https://www.cna.com.tw/news/firstnews/202006075004.aspx.
6 https://www.taipeitimes.com/News/front/archives/2020/12/23/2003749218.

References

Belogianni, K., Ooms, A., Ahmed, H., Nikoletou, D., Grant, R., Makris, D., & Moir, H. J. (2019). Rationale and design of an online educational program using game-based learning to improve nutrition and physical activity outcomes among university students in the United Kingdom. *Journal of the American College of Nutrition*, 38(1), 23–30. https://doi.org/10.1080/07315724.2018.1476929

Dryhurst, S., Schneider, C. R., Kerr, J., Freeman, A. L., Recchia, G., van der Bles, A. M., Spiegelhalter, D., & van der Linden, S. (2020). Risk perceptions of COVID-19 around the world. *Journal of Risk Research*, 23(7–8), 994–1006.

Ezika, E. A. (2020). Use of case stories to explore the contextual application of cardiovascular health knowledge in Nigeria. *Health Education Journal*, 79(5), 607–615. https://doi.org/10.1177/0017896919897411

Fan, K. S., Ghani, S. A., Machairas, N., Lenti, L., Fan, K. H., Richardson, D., et al. (2020). COVID-19 prevention and treatment information on the internet: a

systematic analysis and quality assessment. *BMJ Open*, *10*(9). https://bmjopen
.bmj.com/content/bmjopen/10/9/e040487.full.pdf

Kim, S. (2020). The crisis of public health and infodemic: Analyzing belief structure
of fake news about COVID-19 pandemic. *Sustainability*, *12*(23), 9904. https://
doi.org/10.3390/su12239904

Krause, Freiling, I., Beets, B., & Brossard, D. (2020). Fact-checking as risk
communication: the multi-layered risk of misinformation in times of COVID-
19. *Journal of Risk Research*, *23*(7–8), 1052–1059. https://doi.org/10.1080
/13669877.2020.1756385

Lee, P. H., Yang, Y. W., Wu, H. Y. J., & Liu, W. (2022). The future of Taiwan studies
in the post-covid world': Online series on covid and Governance: Global and social
solidarity. *International Journal of Taiwan Studies*, *5*, 165–180.

Lin, Y-C. J. (2022). Establishing legitimacy through the media and combating fake
news on COVID-19: a case study of Taiwan. *Chinese Journal of Communication*,
15(2), 250–270. https://doi.org/10.1080/17544750.2021.2011343

Martin, C, & MacDonald, B.H. (2020). Using interpersonal communication
strategies to encourage science conversations on social media. *PLOS ONE*, *15*(11),
e0241972. https://doi.org/ 10.1371/journal.pone.0241972

Melki, J., Tamim, H., Hadid, D., Makki, M., el Amine, J., & Hitti, E. (2021).
Mitigating infodemics: The relationship between news exposure and trust and
belief in COVID-19 fake news and social media spreading. *PLOS ONE*, *16*(6),
e0252830. https://doi.org/10.1371/journal.pone.0252830

Phlypo, I., Palmers, E., Janssens, L., Marks, L., Jacquet, W., & Declerck, D. (2020).
The perception of oral health and oral care needs, barriers and current practices as
perceived by managers and caregivers in organizations for people with disabilities
in Flanders, Belgium. *Clinical Oral Investigations*, *24*(6), 2061–2070. https://
doi.org/10.1007/s00784-019-03071-z

Pulido, C. M., Villarejo-Carballido, B., Redondo-Sama, G., & Gómez, A. (2020).
COVID-19 infodemic: More retweets for science-based information on
coronavirus than for false information. *International Sociology*, *35*(4), 377–392.
https://doi.org/10.1177/0268580920914755

Rudd, R., & Baur, C. (2020). Health literacy and early insights during a pandemic.
Journal of Communication in Healthcare, *13*(1), 13–16. https://doi.org/10
.1080/17538068.2020.1760622

Su, Y., Lee, D. K. L., Xiao, X., Li, W., & Shu, W. (2021). Who endorses conspiracy
theories? A moderated mediation model of Chinese and international social media
use, media skepticism, need for cognition, and COVID-19 conspiracy theory
endorsement in China. *Computers in Human Behavior*, *120*(C), 106760. https://
doi.org/10.1016/j.chb.2021.106760

van der Linden, S., Roozenbeek, J., & Compton, J. (2020). Inoculating against fake
news about COVID-19. *Frontiers in Psychology*, *11*. https://doi.org/10.3389/
fpsyg.2020.566790

Walsh, L., Hemsley, B., Allan, M., Dahm, M. R., Balandin, S., Georgiou, A., Higgins,
I., McCarthy, S., & Hill, S. (2021). Assessing the information quality and usability
of my health record within a health literacy framework: What's changed since
2016? *Health Information Management Journal*, *50*(1–2), 13–25. https://doi
.org/10.1177/1833358319864734

Walsh, L., Hill, S., Allan, M., Balandin, S., Georgiou, A., Higgins, I., Kraal, B.,
Mccarthy, S., & Hemsley, B. (2017). A content analysis of the consumer-facing

online information about my health record: Implications for increasing knowledge and awareness to facilitate uptake and use. *Health Information Management Journal, 47*(3), 106-115. https://doi.org/10.1177/1833358317712200

Wingard, R. (2005). Patient education and the nursing process: Meeting the patient's needs. *Nephrology Nursing Journal: Journal of the American Nephrology Nurses' Association, 32*(2), 211–214; quiz 215.

4 "Noise" in Communicating Risk about the COVID-19 Pandemic in Taiwan

The Impact of Uncivil Online Messages

Tsung-Jen Shih

Introduction

Many cyberoptimists believe that social networking sites (SNSs) have great potential to contribute to democracy by increasing people's opportunities to obtain information and express opinions, which are essential components of public engagement (Gil de Zúñiga et al., 2014). SNSs have become an important source of information, with about four in ten Taiwanese now acquiring news from social media platforms (*Taiwan Communication Survey Newsletter*, 2021). Empirical research has also shown that exposure to news on SNSs is positively associated with political expression on social media, which subsequently increased political participation among the Taiwanese (Chan et al., 2017).

However, the freedom to speak out also has negative outcomes. Whereas interpersonal discussion produced the most benefits when the parties involved exchanged opinions rationally, many netizens nowadays are accustomed to using harsh words or tones when discussing social or political issues online, which is exacerbated by the media's increasing use of uncivil language to attract a larger audience. These abusive or uncivil messages have caught researchers' attention (e.g., Anderson et al., 2018; Gervais, 2015; Kim & Kim, 2019) because they jeopardize the opportunity for people to engage in rational discussions that serve as the cornerstone for participatory democracy (Nisbet & Scheufele, 2004; Scheufele, 2000).

Researchers have started to explore the impacts of online incivility, which refers to disrespectful and unnecessary means of expression that impede the function of a democracy, on several attitudinal and behavioral outcomes, including emotions (Kim & Kim, 2019), risk perceptions (Anderson et al., 2014), media perceptions (Anderson et al., 2018), the intention to use uncivil language (Gervais, 2014), political participation (Borah, 2014), and attitude polarization (Kim & Kim, 2019). Others have focused on the prevalence of uncivil information in the media (Coe et al., 2014; Papacharissi, 2004; Sobieraj & Berry, 2011). However, the role of online incivility in the context of a collective problem, such as the COVID-19 pandemic, has not received enough scholarly attention.

It is noteworthy that the networked information environment, where these uncivil messages are circulating, provides not only content for people to make

DOI: 10.4324/9781003286684-4

informed decisions but also cues for people to observe the opinion climate regarding public issues in wider society (Neubaum & Krämer, 2017). Online incivility, therefore, can affect people's collective efficacy, referred to as others' willingness to cooperate. Such an impersonal influence transforms online incivility from an opinion expression variable at the individual level to a concept with collective implications.

Furthermore, in light of the detrimental effects of uncivil messages (e.g., Borah, 2014), it will be enlightening to explore what mechanisms may mitigate the negative influences of online incivility. Among various factors, interpersonal discussion is likely to neutralize the vicious consequences of uncivil messages because it encourages cognitive elaboration and facilitates the rational deliberation of issues (Sotirovic & McLeod, 2001).

In addition, existing research on risk communication has often examined risk perception as the final dependent variable or focused on its impact on protective behaviors, but scholars have rarely explored whether it is connected with policy support. Researchers have also seldom investigated the relationship between impersonal factors (e.g., collective efficacy) and policy support. This study will address the gaps by examining the associations of these variables with the moderating role of trust, which serves as an essential information shortcut when people are facing complex social issues (Petty & Cacioppo, 1986).

In sum, this study will draw on theories from risk communication, social psychology, and collective actions and will propose an integrative model that incorporates communication and social cognitive variables to predict public support for COVID-19 policies in Taiwan. Specifically, this study will examine the effects of online incivility on personal risk perception, collective efficacy, and, ultimately, policy support, with interpersonal discussion and trust in the government serving as two potential moderators.

Definition and Impact of Incivility Online

Scholars have provided various definitions for incivility. A broad definition came from Papacharissi (2004), who considered incivility as any discussion that impedes democracy. Other scholars have offered more specific definitions by identifying the features of uncivil messages. For example, Coe et al. (2014) defined online incivility as "features of discussion that convey an unnecessarily disrespectful tone toward the discussion forum, its participants, or its topics" (p. 660). This definition emphasizes "disrespect" and "unnecessary" as two distinctive characteristics. The "unnecessary" feature refers to both the content and tone of the discussion. If a message fails to add anything relevant to the original threads of debate and uses hyperbolic language that does not help strengthen its argument, it is unnecessary and can be avoided. The definition also specified the targets of incivility, including the forum that carries the message, the people involved in the exchange of opinions, and the views expressed.

Rösner et al. (2016) proposed two forms of incivility based on the similar criteria outlined by Coe et al. (2014). Uncivil attack posts focus on the entities under attack (e.g., article authors, commentators, and news media). In comparison, uncivil language posts are categorized because of the language used, including words, punctuation, and symbols. Against these backgrounds, incivility may include the following five forms: name-calling, casting aspersions, lying, being vulgar, and using pejorative speech (Coe et al., 2014). This study employs these five categories in its operationalization of incivility.

Online incivility can have significant consequences. Based on social learning theory, individuals learn about behavior by observing other people. This is especially the case when people have a strong desire to be accepted or liked by others. Research has found that those who are exposed to incivility online may learn to use similar aggressive language in their comments, partly because they identify the original posters as role models and partly because they misperceive that uncivil language is the norm for communication in an online environment (Zimmerman & Ybarra, 2016). It is noteworthy that in other studies, this modeling effect only took place when the uncivil messages came from a like-minded political party or media outlet (Gervais, 2014, 2015).

Research has also suggested that although exposure to uncivil user comments online does not directly shape risk perception of emerging technology, it strengthens people's original attitudes or predispositions and makes them even more polarized (Anderson et al., 2014). Specifically, people who were less supportive of nanotechnology and were more religious perceived nanotechnology as riskier after exposure to uncivil messages. In contrast, those who were more supportive and less religious saw fewer risks associated with nanotechnology.

Furthermore, uncivil messages online can lead the audience to perceive that society is polarized on the issue under debate (Hwang et al., 2014). Earlier research findings also indicated that incivility on television decreased people's trust in politics (Mutz & Reeves, 2005). Therefore, it is likely that when people are exposed to uncivil messages about COVID-19, they may perceive a greater social divide on the issue, lowering their confidence in others' ability and willingness to fight the pandemic together. The perception of a lack of agreement in society may give rise to a higher level of uncertainty about the pandemic and protective measures, resulting in a hesitancy to support relevant policies (Ding et al., 2011).

Based on the literature, this study proposed the following hypotheses:

H1a: Uncivil messages will be positively associated with the risk perception of COVID-19.
H1b: Uncivil messages will be negatively associated with collective efficacy.
H1c: Uncivil messages will be negatively associated with policy support.

The Role of Interpersonal Discussion

Researchers in political science and communication have long recognized interpersonal discussion as a critical cornerstone of a healthy and functioning democracy (Nisbet & Scheufele, 2004; Scheufele, 2000). Political discussion assumes a vital role because it is associated with various positive attributes necessary for people to fulfill their duties as democratic citizens, including increased political knowledge, political participation, and community integration (Shah et al., 2017).

Interpersonal discussion has its roots in several communication models. For example, the communication mediation model posits that the effect of mass media use on political participation is mediated by interpersonal discussion (Shah et al., 2017; Sotirovic & McLeod, 2001). In other words, political discussion often originates from people's need to understand and interpret media messages, resulting in more participatory behaviors.

More specifically, interpersonal communication can mediate the impact of mass media because it allows people to reflect on media content. As Sotirovic and Mcleod (2001) stated: "Reflecting on news and integrating information from various sources promote a better understanding of the political world and may provide a stronger cognitive base for political participation than factual political knowledge" (p. 273). Many empirical studies have supported this mediating role of interpersonal discussions, especially in Western countries. More evidence, however, has also accumulated in other cultural contexts, including Asia (Chan et al., 2017; Gil de Zúñiga et al., 2019) and the new media platforms (Gil de Zúñiga et al., 2014).

On the other hand, people may consume media content because they anticipate interpersonal discussions with others, an argument in line with the uses and gratification theory (Palmgreen et al., 1985). The theory posits that people use media for an active purpose rather than as passive users, and further discussion serves as a legitimate objective that motivates media use. In the process, people can either pass along the information they acquire in the media, as opinion leaders do, or use the media content as arguments when engaging in conversation with others (Scheufele, 2002). Interpersonal communication, therefore, is both independent of and complementary to mass communication in the theorizing of these models (Chaffee & Mutz, 1988).

Although research about interpersonal communication has been well established in political communication, it is less investigated in the realm of risk communication. As some scholars argued, "our understanding of media influences far outweighs our understanding of interpersonal communication" (Binder et al., 2011, p. 324). It is, therefore, imperative to dig deeper into the role of interpersonal discussion, especially in the areas of science, technology, and risks. The social amplification of risk framework (SARF) provides a pertinent theoretical underpinning for such an investigation (Kasperson et al., 1988). The purpose of the SARF is to explain the gap between people's perceived risk and the objective chance the risk is estimated to take place. The SARF stipulates that people do not always follow the technical definition of risks but rather experience risks in a social context where various "amplification stations," such as mass media, institutions, or social groups, are at work (Binder et al., 2014).

Among the few studies that focus on the role of interpersonal discussion in science or risk communications, Binder et al. (2011) found that the valence of discussion was negatively associated with the perceived risk of a biological research facility and was positively associated with perceived benefits. The fact that people discussed the issue with the facility's supporters led them to see more benefits and fewer risks. The frequency of discussion was also positively related to benefit perception. In another study, however, the impact of interpersonal discussion was small and was more prominent when people made risk judgments about involuntary societal health hazards rather than about personal hazards (Coleman, 1993).

In addition to the direct impacts, interpersonal communication may also work in tandem with media variables in shaping people's attitudes or behaviors. For example, the differential gains model suggests that whereas media use, in general, is positively associated with knowledge acquisition, those who have more discussions tend to gain more knowledge (Scheufele, 2002). Research also identified the complicated interactive relationships between media dependency, media exposure, and interpersonal communication (Morton & Duck, 2001). Specifically, when newspaper dependency is low, newspaper exposure increases the perceived risks of skin cancer in people who do not discuss it with others frequently. These results suggest that interpersonal communication can moderate the impact of media messages on shaping people's risk perception.

As the reviewed literature suggests, most current studies focus on the interaction between a more positive form of media content (i.e., news) and interpersonal discussion. As the types of information have become more multifaceted in the social media environment, it is less clear about the dynamics between interpersonal communication and a more malicious form of information, such as uncivil messages. Will deliberate and rational interpersonal communication compensate for the uncivil information and mitigate its negative impact? Or does interpersonal communication magnify the impact of incivility because people are primed to use similar acrimonious language in their conversations? Based on the literature, this study proposes the following research questions:

RQ1a: Will interpersonal discussion moderate the effect of uncivil messages on the risk perception of COVID-19?

RQ1b: Will interpersonal discussion moderate the effect of uncivil messages on the collective efficacy regarding COVID-19?

Risk Perception and Policy Support

Although scholars have recognized the importance of risk perception, most of the studies are dedicated to uncovering the factors determining how people judge risks. The relationship between risk perception and public support for policies aiming to manage the risks receives insufficient scholarly attention (Gerber & Neeley, 2005; Mayer et al., 2017). Investigating such an association is important because governmental policies represent direct social responses to a dangerous hazard and have the objective of eliminating or mitigating it. How successful these policies can be is predicated on the levels of public compliance. If people do not perceive a certain hazard as threatening, they may not support government initiatives to ameliorate the problem. In other words, risk perception may serve as a prerequisite for policy support. This is in line with some scholars who consider governmental meliorative initiatives as a function of risk perception (O'Connor et al., 1999).

Understanding the predictors of policy support is particularly essential in democratic societies, where governmental initiatives are subject to public scrutiny and decisions. In Taiwan, the government has hosted two referendums since 2018 for the general public to decide whether some policies should be continued or abolished. A large portion of the policies in the referendums was related to science and public health, including the reopening of a nuclear power plant and the import of pork from the United States that contains ractopamine (Focus Taiwan, 2021). Understanding people's risk perception of social hazards, along with proper management of that perception, can have significant implications for effective policymaking.

Although evidence about the relationship between risk perception and policy support is scarce, it is gradually accumulating. For example, research showed that risk perception of climate change, represented by susceptibility and severity, was positively associated with support for relevant policies, such as imposing taxes to reduce carbon emissions (O'Connor et al., 1999). In another study, risk perception of air pollution was not related to support for climate policy, while perceiving global warming as a threat was (Mayer et al., 2017). Regarding nuclear policy, researchers also found that affective risk perception (i.e., worry) was negatively associated with support for nuclear power (Stoutenborough et al., 2013). In Taiwan, the more people thought of climate change as severe and consequential, the less likely they were to support the development of renewable energy as a policy to curb carbon emissions. However, such risk perception was unrelated to the other five climate and energy-related policies in the study (Hsu & Shih, 2015). These results suggest that, in general, risk perception is positively related to policy support, although the relationship may be slightly different depending on the dimensions of risks and the types of policy being measured.

In the context of COVID-19, where people face more immediate, concrete, and personal threats than climate change, researchers found that people with a higher level of risk perception tended to support prevention policies, regardless of whether they were nudges or regulations (Dudás & Szántó, 2021). Based on the literature, this study proposed the following hypothesis:

H2a: Risk perception of COVID-19 will be positively associated with policy support.

Collective Efficacy and Policy Support

The COVID-19 pandemic is a collective issue because the outbreak of the disease is wreaking havoc on a large number of people across the globe, and it will take everybody's effort to contain the spread of the disease. Wright et al. (1990) considered that people engage in collective action when "he or she is acting as a representative of the group and where the action is directed at improving the conditions of the group as a whole" (p. 995). Grappling with the pandemic, therefore, serves as a typical example of collective action.

Based on the resource mobilization theory, whether people take collective action or not depends on their calculation of benefits and available resources (Klandermans, 1984). These available resources include one's own ability to solve the collective problem (i.e., self-efficacy) and other people's willingness to cooperate (i.e., collective efficacy). Bandura (1997) defined collective efficacy as the confidence people have in solving a collective problem through collective actions. In other words, it is the belief that society, as an aggregation of citizens, has both the ability and willingness to perform the collective task. The perception of collective ability plays a more prominent role when the issue at hand requires the effort, coordination, and cooperation of a larger group of social members (Velasquez & LaRose, 2015).

Research on political communication has demonstrated a positive association between collective efficacy and several participatory behaviors (Lee, 2006; van Zomeren et al., 2008; Velasquez & LaRose, 2015). In climate change communication, research has also indicated a positive relationship between collective efficacy and environmentally friendly behaviors (Lubell et al., 2007; van Zomeren et al., 2010). On COVID-19, a study in Spain found that collective efficacy was related to two forms of coping behaviors; it had a direct, positive effect on self-protection behaviors (e.g., purchasing medications in case one got infected) and an indirect effect on physical distancing behaviors (Tabernero et al., 2020).

As the literature reviewed above shows, most studies examining the effects of collective efficacy have focused on its impact on individual behaviors rather than on policy support. A study in India about water conservation is an exception. The study found that the more collective efficacy Indian people had, the more likely they were to engage in protests that demanded safe drinking water and support governmental policies addressing water scarcity (Thaker et al., 2019). Based on the literature, this study proposed the following hypothesis:

H2b: Collective efficacy will be positively associated with policy support.

The Role of Trust

Trust has emerged as an important concept in modern society, where people's lives are deeply intertwined with uncertainties and risks derived from an increasingly complex technical and social system (Luhmann, 1988). As Funtowicz and Ravetz (1993) suggested, people are living in the age of post-normal science where both system uncertainties and decision stakes are high. Trust is especially relevant when the severity, impact, and development of risk are unknown or uncertain, such as the COVID-19 pandemic.

Although specific definitions of trust vary, scholars generally refer to trust as the belief that other people or institutions are willing to act with good intentions or in a mutually beneficial manner (Smith & Mayer, 2018). At the individual decision-making level, people often rely on trust as an information shortcut to form attitudes when they have difficulties understanding complex social risks (Petty & Cacioppo, 1986). Many studies have established a positive relationship between trust in scientists and public attitudes toward various applications of science and technology (Ho et al., 2010; Lee et al., 2005; Liu & Priest, 2009). Specifically, Ho et al. (2011) found that trust in scientists was predictive of experts' support for the federal funding of nanotechnology, suggesting the potential role of trust in shaping people's support for policies.

At the level of collective action, trust also plays an important role because it informs people about others' intentions to engage in the problem-solving process together. Previous research found that, when facing a social dilemma, people were more likely to cooperate when the mutual trust was high (De Cremer & Stouten, 2003). Studies have also established a positive relationship between trust in the government and policies aiming to address collective problems, such as climate change (Fairbrother, 2016; Zannakis et al., 2015).

In addition to the direct effects, trust may have an interactive relationship with risk perception in shaping individual behaviors and policy support. As mentioned earlier, trust involves the belief that other people or institutions will serve common interests. When people are facing risks, such as the COVID-19 pandemic, those who trust the government more will tend to believe that it will take good care of the general public and solve the problem, resulting in a higher level of policy support. This reasoning is echoed by researchers who argued that community members were more likely to abide by community rules if their trust was high because they believe that the authorities will act on behalf of people's interests (Tyler & Blader, 2013). Since empirical research in this area is very limited, this study will use a research question to explore the interactive relationship between risk perception and trust.

RQ2a: Will trust moderate the effect of risk perception on policy support?

Trust may also have a dynamic relationship with collective efficacy. Specifically, different combinations of trust and efficacy may result in different participatory behaviors (Gamson, 1968; Thaker et al., 2019). Whereas high efficacy and low trust drive a more dramatic form of participation (e.g., protests), citizens with high trust and efficacy tend to engage in more conventional forms of participation, such as voting. On the other hand, those who have high trust and low efficacy are likely to support government policies because they believe the government will serve them well, but, at the same time, they do not feel confident enough to change the political status quo. Finally, people who are low in trust and efficacy tend to be politically apathetic. Empirically, Thaker et al. (2019) found that collective efficacy increased support for water conservation policies when individuals had low trust in the government. However, they failed to observe this positive relationship among people who trusted the government more. Again, because there is a lack of research in this area, this current study proposed the following research question:

RQ2b: Will trust moderate the effect of collective efficacy on policy support?

In general, the analytical framework of this study is illustrated in Figure 4.1.

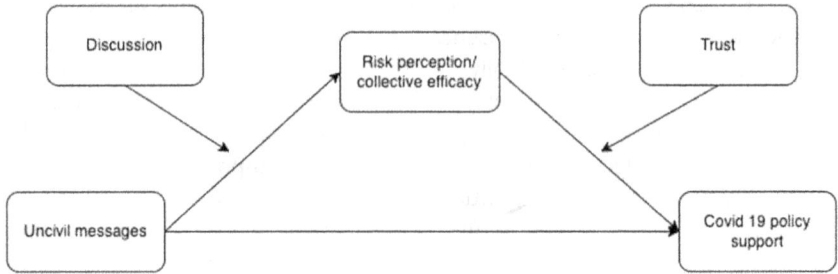

Figure 4.1 Research framework

Methods

Survey Procedures

This study conducted a representative survey of Taiwanese adults above 18 years old. The survey was conducted between March 2 and March 10, 2020, via landlines and cellphones. The landline respondents were selected through a stratified and clustered multistage sampling process based on a computer-assisted telephone interview (CATI) system. The CATI program employed the random digit dialing approach and generated the last two digits of the selected phone numbers. This study compared the survey's demographic features with the statistics released by the Taiwanese Ministry of the Interior. After being weighted by the raking ratio estimation, gender ($X^2 = 0.001$, $p > .05$), age ($X^2 = 1.711$, $p > .05$), education ($X^2 = 1.057$, $p > .05$), and area of residence ($X^2 = 5.045$, $p > .05$) were not statistically different from the national data.

The cellphone sample was selected based on the "Allocation of Telecommunications Numbers" principles released by the Taiwanese National Communication Committee (NCC). In Taiwan, the first five digits of the cellphone numbers were assigned by the NCC to each telecommunication company. The study drew a random sample of cellphone numbers based on the first five digits and randomly generated the last five digits.

The total sample size of the study was 1,068 (872 via landline and 201 via cellphones). The margin of error is ±3.0% based on the 95% confidence level.

Measurements

Policy support. This study measured the concept with three items adapted from the actual policies enacted by the Taiwanese government in response to the COVID-19 outbreak. The respondents indicated their levels of agreement with the following statements: (1) "Masks should be reserved for those who are in greater need, such as the first responders and the socially disadvantaged"; (2) "The government should not limit the number of masks people can buy"; and

(3) "The government should not prohibit the manufacturers from exporting the masks they produced." The answers ranged from "strongly disagree" (coded as 1) to "strongly agree" (coded as 5). This study first reverse-coded the second and third items and then averaged all three variables to form a scale of policy support (M = 4.43, SD = 0.72, Cronbach's α = 0.52).

Uncivil messages exposure. This study measured the concept by asking whether the respondents had seen the following types of messages on social media: (1) name-calling, which refers to disparaging words targeting a person or group of people; (2) casting aspersions, which refers to posts or comments that attack others' opinions, policies, or behaviors; (3) pejorative speech, which refers to posts or comments that show contempt to others' opinions; (4) lying, which refers to posts or comments that accuse others of lying without any evidence; and (5) vulgar language, including expletives or profanities. The responses were coded "1" if the answer was "yes" and "0" if the answer was "no." This study added up all five scores to form an index that ranged from 0 to 5, with a higher value indicating more exposure to uncivil messages on social media (M = 1.38, SD = 1.87, KR-20 = 0.89).

Risk perception. The concept was operationalized as the subjective evaluation of the respondents' probability of contracting COVID-19. The respondents indicated their levels of agreement with two statements: (1) "How likely do you think you will be infected by the coronavirus that causes the outbreak, compared with other people in Taiwan?" and (2) "How likely do you think you will be infected by the coronavirus that causes the outbreak compared with people in other countries?" The respondents answered these two questions on a five-point Likert scale that ranged from 1 (very unlikely) to 5 (very likely). This study added up and averaged the two items to form a scale of risk perception of COVID-19 (M = 2.22, SD = 0.91, r = .58, p < .01).

Trust. This study used two items to measure people's trust in the government. The respondents indicated their levels of agreement with the following two statements: (1) "Do you trust the government's ability to handle the COVID-19 pandemic?" and (2) "Do you trust the information that the government releases about the COVID-19 pandemic?" The respondents answered these two questions on a five-point Likert scale that ranged from 1 (do not trust at all) to 5 (trust very much). This study added up and averaged the two items to form a scale of risk perception of COVID-19 (M = 4.40, SD = 0.78, r = .72, p < .01).

Collective efficacy. This study used a single-item measure that asked the respondents about their levels of agreement with the following statement: "How confident you are that most Taiwanese people can comply with the preventive measures suggested by the government?" The respondents answered the questions on a five-point Likert scale that ranged from 1 (do not have any confidence at all) to 5 (have a lot of confidence) (M = 3.80, SD = 1.10).

Discussion. This study used a single-item measure that asked the respondents about how frequently they discussed the COVID-19 pandemic with others, including face-to-face and virtually. The respondents indicated their frequency on a four-point scale that ranged from 0 (never) to 4 (often) (M = 2.63, SD = 1.15).

This study also controlled age (M = 47.38, SD = 16.93), gender (male = 48.9%), education (median = high school or vocational school, 27.6%), and social media use (M = 2.03, SD = 0.84, Cronbach's α = .66). Social media use was measured by four items that asked how frequently people (1) obtained information about COVID-19 on SNSs; (2) obtained information about COVID-19 through instant messengers (IMs); (3) shared, responded, or commented on information about COVID-19 on SNSs or IMs; and (4) searched for information about COVID-19 through governmental mobile applications or websites. The answers were measured on a four-point scale that ranged from 0 (never) to 4 (often).

Results

Descriptive Analysis

During the COVID-19 pandemic, Taiwanese people relied mainly on television to obtain information about the disease. About three-quarters of the respondents mentioned television as their main source of information (73.7%). Many Taiwanese people acquired information from social media (44.5%) and instant messaging platforms (34.5%), whereas relatively few people used smartphone apps to receive information (11.8%). Furthermore, only 4% of the respondents shared, replied, and commented on social media messages. The pandemic has become an important topic of discussion in people's daily lives as 61.4% of the respondents reported talking about this issue with others "sometimes" or "frequently."

Uncivil online messages were not uncommon to the Taiwanese public. The form of incivility that people encountered most frequently online was "casting aspersions" that attacked others' opinions, policies, or behaviors (30.3%), followed by "pejorative speech" that showed contempt for others' opinions (29.6%). Furthermore, about a quarter of Taiwanese respondents saw "name-calling" (27.7%), "accusing others of lying" (27.1%), and "vulgar language" (23.6%) when they were online.

In addition, although 78.6% of Taiwanese respondents felt worried about the pandemic, very few people considered themselves vulnerable to the disease. Only 22% of people thought they were likely or very likely to contract the virus compared to other people in Taiwan. The proportion was even lower when the base of comparison was people in other countries (16%).

Among the four policy statements asked in the survey, Taiwanese people supported three of them. Almost everybody (97.7%) agreed that the limited number of masks at the onset of the COVID-19 outbreak should be reserved for first responders and the socially disadvantaged. People also highly supported the government's mask rationing policy (87.3%) and export ban (87%). However, people were hesitant about the policy that asked healthy citizens not to wear a mask (79% disagreed). In general, the government enjoyed a high level of trust from the public concerning its ability to deal with the pandemic (92%) and the information it released (92.6%).

Hypothesis Testing

In order to test the hypotheses and research questions, this study employed the PROCESS macro developed by Hayes (2018). The macro used the bootstrapping approach to test mediation, moderation, or moderated mediation, which has fewer restrictions about the distribution of variables. This study used model 21 in the macro, which allows researchers to test a mediation relationship with two moderators.

H1a posited that uncivil messages and risk perception of COVID-19 would be positively related. The results, as presented in Table 4.1, indicated that the two variables were not associated with each other in a statistically significant manner ($\beta = .0391$, $p > .05$). **H1b** stipulated a negative association between uncivil messages and collective efficacy. According to Table 4.2, exposure to uncivil messages on social media did not either increase or decrease people's perceived collective efficacy ($\beta = -.1008$, $p > .05$). **H1c** hypothesized that uncivil messages would be negatively associated with policy support. The results, however, indicated that online incivility increased policy support in both the risk perception model ($\beta = .0275$,

Table 4.1 Moderated Mediation Model for Risk Perception

	Coefficients	SE
Mediator Model (Risk Perception)		
Age	.0018	.0020
Female	−.0311	.0686
Education	.0506*	.0254
TV use	−.0971**	.0365
Social media	.0282	.0408
Discussion	.0647*	.0318
Uncivil messages	.0391	.0462
Discussion × uncivil messages	.0364*	.144
Dependent variable model (policy support)		
Age	−.0028*	.0014
Female	.0288	.0383
Education	.0249	.0171
TV use	.0370	.0249
Social media	−.0260	.0267
Risk perception	.3780**	.1090
Uncivil message	.0275*	.0111
Trust	.6706**	.0621
Risk perception × trust	−.0749**	.0245
R square	29.97%	

**$p < .01$. *$p < .05$.

Table 4.2 Moderated Mediation Model for Collective Efficacy

	Coefficients	*SE*
Mediator Model (Collective Efficacy)		
Age	.0015	.0025
Female	−.0311	.0686
Education	−.1262**	.0312
TV use	.1549**	.0444
Social media	.0324	.0498
Discussion	−.0384	.0391
Uncivil messages	−.1008	.0567
Discussion × uncivil messages	.0236	.177
Dependent variable model (policy support)		
Age	−.0031*	.0014
Female	.0338	.0376
Education	.0175	.0171
TV use	.0584*	.0244
Social media	−.0181	.0263
Collective efficacy	−.3747**	.0831
Uncivil message	.0240*	.0108
Trust	.2462**	.0664
Collective efficacy × trust	.0775**	.0188
R square	30.58%	

**$p < .01$. *$p < .05$.

$p < .05$) and the collective efficacy model ($\beta = .0240$, $p < .05$). Therefore, H1a, H1b, and H1c were not supported.

RQ1a investigated whether interpersonal discussion may moderate the effect of uncivil messages on the risk perception of COVID-19. The results in Table 4.1 showed that the interactions between discussion and uncivil messages were statistically significant ($\beta = .0364$, $p < .05$). As shown in Figure 4.2, for those who did not frequently have discussions with others, exposure to uncivil messages was not related to risk perception ($\beta = −.0027$, $p > .05$). However, exposure to uncivil messages increased risk perception when people were engaged in interpersonal discussion more frequently ($\beta = .1066$, $p < .01$).

RQ1b investigated whether interpersonal discussion may moderate the effect of uncivil messages on people's perceived collective efficacy. The results indicated that the interaction effect between discussion and uncivil messages was not statistically significant ($\beta = .0236$, $p > .05$).

H2a posited that risk perception would be positively associated with policy support. Based on Table 4.1, the more people perceived themselves to be vulnerable to COVID-19, the more likely they were to support relevant governmental policies ($\beta = .3780$, $p < .01$). On the other hand, H2b posited that collective

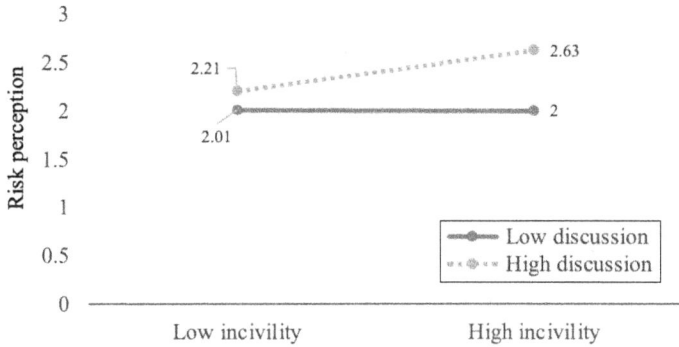

Figure 4.2 Interaction effect between incivility and discussion on risk perception

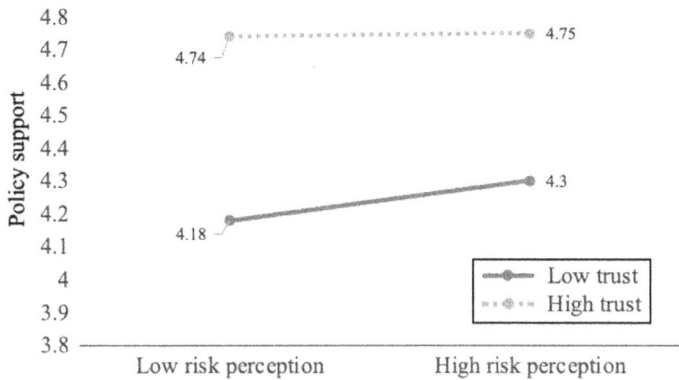

Figure 4.3 Interaction effect between risk perception and trust on policy support

efficacy would be positively associated with policy support. Although the relationship between the two variables was statistically significant, it was a negative association. The more collective efficacy people had, the less likely they were to support governmental policies ($\beta = -.3747$, $p < .01$). Therefore, while H2a was supported, H2b was not.

RQ2a examined whether the trust would moderate the effect of risk perception on policy support. The results showed that the moderation effect was statistically significant ($\beta = -.0749$, $p < .01$). Risk perception was positively associated with policy support when the trust was low ($\beta = .0783$, $p < .01$). When people had high levels of trust in the government, the two variables were not related ($\beta = .0034$, $p > .05$). Figure 4.3 provided a visual illustration of the interaction pattern.

RQ2b examined whether the trust would moderate the effect of collective efficacy on policy support. The results showed that the moderation effect was

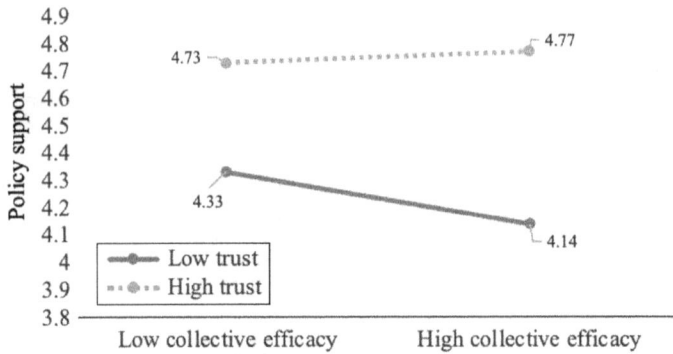

Figure 4.4 Interaction effect between collective efficacy and trust on policy support

also statistically significant (β = .0775, p < .01). As illustrated in Figure 4.4, when people had high levels of trust in the government, collective efficacy and policy support were not related, and the moderation effect was statistically significant (β = .0126, p > .05). However, for people who did not trust the government, the two variables were negatively associated with each other (β = −.0649, p < .01).

Discussion

Drawing upon a representative survey of data collected at the early stage of the COVID-19 pandemic in Taiwan, this study examined the impact of a unique feature in the modern communication environment—uncivil messages—on the public's reaction to the disease, including risk perception, the perception of collective efficacy, and policy support. Descriptive results showed that Taiwanese people, in general, had low-risk perception because of the low number of confirmed cases locally at the time the survey was conducted, but they were very worried about COVID-19. In other words, although people cognitively perceived themselves as unlikely to contract the virus, they had quite a strong emotional response to it.

It is interesting to find out that uncivil messages prompted people to support policies aiming to mitigate the pandemic. The finding pointed to a possibility that the target of the uncivil messages may not be the government. For example, in early February 2020, people surged to purchase toilet paper after the spread of an online rumor, which stated that raw materials used to manufacture toilet paper were being diverted to make masks (Pan, 2020). Many netizens were criticizing the irrational behaviors online rather than blaming the government.

The findings also showed that uncivil messages did not directly shape people's risk perception of COVID-19, a result consistent with previous research (Anderson et al., 2014). However, the results indicated that the effect of uncivil messages on risk perception varied depending on how frequently people had discussions. Uncivil messages only increased risk perception for those who frequently talked about the pandemic with others.

One explanation lies in the increasing trend for the media, both traditional and online, to use strong and bitter language to attract a larger audience (Sobieraj & Berry, 2011). Although the strategy is useful in driving user visits and spawning discussions, it can also lead the audience to perceive more media bias, have more emotional arousal, and lose trust in the government (Anderson et al., 2018; Borah, 2014; Gervais, 2015; Kim & Kim, 2019; Mutz & Reeves, 2005). As emotions and trust play an important role in shaping risk perception, the discussion that has its root in uncivil messages can make people feel more susceptible to COVID-19.

Another explanation may be related to the role of issue concern. People who are more concerned about an issue, including COVID-19, may have a stronger propensity to discuss it with others (Southwell & Yzer, 2009). As previous literature has suggested, uncivil messages have a polarizing effect that separates people further along the line of pre-existing attitudinal differences (Anderson et al., 2014). Those who are more concerned about COVID-19 may perceive the pandemic as even more threatening after exposure to uncivil messages.

In line with the existing literature, this study identified a positive relationship between risk perception and policy support. However, the results deviated from previous studies in finding a negative association between collective efficacy and policy support. This negative association may be attributed to the "free-rider" effects observed in some studies about collective actions. The collective interest model posits that people are more likely to engage in collective efforts when they perceive that the value of participation outweighs that of non-participation (Lubell et al., 2007). It is noteworthy that the policies of the Taiwanese government in the early stage of the pandemic were primarily about the allocation and rationing of masks (Su et al., 2020). These restrictions imposed by the government ran counter to the public's need to purchase a sufficient number of masks for self-protection, which increased the cost of compliance with the policies. The rising costs, coupled with the perception that the pandemic will not be ended with the efforts of a single individual, prompted people with high collective efficacy to become free riders. A Taiwanese study has confirmed the free-rider effect by showing a negative association between collective efficacy and mitigation behaviors related to climate change (Shih, 2017).

The interaction between risk perception and trust also warrants discussion. Specifically, risk perception increased policy support when trust in the government was low. Although people who trusted the government were more supportive of the policies, compared with people who had a low trust, risk perception did not factor in as a moderator of the relationship between trust and policy support. These findings may be explained by the concept of the ceiling effect, where people with high trust levels were already supportive of the policies, and risk perception was not able to have an additional impact. In contrast, risk perception had more room to affect compliance with policies for people whose trust levels were low. Furthermore, under an unusual circumstance, such as the COVID-19 pandemic, policy support may be less of a function of individual psychological factors (e.g., trust) than the perception of how threatening the disease was, especially when the government enacted stringent policies in response to the pandemic (Jørgensen et al., 2021).

This study also found a significant interaction between the effect of trust and collective efficacy on policy support. Policy support was the highest for people who had both high trust and collective efficacy. Additionally, collective efficacy did not add additional predictive power to policy support on top of trust. Both of the findings were consistent with those in previous research (Thaker et al., 2019). However, this study deviated from Thaker et al. (2019) in that collective efficacy decreased policy support for people with low levels of trust.

The disparity may result from the difference in the topics under examination. Water conservation and the effectiveness of policies that may solve the problem of water scarcity were relatively familiar to the general public in Thaker et al.'s (2019) study context. In contrast, COVID-19 was an emerging disease about which many uncertainties existed, including the origins of the virus, solutions, and evolution of the pandemic, especially at the early stage of the outbreak. It is therefore likely that people were less certain about the effectiveness of government policies in mitigating the pandemic, that is, people had low response efficacy (Choi & Hart, 2021). When people did not perceive the potential solutions to be effective, they would still comply with government policies, considering other people to be less cooperative (i.e., low collective efficacy). However, they could shift the onus of action to other people if the perceived collective efficacy was high, resulting in low policy support.

In fact, the interaction pattern fits Gamson's (1968) argument that people with high collective efficacy and low trust are most likely to engage in dramatic forms of mobilization, such as protests, rallies, strikes, or boycotts. The theorizing implies that this group of people was not satisfied with the policies aiming to solve the collective problems and intended to modify them by actively participating in the policymaking process. In other words, those who had low trust and high collective efficacy were the least supportive because they considered themselves capable of ameliorating the policies.

Before presenting the contributions and implications of this study, it is necessary to discuss the caveats that may influence the interpretation of the results. First, this study was conducted in March 2020 when the COVID-19 outbreak had just started. Public reactions to the pandemic and the strategies deemed effective to curb the spread of the virus may well have been different as the circumstances changed over time, and so, too, are the relationships of variables examined in this study. Second, this study failed to enquire about the content and valence of the uncivil messages people were exposed to. One experimental study has suggested that exposure to uncivil messages from like-minded sources may have different consequences than non-likeminded sources (Gervais, 2014). It is worthwhile for future research to keep exploring the role of the valence of incivility.

Conclusion

Since the outbreak of the COVID-19 pandemic, countries and international governing bodies, such as the World Health Organization, have paid considerable attention to the issue of disinformation (World Health Organization,

2020). However, another form of ill-qualified information is also pervasive on the Internet—uncivil messages, which may have remarkable impacts on a wide array of elements in the risk communication process, including attitudinal and behavioral responses to the disease and relevant mitigation policies. The role of uncivil messages, therefore, warrants more scholarly attention.

This study proposed a framework that integrates communication variables (i.e., exposure to uncivil messages and interpersonal discussion) with social cognitive variables (i.e., collective efficacy and trust). The results indicated that these variables functioned linearly and interactively in shaping public support for COVID-19-related policies. This integrated model contributed to our understanding in three areas. First, most studies in risk communication either treat risk perception as the final dependent variable or focus more on its predictive power on individual behaviors. As Gerber and Neeley (2005) pointed out, "relatively less attention has been devoted to explaining whether perceived risk systematically shapes an individual's views of public policies designed to manage possible hazards" (p. 397). This study expands on current literature by investigating the link between risk perception and policy support.

Second, the current study examined collective efficacy as a consequence of exposure to online incivility, which is also an area that warrants more scholarship. Collective efficacy is an important concept in social cognitive theory, but it is explored less frequently than the other two similar concepts—self-efficacy and response efficacy. It is particularly relevant when it comes to a collective problem, such as the COVID-19 pandemic. As most studies about online incivility emphasized its effects on individual perception and reactions, this study expands its applicability to the field of collective action.

Third, this study also attested to the importance of attending to the dynamics between mediated and interpersonal communication. The finding indicated that the effect of uncivil messages was amplified by the frequency of discussion, which suggests that interpersonal discussion may not live up to its expected function of facilitating rational deliberation and crystallizing confusion. The findings also suggest that different "amplifying stations," as stipulated in the SARF, may work interactively with each other in shaping risk perception.

On top of the theoretical contributions, the results of this study provided important practical insights for policymakers and risk communication professionals. First, to ensure information transparency and increase the efficiency of public communication, the government has adopted a variety of approaches to communicate with people, especially in the online realm. However, people did not seem to keep up with the new media platforms the government was using, as most Taiwanese people still obtained their disease-related information from television. The government may want to make greater efforts to promote the new platforms or distinguish the functions of different information channels to strengthen the efficiency of communication.

Second, the fact that collective efficacy engendered a free-rider phenomenon suggested that the concept may not always lead to a stronger agreement with policies. Collective efficacy may be counter-productive when the policies are contradictory to people's need for self-protection in an uncertain and emergent situation, such as the COVID-19 pandemic. The government should also pay special attention to people who had low trust in them but high collective efficacy because this was the group that was least supportive of government policies. This is also the group that tended to resort to more dramatic social actions in response to the unsatisfactory policies.

References

Anderson, A. A., Brossard, D., Scheufele, D. A., Xenos, M. A., & Ladwig, P. (2014). The "nasty effect:" Online incivility and risk perceptions of emerging technologies. *Journal of Computer-Mediated Communication*, *19*(3), 373–387. https://doi.org/10.1111/jcc4.12009

Anderson, A. A., Yeo, S. K., Brossard, D., Scheufele, D. A., & Xenos, M. A. (2018). Toxic talk: How online incivility can undermine perceptions of media. *International Journal of Public Opinion Research*, *30*(1), 156–168.

Bandura, A. (1997). *Self-efficacy: The exercise of control*. Freeman & Co.

Binder, A. R., Cacciatore, M. A., Scheufele, D. A., & Brossard, D. (2014). The role of news media in the social amplification of risk. In H. Cho, T. Reimer, & K. A. McComas (Eds.), *The SAGE Handbook of Risk Communication* (pp. 69–85). Sage.

Binder, A. R., Scheufele, D. A., Brossard, D., & Gunther, A. C. (2011). Interpersonal amplification of risk? Citizen discussions and their impact on perceptions of risks and benefits of a biological research facility. *Risk Analysis: An International Journal*, *31*(2), 324–334.

Borah, P. (2014). Does it matter where you read the news story? Interaction of incivility and news frames in the political blogosphere. *Communication Research*, *41*(6), 809–827.

Chaffee, S. H., & Mutz, D. (1988). Comparing mediated and interpersonal communication data. In R. P. Hawkins, J. M. Wiemann, & S. Pingre (Eds.), *Advancing communication science: Merging mass and interpersonal processes* (pp. 19–43). Sage.

Chan, M., Chen, H.-T., & Lee, F. L. (2017). Examining the roles of mobile and social media in political participation: A cross-national analysis of three Asian societies using a communication mediation approach. *New Media & Society*, *19*(12), 2003–2021.

Choi, S., & Hart, P. S. (2021). The influence of different efficacy constructs on energy conservation intentions and climate change policy support. *Journal of Environmental Psychology*, *75*, 101618. https://doi.org/10.1016/j.jenvp.2021.101618

Coe, K., Kenski, K., & Rains, S. A. (2014). Online and uncivil? Patterns and determinants of incivility in newspaper website comments. *Journal of Communication*, *64*(4), 658–679. https://doi.org/10.1111/jcom.12104

Coleman, C.-L. (1993). The influence of mass media and interpersonal communication on societal and personal risk judgments. *Communication Research*, *20*(4), 611–628.

De Cremer, D., & Stouten, J. (2003). When do people find cooperation most justified? The effect of trust and self–other merging in social dilemmas. *Social Justice Research*, *16*(1), 41–52.

Ding, D., Maibach, E. W., Zhao, X., Roser-Renouf, C., & Leiserowitz, A. (2011). Support for climate policy and societal action are linked to perceptions about scientific agreement. *Nature Climate Change, 1*(9), 462–466.

Dudás, L., & Szántó, R. (2021). Nudging in the time of coronavirus? Comparing public support for soft and hard preventive measures, highlighting the role of risk perception and experience. *PLoS ONE, 16*(8), e0256241. https://doi.org/10.1371/journal.pone.0256241

Fairbrother, M. (2016). Trust and public support for environmental protection in diverse national contexts. *Sociological Science, 3*, 359–382.

Focus Taiwan. (2021). *Taiwan's upcoming referendums: What are they all about?* Retrieved January 14 from https://focustaiwan.tw/politics/202112160022

Funtowicz, S. O., & Ravetz, J. R. (1993). Science for the post-normal age. *Futures, 25*(7), 739–755.

Gamson, W. A. (1968). *Power and discontent.* Dorsey.

Gerber, B. J., & Neeley, G. W. (2005). Perceived risk and citizen preferences for governmental management of routine hazards. *Policy Studies Journal, 33*(3), 395–418.

Gervais, B. T. (2014). Following the news? Reception of uncivil partisan media and the use of incivility in political expression. *Political Communication, 31*(4), 564–583. https://doi.org/10.1080/10584609.2013.852640

Gervais, B. T. (2015). Incivility online: Affective and behavioral reactions to uncivil political posts in a web-based experiment. *Journal of Information Technology & Politics, 12*(2), 167–185.

Gil de Zúñiga, H., Diehl, T., Huber, B., & Liu, J. H. (2019). The citizen communication mediation model across countries: A multilevel mediation model of news use and discussion on political participation. *Journal of Communication, 69*(2), 144–167.

Gil de Zúñiga, H., Molyneux, L., & Zheng, P. (2014). Social media, political expression, and political participation: Panel analysis of lagged and concurrent relationships. *Journal of Communication, 64*(4), 612–634.

Hayes, A. F. (2018). *Introduction to mediation, moderation, and conditional process analysis: A regression-based approach.* Guilford Publications.

Ho, S. S., Scheufele, D. A., & Corley, E. A. (2010). Making sense of policy choices: Understanding the roles of value predispositions, mass media, and cognitive processing in public attitudes toward nanotechnology. *Journal of Nanoparticle Research, 12*(8), 2703–2715.

Ho, S. S., Scheufele, D. A., & Corley, E. A. (2011). Value predispositions, mass media, and attitudes toward nanotechnology: The interplay of public and experts. *Science Communication, 33*(2), 167–200.

Hsu, M. L., & Shih, T. J. (2015). Patterns of public support for policies related to climate change. *Chinese Journal of Communication Research, 28*, 239–278.

Hwang, H., Kim, Y., & Huh, C. U. (2014). Seeing is believing: Effects of uncivil online debate on political polarization and expectations of deliberation. *Journal of Broadcasting & Electronic Media, 58*(4), 621–633.

Jørgensen, F., Bor, A., & Petersen, M. B. (2021). Compliance without fear: Individual-level protective behaviour during the first wave of the COVID-19 pandemic. *British Journal of Health Psychology, 26*(2), 679–696.

Kasperson, R. E., Renn, O., Slovic, P., Brown, H. S., Emel, J., Goble, R., Kasperson, J. X., & Ratick, S. (1988). The social amplification of risk: A conceptual framework. *Risk Analysis, 8*(2), 177–187.

Kim, Y., & Kim, Y. (2019). Incivility on Facebook and political polarization: The mediating role of seeking further comments and negative emotion. *Computers in Human Behavior, 99*, 219–227. https://doi.org/10.1016/j.chb.2019.05.022

Klandermans, B. (1984). Mobilization and participation: Social-psychological expansions of resource mobilization theory. *American Sociological Review, 49*(5), 583–600.

Lee, C.-J., Scheufele, D. A., & Lewenstein, B. V. (2005). Public attitudes toward emerging technologies: Examining the interactive effects of cognitions and affect on public attitudes toward nanotechnology. *Science Communication, 27*(2), 240–267.

Lee, F. L. (2006). Collective efficacy, support for democratization, and political participation in Hong Kong. *International Journal of Public Opinion Research, 18*(3), 297–317.

Liu, H., & Priest, S. (2009). Understanding public support for stem cell research: Media communication, interpersonal communication and trust in key actors. *Public Understanding of Science, 18*(6), 704–718.

Lubell, M., Zahran, S., & Vedlitz, A. (2007). Collective action and citizen responses to global warming. *Political Behavior, 29*(3), 391–413.

Luhmann, N. (1988). Familiarity, confidence, trust: Problems and alternatives. In D. Gambetta (Ed.), *Trust: Making and breaking cooperative relations* (Vol. 6, pp. 94–108). Basil Blackwell.

Mayer, A., Shelley, T. O. C., Chiricos, T., & Gertz, M. (2017). Environmental risk exposure, risk perception, political ideology and support for climate policy. *Sociological Focus, 50*(4), 309–328.

Morton, T. A., & Duck, J. M. (2001). Communication and health beliefs: Mass and interpersonal influences on perceptions of risk to self and others. *Communication Research, 28*(5), 602–626.

Mutz, D. C., & Reeves, B. (2005). The new videomalaise: Effects of televised incivility on political trust. *American Political Science Review, 99*(1), 1–15.

Neubaum, G., & Krämer, N. C. (2017). Opinion climates in social media: Blending mass and interpersonal communication. *Human Communication Research, 43*(4), 464–476.

Nisbet, M. C., & Scheufele, D. A. (2004). Political talk as a catalyst for online citizenship. *Journalism & Mass Communication Quarterly, 81*(4), 877–896.

O'Connor, R. E., Bard, R. J., & Fisher, A. (1999). Risk perceptions, general environmental beliefs, and willingness to address climate change. *Risk Analysis, 19*(3), 461–471.

Palmgreen, P., Wenner, L. A., & Rosengren, K. E. (1985). Uses and gratifications research: The past ten years. In K. E. Rosengren, L. Wenner, & P. Palmgreen (Eds.), *Media gratifications research: Current perspectives* (pp. 11–37). Sage.

Pan, J. (2020). *Virus Outbreak: Women sparked panic buying of toilet paper: Officials.* Retrieved January 17 from https://www.taipeitimes.com/News/taiwan/archives/2020/02/12/2003730827

Papacharissi, Z. (2004). Democracy online: Civility, politeness, and the democratic potential of online political discussion groups. *New Media & Society, 6*(2), 259–283.

Petty, R. E., & Cacioppo, J. T. (1986). The elaboration likelihood model of persuasion. In L. Berkowitz (Ed.), *Advances in experimental social psychology* (Vol. 19, pp. 123–205). Academic Press.

Rösner, L., Winter, S., & Krämer, N. C. (2016). Dangerous minds? Effects of uncivil online comments on aggressive cognitions, emotions, and behavior. *Computers in Human Behavior, 58*, 461–470. https://doi.org/10.1016/j.chb.2016.01.022

Scheufele, D. A. (2000). Talk or conversation? Dimensions of interpersonal discussion and their implications for participatory democracy. *Journalism & Mass Communication Quarterly, 77*(4), 727–743.

Scheufele, D. A. (2002). Examining differential gains from mass media and their implications for participatory behavior. *Communication Research, 29*(1), 46–65.

Shah, D. V., McLeod, D. M., Rojas, H., Cho, J., Wagner, M. W., & Friedland, L. A. (2017). Revising the communication mediation model for a new political communication ecology. *Human Communication Research, 43*(4), 491–504. https://doi.org/10.1111/hcre.12115

Shih, T.-J. (2017). How message framing and presentation affect pro-environmental behavioral intentions: A dual-pathway model perspective. *Journal of Communication Research and Practice, 7*(1), 5–36.

Smith, E. K., & Mayer, A. (2018). A social trap for the climate? Collective action, trust and climate change risk perception in 35 countries. *Global Environmental Change, 49*, 140–153. https://doi.org/10.1016/j.gloenvcha.2018.02.014

Sobieraj, S., & Berry, J. M. (2011). From incivility to outrage: Political discourse in blogs, talk radio, and cable news. *Political Communication, 28*(1), 19–41.

Sotirovic, M., & McLeod, J. M. (2001). Values, communication behavior, and political participation. *Political Communication, 18*(3), 273–300.

Southwell, B. G., & Yzer, M. C. (2009). When (and why) interpersonal talk matters for campaigns. *Communication Theory, 19*(1), 1–8.

Stoutenborough, J. W., Sturgess, S. G., & Vedlitz, A. (2013). Knowledge, risk, and policy support: Public perceptions of nuclear power. *Energy Policy, 62*, 176–184.

Su, V. Y.-F., Yen, Y.-F., Yang, K.-Y., Su, W.-J., Chou, K.-T., Chen, Y.-M., & Perng, D.-W. (2020). Masks and medical care: Two keys to Taiwan's success in preventing COVID-19 spread. *Travel Medicine and Infectious Disease, 38*, 101780. https://doi.org/10.1016/j.tmaid.2020.101780

Tabernero, C., Castillo-Mayén, R., Luque, B., & Cuadrado, E. (2020). Social values, self- and collective efficacy explaining behaviours in coping with Covid-19: Self-interested consumption and physical distancing in the first 10 days of confinement in Spain. *PLoS ONE, 15*(9), e0238682. https://doi.org/10.1371/journal.pone.0238682

Taiwan Communication Survey Newsletter. (2021). *Overview of social media use statistics from 2016 to 2020.* Retrieved January 18 from https://crctaiwan.dcat.nycu.edu.tw/ResultsShow_detail.asp?RS_ID=135

Thaker, J., Howe, P., Leiserowitz, A., & Maibach, E. (2019). Perceived collective efficacy and trust in government influence public engagement with climate change-related water conservation policies. *Environmental Communication, 13*(5), 681–699.

Tyler, T., & Blader, S. (2013). *Cooperation in groups: Procedural justice, social identity, and behavioral engagement.* Psychology Press.

Van Zomeren, M., Postmes, T., & Spears, R. (2008). Toward an integrative social identity model of collective action: A quantitative research synthesis of three socio-psychological perspectives. *Psychological Bulletin, 134*(4), 504–535.

van Zomeren, M., Spears, R., & Leach, C. W. (2010). Experimental evidence for a dual pathway model analysis of coping with the climate crisis. *Journal of Environmental Psychology*, *30*(4), 339–346.

Velasquez, A., & LaRose, R. (2015). Youth collective activism through social media: The role of collective efficacy. *New Media & Society*, *17*(6), 899–918.

World Health Organization. (2020). *Managing the COVID-19 infodemic: Promoting healthy behaviours and mitigating the harm from misinformation and disinformation*. Retrieved January 10 from https://www.who.int/news/item/23 -09-2020-managing-the-covid-19-infodemic-promoting-healthy-behaviours-and -mitigating-the-harm-from-misinformation-and-disinformation

Wright, S. C., Taylor, D. M., & Moghaddam, F. M. (1990). Responding to membership in a disadvantaged group: From acceptance to collective protest. *Journal of Personality and Social Psychology*, *58*(6), 994–1003.

Zannakis, M., Wallin, A., & Johansson, L. O. (2015). Political trust and perceptions of the quality of institutional arrangements: How do they influence the public's acceptance of environmental rules. *Environmental Policy and Governance*, *25*(6), 424–438.

Zimmerman, A. G., & Ybarra, G. J. (2016). Online aggression: The influences of anonymity and social modeling. *Psychology of Popular Media Culture*, *5*(2), 181–193.

5 A Sense of *the Public*
Japan and Vietnam

Vu Le Thao Chi

Introduction

Japan and Vietnam offer contrasting images of different economies, cultures, and governance styles. Both were at high risk, given their proximity to China during the initial stage of the coronavirus pandemic. The increasing age of the population (Japan, 30% and Vietnam, 11%) and densely populated cities put the two countries in a precarious position if the virus spreads unchecked. However, Japan and Vietnam continue to exhibit two entirely different approaches to curbing the spread of the coronavirus—Vietnam has a monolithic, top-down style, and Japan is more moderate, leaving its citizens a greater margin of freedom to choose their actions. Both approaches yielded similar positive results in the first year of the pandemic. They then began showing the contrasting outcomes soon afterwards.

The chapter is an interpretative foray into the people's narratives: the grasp of the pandemic in the vernacular language of Japanese and Vietnamese people. The Japanese are conscious of the threat of the coronavirus in their everyday lives and of the need to learn how to protect themselves from it. In contrast, the Vietnamese are less responsive to the threat of the virus and more responsive to the government's orders.

The narratives of these two groups also reveal how they see *the public*, which results from the long tradition of authority relationships and the recent past in each country. For the Japanese, *the public* is a specific space where social norms govern people's behavior in *others'* presence. The sense of public is the sense of *others* in the Japanese consciousness. It reaches the everyday life practices of individuals through sets of manners, rules, and etiquette, which they observe in a public space. The absence of a national crisis since 1945 frees people from the pressure of acting in the name of Japan as a whole. On the other hand, the Vietnamese sense of *the public* is awakened whenever they are reminded of the recent history of unification as a whole. They readily allow this sense to sweep away their individual or communal inclinations under the circumstances perceived as a national threat. Likewise, the government readily resorts to wartime rhetoric as it animates this sense.

The chapter argues that the Japanese and the Vietnamese perceptions of *the public* through the pandemic can help us to capture the differences in each respective government's style and other areas of policy concerns.

DOI: 10.4324/9781003286684-5

Research Method

From March 31 to April 30, 2020, I circulated a set of four questions among 22 Vietnamese (from 10 years old to 70 years old) and 26 Japanese (from 18 to 73 years old) by email, by text messages (Line, Facebook messenger, Viber), or by video phone calls. That is when both the Japanese and Vietnamese were under movement restrictions: the first State of Emergency, Japan, and social quarantine on a national scale, Vietnam. The four questions (in Vietnamese, English, and Japanese) are:

1. What do you think of the coronavirus?
2. How does this pandemic affect the way you think about *other* risks?
3. What concerns you the most now in your everyday life?
4. What do you think about life?

The questions were open-ended. I hoped to give the respondents freedom to interpret the questions however they saw fit, thereby encouraging them to express what they thought freely without my prompting. For that purpose, I avoided more structured questions. Some informants "poured out" their thoughts in one long paragraph instead of answering questions one by one. Their narratives reveal what popped up in their minds, their concerns, and their priorities in everyday lives.

These informants are "historical agents" of not only this unique historical moment. Their narratives and their behaviors are also reflective of "larger historical forces"—a past that they may have never lived in a way that makes sense to them. "Historiciz[ing] these narratives" within "larger historical forces" (Maynes et al., 2008, p. 45) helps to explain why the Japanese and Vietnamese think, behave, and narrate the way they do. The research is not predictive but explanatory and interpretive.

How Japan and Vietnam Responded to the Coronavirus Pandemic

A Snapshot of the Coronavirus Pandemic in the Two Countries

Japan and Vietnam exhibited remarkable similarities in the spreading patterns in their first year (early 2020 ~ early 2021) despite the wide gap in the total number of infections (over 400,000 in Japan and 2,000 in Vietnam as of early March 2021) and the total deaths (approaching 9,000 during March 2021 in Japan and 35 from September 2020 until May 2021 in Vietnam) (Worldometers. Info, n.d.).

When Japan entered its fourth wave (mid-March 2021), Vietnam still enjoyed the success of its zero-COVID strategy with no additional death and new infections were mainly detected at entry points. The victorious narrative of Vietnam stumbled exactly on April 27 when they found new untraceable cases in Ho Chi Minh. That marked the beginning of the fourth wave, the longest and the most devastating for Vietnam, especially Ho Chi Minh, the country's financial center.

The round lasted until September, and the fifth wave quickly followed it, adding more than 1 million new cases within only half a year (1,065,469 in Vietnam compared to Japan's *total* of 1,725,901 since March 2020). Vietnam toppled Japan in the total deaths (23,476 in Vietnam compared to 18,336 in Japan) (Worldometer.info, n.d.). Japan, meanwhile, also experienced the worst phase in August 2021 during its fifth wave, with daily infections reaching as many as 26,184 cases a day (August 22), although the daily death rate did not change. The number of infections in Japan started declining from September 2021 and continued so long after the State of Emergency was lifted in the entire country at the end of September, which surprised even local experts and policymakers. At the time of this writing (November 18, 2021), the daily infection is 163 and 5 deaths (NHK n.d., retrieved 2021, November 19), compared to 10,209 infections and 139 deaths in Vietnam (VnExpress, n.d.).

Vietnamese Government: Monolithic Measures and Wartime Rhetoric

From the beginning of the coronavirus outbreak, Vietnam has been immensely swift and efficient in its response. As early as January 3, 2020, the General Department of Preventive Medicine (Ministry of Health) issued a document requesting increased medical surveillance at all border entries in the country against the threat of "pneumonia caused by an as-yet-to-be-identified virus from China" (General Department of Preventive Medicine, 2020). At that time, there was still not even one infection reported in the country. On January 21, the first two cases of infection (both from Wuhan) were detected. Vietnam took no time to enforce its preparation to fend off further penetration of the virus into the population.

The persistent use of wartime rhetoric marked the government's determination to wage an all-out war against the coronavirus. On January 27, Prime Minister Nguyen Xuan Phuc, in his emergency meeting with the heads of ministries, requested the officials in charge to "fight the virus as if we were fighting a foreign enemy (chống dịch như chống giặc)" (MOH, 2020a). On March 8, after the 17th infection case following 16 days without a new patient, Deputy Prime Minister Vu Duc Dam stated: "We have won the opening operation in the initial phase of the battle. In reality, the virus has penetrated our country and is ready to 'ambush' us […] We have to win the whole battle" (MOH, 2020b). On March 30, General Secretary of the Communist Party, Nguyen Phu Trong, in his address to call for a "social quarantine of national scale" (giãn cách toàn xã hội), stated that "Every Vietnamese citizen is a soldier fighting the pandemic." On April 1, Nguyen Xuan Phuc reiterated the message: "Everyone, every household, every business, every neighborhood, every village, every commune, every district, every province, every city is a fortress against the pandemic." On May 21, after more than a month without a new case in the country, the Deputy Prime Minister said, "We have not won the pandemic. We have only succeeded in getting the pandemic under control […] this battle continues" (MOH, 2020c).

The newly elected Prime Minister, Pham Minh Chinh, continued the rhetoric of "fighting the virus as if we were up against a foreign enemy" throughout the fourth wave of the pandemic.

The government is not alone in the use of wartime rhetoric. People translated these messages into popular slogans on social media and on the streets: "Stay still when the Fatherland needs you to." That is an adaptation of the slogan "Stand up when the Fatherland needs you to," which was used during the Vietnam War when the government implemented a campaign to mobilize the youth to the forefront of the war for the country's unification.

The Military Plays a Pivotal Role

An unprecedented and monolithic measure that the Communist Party adopted in response to the coronavirus included the military's involvement from the very beginning. On February 2 (10 days after the first infection), the Ministry of Defense organized a large-scale military drill to prepare for the five-level worst-case scenario, which ranged from the initial virus infection in the country to the highest-level scenario where there were 3,000 to 30,000 infections including military units.

Soon after the drill, the government dispatched soldiers to entry points (airports and border posts along the borders with Laos, Cambodia, and especially China) to enforce tighter control over people's inflow. The government also mobilized soldiers to each locality to man temporary quarantine centers. The centers multiplied quickly in many of the country's main cities after the government imposed a mandatory 14-day quarantine on all people entering Vietnam starting from March 21. On March 22, it stopped receiving all foreign citizens.

The number of people under strict medical surveillance at these quarantine centers was as high as 50,000 by the end of March. Accommodation and food were free until August 31, 2020. To justify this generosity, Colonel Ha The Tan reasoned that supporting 10,000 people under quarantine was still cheaper than treating 1,000 patients (Hoang Phuong & Viet Tuan, 2020).

At the beginning of the third wave of the coronavirus, on February 16, 2021, Senior Lieutenant Tran Don, Deputy Minister of Defense, said: "the military is now activated in a war-time mode to fight the virus" (Hoang Thuy, 2021).

During the fourth wave, the Communist government mobilized 137,058 troops (63,958 regular soldiers and 73,100 militias) to Ho Chi Minh City, the epicenter of the pandemic, to enforce the implementation of Directive 16 (Figure 5.1). That is considered the largest deployment of Vietnam after the end of the war in 1975 (Huu Cong et al., 2021).

Exhaustive Tracing System

At a glance, Vietnam's measures are no different from those in many other countries, including contact tracing, cluster-avoiding strategy, and lockdown.

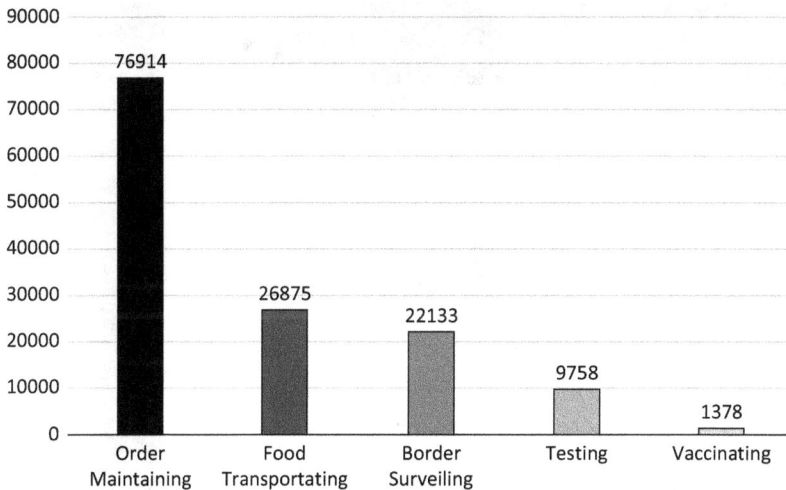

Figure 5.1 The five tasks that the soldiers and militias were in charge of during the fourth wave (reproduced from Huu Cong et al., 2021).

However, a closer look at their implementation reveals how exhaustive and thorough each measure is.

The most impressive measure was the tracing system that the government enacted at every local medical facility in the country at the beginning of the pandemic (Figure 5.2). Unlike Japan, Vietnam did not have a specific definition of "close contact" or "cluster." Nonetheless, an infected person was required to report everyone else with whom they came into contact and every place they had been to.

This information was made public on social media to facilitate tracing efforts. Usually, the number of people traceable (F1–F5) was exceptionally high. For example, in Quang Ninh Province, 18 new cases were found on January 29, 2021. By January 30, the authority identified 23,600 people, ranging from F1 to F4 (Minh Cuong, 2021). In addition, although the Communist government refrained from resorting to a national/regional lockdown, it enforced smaller-scale lockdowns (apartment blocks, neighborhoods, villages, or cities) and shutdowns (applied to service facilities or offices) if an infected person was found or if the place was in the infected person's paths.

These small-scale lockdowns often took the Vietnamese by surprise. One infected individual can turn the everyday lives of thousands of others upside down, especially in large apartment complexes in big cities such as Ho Chi Minh and Hanoi. However, people did not show any resistance to these coercive measures. Their reaction was a re-enactment of the end of the protracted war of unification: When the government lifted a lockdown order, people grabbed the national red flags and ran around, sharing not only the relief but also the joy with one another.

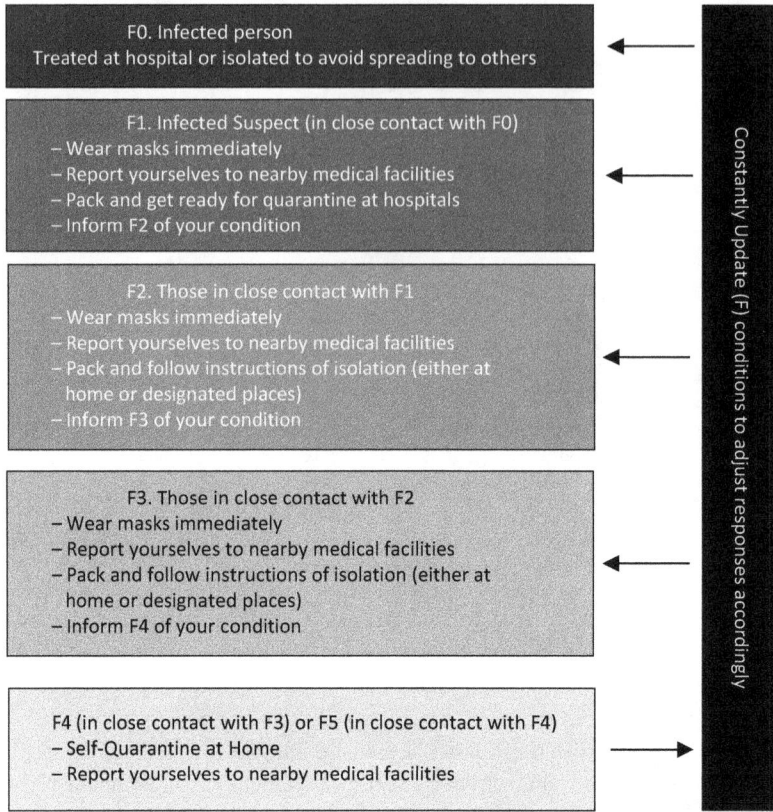

Figure 5.2 Coronavirus tracing guideline from the Ministry of Health, Vietnam (the graphic chart was acquired from Truong Quang Dat, M.D. (Binh Dinh Medical College, Vietnam) on March 23, 2020. Similar charts are seen at every local medical facility across the country).

The Fourth Wave

The fourth wave took Vietnam by storm and engulfed the country in the worst medical crisis since. The central government focused its draconian measures upon Ho Chi Minh while leaving other localities a large margin of autonomy to respond to the COVID-19 depending on the seriousness of the situation. Here is the timeline of restrictions implemented in Ho Chi Minh since May 2021 (see the appendix for the restriction orders).

- May 31: the City applied the Government Directive 15 for 15 days and later extended the application until June 29.
- June 19: the City issued Directive 10 to supplement Directive 15.

- July 9: the City applied Directive 16 (Social Quarantine of the entire city) and extended the application four times until September 31.
- August 23: the government sent soldiers and militias to the City.
- September 31: Directive 16 lifted.

Penalties for the violations stretched from US$50 fine for "unnecessary outings" to US$2000 for operating "unnecessary business." The list of penalties was posted in public space for people to observe in addition to the message 5K— Mask-wearing, Sanitizing, Distancing, No gathering, Medical reporting (Khẩu trang, Khử khuẩn, Khoảng cách, Không tập trung, Khai báo y tế). After one week of implementing Directive 16 in Ho Chi Minh, the authorities caught 3,931 people violating the rules and collected 16 billion VND ($800,000) (Le Trai, 2021).

As the coronavirus started spreading to most of the provinces and cities following the lifting of lockdown in Ho Chi Minh, the Vietnamese government issued Resolution 128 on October 18, 2021, to provide provisional regulations on "Safety, flexibility, and Effective Control of COVID-19." This move marked the shift from a zero-COVID strategy to "safe adaption to the pandemic with vaccination being the key to help the country gradually resume social and economic activities" (Quang Minh, 2021).

Japan and Its Moderate Approach

By contrast, the Japanese government adopted a surprisingly moderate approach to prevent and contain the pandemic in a country that usually receives millions (JTB Tourism Research & Consulting Co., 2021) of visitors from China annually. There have been no stringent measures such as community lockdown and mandatory quarantine, except for the State of Emergency declaration on April 7, 2020, and on January 7, 2021. Even that Emergency declaration fell short of enforcing a large-scale lockdown.

Neither did Japan close its country entirely. Instead, it implemented gradual responses with a travel ban or travel restrictions on people coming from affected countries. Nor did it implement preventive measures at entry points (e.g., a mandatory quarantine). Japan also concentrated on a cluster strategy and contact tracing with unambiguous definitions. "Close contact" was defined as those who came into contact with the infected person two days before the infected person began showing the symptoms and were exposed for more than 15 minutes within a 1-m distance (NHK, 2020a). A place was considered a "cluster" if more than five people were infected on the same premises (Ministry of Health, Labor and Welfare, 2020).

On April 7, Prime Minister Abe declared the State of Emergency, Japan's first drastic move after escalating pressure from its people demanded a more decisive intervention from the government after a spike in the number of infections in March 2020. One crucial point is that the Japanese Prime Minister does not have the legal authority to impose a drastic measure like lockdown, as seen in many other countries. The PM needs the Diet's approval less than a month before the emergency declaration.

In his speech, Abe also repeatedly emphasized that the State of Emergency was not "a lockdown" to assure his people of the country's long-held democratic values and fundamental civil rights. Legal enforcement of the State of Emergency was also largely limited. The power that the State of Emergency granted the local governments was that they could legally and forcefully expropriate land or buildings for medical purposes, overriding the owners' objections in the event of an influx of infected patients. In addition, local (prefectural) governors could only "*request*" the residents to stay at home, and businesses deemed non-essential (e.g., pachinko parlors) closed. No penalty was imposed in case of violation, although the governors might "make public" the names of businesses refusing the request. The government largely relied on people's behavior in public spaces, as Abe explained in his speech:

> We, especially young fellows, have to think that every one of us may be the infected person. When we go out, please avoid crowded places, keep a distance from others, and wear a mask. By doing so, we are protecting other people's lives. By doing so, we are protecting our own lives.
>
> (Abe, 2020)

Not many Japanese, including the media, paid much attention to the message, or they just mentioned it in passing.

The contrast in Vietnam is striking. One week before that, a message with the opposite content went viral on the social networks in Vietnam: "Treat all your friends, relatives, and those with whom we come in contact as infected people. Only by so doing can we fight this virus." The message was allegedly sent by Vu Duc Dam, the Deputy PM, the Head of the National Steering Committee for COVID-19 Prevention and Control, and the COVID-19 Response Steering Committee. Even though the message was a hoax, its content still resonated among many Vietnamese. On June 18, 2021, Ho Chi Minh CDC (Center for Disease Control and Prevention) made official a similar message: "Treat people you come in contact as if they were F0 (the infected) in order to seriously adopt protection measures" (Tuan Kiet, 2021).

In Japan, Abe's successor, Suga Hideyoshi, delivered a similar message as Abe's, although in a different tone, to the young Japanese on January 6, 2021, in declaring the second State of Emergency, applicable to Tokyo and ten prefectures:

> Even when you get infected, not many of you will show any severe symptoms. However, the reality is that there is a connection between your being infected and the current wave of infection. I would like you to act accordingly to protect precious lives, including that of your parents, your grandparents, and your friends.
>
> (Suga, 2021)

On the same day, the Diet passed two bills, allowing the authorities to levy financial punishments on the individuals and businesses that violated the government's antivirus measures. In the areas under the State of Emergency, businesses refusing to cooperate with orders to shorten their hours or shut down for a designated period faced a ¥300,000 fine. Even in the areas where the State of Emergency had not been declared, the legislation also allowed local authorities to inspect businesses during a Stage 3 alert, one level away from the maximum, to ensure that they shortened their service hours. Those who refused to do so would face a ¥200,000 fine. In addition, under the new revisions to the Infectious Disease Law, those infected who refused orders to be hospitalized could be fined up to ¥500,000. Furthermore, those infected who refused to cooperate with public health officials in tracking their infection route could face a ¥300,000 fine for more (Johnston, 2021). These efforts to increase rule enforcement showed the determination of the new administration to curb the pandemic.

However, both Abe and Suga were criticized for their delayed responses to the pandemic, regarding the timing of the State of Emergency. Two independent surveys by *the Mainichi Shimbun* in April 2020 and January 2021, soon after the two emergency declarations, showed similar results: 70% and 71% of the surveyed thought that the declarations came out too late, while only 22% and 18% thought that the timing was appropriate (Hirata, 2020, Ito, 2021).

Surprisingly, given the government's moderate approach and the fact that people still had freedom of mobility, the total infections dropped sharply within a month: from around 500 cases per day in April 2020 down to around 20 cases in the second half of May 2020, and from 7–8,000 cases per day throughout December 2020 and January 2021 down to around 1,500 cases by the second week of February 2021 (Worldometers.info, n.d.).

A dramatic increase in the number of cases per day occurred between April and December. Many reasons were conceivable. For one, people became laxer. The cold weather hit some regions. The weather is accounted for the second and third waves in many regions. Still, another reason for Japan's increase was the Go-to-Travel campaign—a government subsidy program—encouraging domestic travel (up to 50% expense coverage) to help boost the economy. While the government has said there was no evidence that its "Go-To"-Travel campaign spread the coronavirus, Suga suspended it in late December (Swift, 2021).

During the first wave, the sharp drop could be attributed to a steep decrease in people's mobility. In some major areas such as Osaka and Tokyo's Ginza, the reduced mobility was down to 70–80% as "requested." On the other hand, in the third wave, the decline in people's mobility was nowhere near the target of 70–80%. One of the Declaration's targets was the shortened business hours of drinking places where people were often oblivious to the necessary precautions against the spread. On December 23, 2020, the government report showed that the number of infections concentrated in drinking places and the increase here was closely related to a similar rise in the infections within the family (NHK, 2020b). Go-to-Eat Campaign, the accompaniment of Go-to-Travel Campaign, was part of the blame.

One reasonable argument is that the people, not the government, should get the credit for the drop in infections because they are the ones who have accustomed themselves to the "new normal" with mask-wearing and hygiene routines, with 3-M avoiding (*San-mitsu*: a closed gathering, a close contact, and a closed space) and, for Tokyo, 5-S (*Go-shop for a group dining*: a small size, small servings, small voices, a short period, and frequent disinfection and use of masks) rules.

The Narratives Speak Volumes

Differences in the narratives of the Japanese and Vietnamese in this study are expected. The notable points are how they express what they want to say in the short answers, what the short narratives represent, and why the differences exist.

Health Concerns Regarding the Coronavirus

According to the Opinion Poll conducted by YouGov.com on April 6, 2020, regarding people's fear of catching the coronavirus, most of the Vietnamese and Japanese in the poll expressed a similar fear of the virus, with 85% (Japanese) and 88% (Vietnamese) reporting that they are "very" or "somewhat" scared that they will contract the coronavirus (Smith, 2020a). This result was expected, given the increase in the number of infections (the first wave) around the same period in the two countries.

However, the narratives I collected illustrate how differently the Vietnamese and Japanese elaborate on their concerns.

It is evident, from Table 5.1, that regardless of their age differences, the Japanese are a great deal more concerned about their health and the presence of the virus (32 mentions in the answers to all four questions) than the Vietnamese (with only 10). Among the Japanese, 18 out of 26 offer "health" to Question 3: "What concerns you the most in your everyday life?" Only seven out of 22 Vietnamese do so. Interestingly, too, the Japanese express health concerns in more than one place. Four of them raise concerns in the answers to two of the four questions, and five of them mention the concerns in answers to three questions. Also, two of them answer in one paragraph where the health concern

Table 5.1 Where the Health-Related Answers Appear

	Vietnamese (22)	Japanese (26)
No mention at all	13	5
In the answer to Question 1	2	7
In the answer to Question 2	1	7
In the answer to Question 3	7	18
In the answer to Question 4	0	0
In one paragraph to respond to all four Questions	*0*	*2*

Note: The answers regarding *health*, *infection*, *safety*, and *danger* are health related.

Table 5.2 Concerns about Health and Infection

	Vietnamese		Japanese	
	Frequency	No. People	Frequency	No. People
Concerns about Health	8	6	8	7
Health in general	5	4	5	5
Health of their own	0	0	1	1
Health of family	1	1	2	2
Health of relatives and close ones	2	2	0	0
Concerns about Infection	8	5	35	16
Infection in general	8	5	11	8
I become infected	0	0	13	10
Family become infected	0	0	9	8
Relatives and loved ones become infected	0	0	3	3
Others (I spread to others)	0	0	4	4

dominates. Of the 22 Vietnamese, 13 (59%) do not mention any health concerns, compared to 5 out of 26 (19%) among the Japanese.

There is little difference between the two groups when they discuss *health*, with 6 Vietnamese and 7 Japanese mentioning *health* (Table 5.2). However, when it comes to *infection*, the contrast between the two groups begins to emerge. Only five Vietnamese mention the term *infection* generally in their answers in the same way they mention *health*. Meanwhile, 16 Japanese are more preoccupied with *infection* than *health*, with ten worrying about themselves being infected, eight about their family members becoming infected, and three expressing a similar concern for their relatives and loved ones. Curiously enough, four Japanese are also nervous about becoming the source of infection for others in addition to the fear of becoming infected.

Tables 5.3 and 5.4 provide a more complex perspective on how each group perceives the virus. In Table 5.3, only one Vietnamese utters her surprise at the event, saying, "I have never seen anything on this scale." Three others state that they are not surprised at the event. Two male respondents even provide an identical answer: "This (pandemic) is a matter of fact." Two state that this virus is "not dangerous," and therefore believe that they are not affected by it: "The virus is more dangerous than flu, but it is not that problematic to young people except for the elderly and children. In fact, I am not bothered by this" (F, 27).

The words *dangerous* or *danger* appear more often in their narratives than in the Japanese narratives: "This virus is a danger" or "This is a dangerous virus." However, they are less expressive about their emotions. The words like *scary/scared* appear only once in all the narratives. One Vietnamese (F, 39) indicates that she is worried and stressed out but adds: "not to the point of becoming pessimistic and skeptical about life."

Table 5.3 Vietnamese Perception of the Coronavirus

Surprised (2)	Not Surprised (3)	Anxiety (6)	Lesson (6)	Not Affected (2)
I have never seen anything on this scale. The most influential event	Not (really) surprised A natural thing Part of life	Danger Dangerous (2) Ferocious Disaster Unpredictable Worried Stressed	An opportunity for reflection A lesson to learn Punishment on the human being A second chance A gift from God A challenge	Not too dangerous More dangerous than flu but not that worrisome

Table 5.4 Japanese Perceptions of the Coronavirus

Surprised at the Event (5)	Anxiety (15)	Not Affected (2)
Didn't expect this (2) Was surprised (2) Didn't imagine this (2)	Scary (3) I am scared (2) Scary thing scariest Anxious I don't like it Anxiety (8) Great anxiety Worried (5) Threat More dangerous than flu I am not too sure about this (2) Menace (2) I am afraid (2) Threatened I am infuriated Unsafe This doesn't look good	Not dangerous Not afraid

Interestingly, instead of seeing this as a threat, six Vietnamese view the virus as *an opportunity* or *a lesson* to reflect on their way of living in their answer to Question 1: What do you think of the virus?

An opportunity for the world to reflect on its operations.

(F, 39, real estate manager)

A lesson in business and personal life.

(F, 39, owner of a resort hotel)

A challenge to our perception and our awareness.

(M, 30, IT specialist)

A gift from God, an opportunity for us to live slowly [...] It is part of our life.

(M, 18, disabled, bedridden)

A punishment toward humans for what they have been doing to the world and nature.

(M, 29, Education worker)

A second chance for humankind

(F, 19, studying in Japan)

The Japanese narratives offer almost opposite reactions. They respond directly to the virus, though less definitive—with the frequent appearance of "maybe" (kamoshirenai) or "I don't know" (wakaranai) compared to the Vietnamese responses.—They are more expressive of their *feelings* towards the virus. The word *dangerous* (virus) appears only once. Instead, a wide range of words fill their narratives describing their emotions towards the virus (Table 5.4): *scared, anxious, worried, menace, infuriated, threatened, not too sure, unsafe*. Five of them are *surprised* at this development. Only two in their early 20s express that they are not affected by nor concerned about the virus.

Order of "Concerns" in Their Everyday Life

In responding to Question 3, "What concerns you the most in your everyday life?," most Japanese (23 of 26) mention health—their own and others. The *infection* and *health* appear first in their responses. Of the 23, ten state *health* as their primary concern. There is a discrepancy between the younger and the older groups in their additional problems. Five younger ones are concerned about how to better adapt themselves to work, and one male is worried especially about his job-hunting (M, 23). Another (M, 21) is worried about his mother's financial situation, while three in their 70s express worries about the social impact of the virus.

Among the Vietnamese, the primary concerns are more diverse and in an entirely different order. Three say that their priorities in life remain unaffected. Their main priorities remain the same: livelihood and family (M, 28), finishing school, and job-hunting (F, 26).

Nine of the respondents express health concerns. Then, they add that it is not their health but the health of others—including parents and children—that they are concerned about. Two are worried about how to adjust to the new tempo of everyday life: "How to keep up daily routine, including the time to work and rest, what to cook for two meals a day?" (F, 39). Four of them are anxious about *when* they can go back to *the old normal*, "When will the pandemic be over?"

(two in their 70s); "When can I travel again?" (M, 29); and "When can I go back to school?" (M, 10 years old).

Through this pandemic, they have come to realize that "Life is short" (M, 55; F, 70; M, 29; F, 19), "Life is evanescent" (F, 70; F, 39), or "Life is full of miseries" (F, 39). What they are most concerned about is how they can revise the meaning of their lives through this pandemic and beyond.

Feelings towards the Government

A survey conducted by YouGov.com (Smith, 2020b) shows that 97% of the Vietnamese expressed that the government was managing the coronavirus very well or somewhat well, as of June 23, 2020. That figure has remained over 90% since the end of March. In contrast, a similar figure in Japan was as low as 42%, as of May 4, a slight improvement over 31% on April 6, one day before Japan declared a State of Emergency.

This discrepancy between the Japanese and Vietnamese attitudes is also found in how they voice their feelings toward their governments. Below are unsolicited expressions responding to the four questions. Consistency in their respective attitudes is noticeable.

First, among the Vietnamese responses, the pride in their government is clear:

> For so long, people have lost their trust in the regime. However, through this pandemic, and through how the government has responded to the pandemic, everyone just realizes it is a pride to be a citizen of a Vietnam of resilience, invincibility, and benevolence.
>
> (F, 70)

> I sent 15 cloth masks to my friend living in France. She was wearing it today. The virus made me proud of Vietnam for the first time in life.
>
> (F, 39)

> I have never seen such solidarity among the Vietnamese. I heard about it, and I read about it. But now I can see with my own eyes and even feel it... I just hope many people can come to realize how benevolent our country is to appreciate more what the country has done for us.
>
> (F, 32)

The pride and trust in, or an almost reverent attitude toward, the Communist government are evident among these three individuals, despite the age differences. The narrative of the senior respondent (F, 70) suggests that their trust is not new and may have been lost but has now returned to the Vietnamese. Likewise, the younger ones' narratives are full of a newly-found pride in the country and the people's solidarity. The difference stems from the older generation's wartime difficulty and its absence among the younger generation.

This generational difference, however, should not obscure a common thread running through them. As will be discussed shortly, the thread is about the way the old and the young act, and relate, among others, mostly strangers.

By contrast, the Japanese, especially among the younger ones, express a more skeptical view toward the government. The sentiment, expressed in "This is a good chance to review how good our leaders are" (M, 23), is common. A male (39), infected in December 2020, has this to say:

> Reliance on the central government declined further because of their inadequate responses. [...] The younger generation, in particular, can no longer have the idea of relying on the central government for solving a problem.

In his answers *after* the recovery, to the same set of questions in January 2021, his view towards the government remains the same: "The government acts too slow. There is nothing we can do but rely on ourselves." That skepticism toward the government is everywhere:

> What is taking them so long? Why is Japan still making their employees go to work and take public transport amidst this global pandemic? Aren't they paying attention to situations abroad?
>
> (M, 19)

> So what is the government doing? Can they not handle things like the United States or other countries do? I thought it would not happen in this country [...] I think Abe-san, Koike (Governor of Tokyo) san should stand firm and not nervous about people's resistance. I want them, instead of telling people to refrain, to tell people what to do more specifically.
>
> (F, 22)

A senior respondent (M, 75) presents a more sarcastic view: "This could pose a bad example of a dictatorship being better at managing crises than a democratic system." The criticisms and sarcasm notwithstanding, I detect the confidence the Japanese have in *themselves* and the unspoken confidence in not feeling alone among others.

I conducted a follow-up survey (minus the fourth question, "What do you think about life?"), in June 2021 among 24 Vietnamese (16~58 years old) and 13 Japanese (19~61). Japan was at the declining phase of the fourth wave, and Vietnam, especially Ho Chi Minh, was finally hit hard by the pandemic. The contrast in the two groups' responses ceases to be apparent as both speak more about their daily concerns such as health, infection, family, jobs, among others. The coronavirus is no longer as distant in Vietnamese everyday life, which was evident in their answers in the first survey, even for those living away from Ho Chi Minh. Nonetheless, no complaint is spotted against coercive measures by the Vietnamese government.

> The situation has become unnerving and complicated as the infections increase so fast. But this small country is trying hard every second, every minute. Vietnam and we will win the pandemic.
>
> (F, 18, Binh Dinh Province)

In Vietnam and Japan, as elsewhere, the behaviors of the individuals play an important role throughout the pandemic. A single individual's reckless behavior could generate unintended consequences for many others, including those he or she may not know. By that same token, the citizens' behaviors contributed significantly to the successful containment of the virus in Japan and Vietnam over the three waves in 2020 and 2021.

A point to note here is that Vietnamese and Japanese exhibited two distinct behavior patterns. The Vietnamese are responsive and compliant to the government's orders, even when exposing their personal information. The Japanese, on the other hand, are cautious and responsive more directly to the threat of the virus.

There is a degree of uniformity in each of the Vietnamese and Japanese reactions. That uniformity hints at a more underlying difference between the two groups' perceptions of others beyond the pandemic context. The difference is noticeable in how they see and act among others. The different views of the public in their lives among the Vietnamese and the Japanese need a closer examination.

A Sense of *the Public* among the Vietnamese and the Japanese

For the Vietnamese, the term *the public* (*công cộng* or just *công*) in their everyday life frequently carries negative connotations: something or someplace undesirable and of dubious quality. The examples are many including public buses (*xe buýt công cộng*), public hospital (*bệnh viện công*), public services (*dịch vụ công*), and especially public toilets (*nhà vệ sinh công cộng*). People usually shy away from making use of these services. If they are out in public, they typically become more guarded, as they regard others as a threat and an intrusion. *The public* becomes a lesser threat when the Vietnamese are aware of a shared national sentiment such as patriotism. Such sentiment usually emerges during times of war or celebration, such as international soccer matches.

In contrast, the sense of *public* is deeply ingrained in Japanese everyday life. Since childhood, each Japanese is trained to nurture a *public mind*, or *spirit* (koukyoushin) to co-exist with *others* in the public space. *The public* is associated with specific open areas such as trains, *onsen*, and waiting rooms, among others. While in a *public space*, the Japanese place themselves in a deferential position, even being a potential offender, and try to observe rules–manners–etiquettes in order *not-to-become-a-nuisance-to-others* (meiwaku kakenaiyouni).

In short, the Vietnamese are more guarded against the presence of *others*, while the Japanese are more conscious of the impact of their presence on *others*. These perceptions of others, *the public*, are rooted in the history and context of each country.

Vietnamese Communal Consciousness

Interestingly enough, *others*, if translated into Vietnamese, mean *different people* (*người khác*). Depending on the context, *others* can be more specific—strangers (*người lạ*), outsiders (*người ngoài*), and non-blood-related people (*người dưng*). Anyone is among others, as defined above, when he or she is with those who do not share a membership (workplace, neighborhood, or birthplace) or kinship (family or extended family). The perception of such others, in turn, offers the "reference point for Vietnamese behavior," whose formation is traceable, according to an observer, to the long history of traditional village life" (Nguyen, 2003, p. 102).

Vietnamese villages were bamboo fortresses, a "state within a state," and "each village struck its own drum" and worshiped its own deities. Their economy was mostly self-sufficient and found little cause for contact with outsiders. The villages were also administrative links to the central government as they served to collect taxes and prepare the land and other registrations. The village heads (usually landowners) were the managers of this link.

Within this relative autonomy of village life, interdependence emerged between the village heads and the villagers (mostly tenant farmers). The former relied on the latter for sustained agricultural production and the latter on the former for various means and ways for securing subsistence. James Scott (1976) calls this asymmetrical reciprocity a "moral economy."

Such a practice of reciprocity operated within the well-defined boundary of a village. Over time, the practice instilled and reinforced in the villagers a dichotomy of "us" vs. "them." People coming from outside and planning to stay in a village (unsettled farmers) were considered khách hộ (guests) or ngoại tịch (outsiders). They were not an integral part of the communal (village) reciprocity and were without access to collective assets such as communal land (Nguyen, 2003, p.114).

One clarification: *communal* here indicates that the shared sense of local origin (community membership) is the prerequisite for benefiting from communal reciprocity. This differs from the modern notion of *public*, which is a membership-free notion. To borrow from Erving Goffman, "it is the realm of 'unfocused' interactions between *anonymous* strangers" (Goffman, 1971, p. 219, Italics added). What matters is not so much who is interacting with whom but where the interactions take place.

This *communal* mind—an understanding that emphasizes membership or a shared sense of belonging or origin—still dominates Vietnamese consciousness. The prolonged war of independence and unification stretching over 30 years reinforced this sense of membership, that of Vietnam. This reinforcement deepened both suspicions of others' intrusion and reliance on anyone who was even remotely intimate.

The expectation of communal reciprocity has thus found its way into Vietnamese daily wisdom. Unwritten rules of behavior place one's personal connection with others prominently as in the "Rule of 4-C" (*con cháu các cụ* = You have to be a descendant of some big guy) or "Rule of 4-E" (*hậu duệ, quan hệ, tiền tệ trí tuệ* = Rule of Survival in Descending Order of Importance:1 a descendant of someone big, 2 good connection, 3 money, and 4 ability) (Vu, 2021).

The dominance of personal ties—or collectively, communal ties—survived even the prolonged collective farming period, from 1955 for the North and the South from 1976 until 1986. The agricultural cooperatives' intrusion did little to alter the Vietnamese inclination to seek and guard their communal reciprocity. After all, an agricultural cooperative was a cluster of old villages preserving their original boundaries. The consequences spread into many dimensions of villagers' lives.

> Cooperatives in the North developed from a pure production unit into a social, economic, and quasi-political entity. During wartime, they were turned into strategic units and took upon themselves many non-economic functions. [Especially] when the cooperative coincided with the area of a village, the distinction between economic and politico-administrative management virtually disappeared even though legally they remained two separate entities.
>
> (United Nations Development Programme,
> *Report on the Economy of Vietnam*, quoted in Vu,
> 2020, p. 54)

With the basic continuity from the past intact, the cooperative's mode of agricultural production provided little or no work incentive for the farmers. The farmers received points for the hours they put into production and had no authority to distribute or market their products. The assignments of work "points" and the distribution of goods and services, which the villagers procured using the points, remained in the hands of the cooperative's officials, leaving the farmers with a limited sense of earning from their invested labor.

The rate of collectivization of the farmers reached nearly 100% by the early 1960s. However, that development was attributable to the worsening of the war in the early 1960s, which began to show signs of protracted confrontation with the United States and its allies around the 1964/65 juncture. The agricultural cooperatives ceased to be mere production units and were transformed into an integral part of the war effort.

An unexpected twist is that the cooperatives reinforced communal ties among the villagers as they, inspired by patriotism, helped to mobilize village youths for the battlefront. The efficacy of their efforts, ironically, took the form of the stream of casualties among their friends, relatives, and family members in the village. The villagers' experience with the cooperatives became indistinguishable from that of surviving the war (Vu, 2020, pp. 54–55).

The farmers exhibited two contradictory patterns of behavior in response to the cooperatives. On the one hand, they worked only half-heartedly in a collectivized farmland. Nowhere else could Olson's description of the difficulties accompanying the production of "collective goods" be so applicable than the farmers in the agricultural cooperatives (Olson, 1971). Instead, they spent most of their time and labor working on their private land (5% land = *dat nam phan tram*), which the collective's authority set aside for the farmers to grow vegetables or livestock (pigs or chickens) for household consumption.

On the other hand, the state control of the distribution of goods threw farmers into fierce competition as they sought to secure necessary and scarce commodities for their families at the state-owned stores. The state-owned stores, public in the sense that they were open to everyone regardless of the village (or collective) affiliations, caused divisive competition for survival among the farmers of the collectives. Popular sayings reflect this competition: *A buffalo coming late has only muddy waters* (*trâu chậm uống nước đục*), and *You go, then you lose your seat* (*đi mất chỗ*).

The only situation that helped the villagers transcend their divisive drive was when an overarching plea, such as the war for the country's unification, swept through their communities. In the absence of that plea, the *public spaces* were the arena where everyone was a stranger and free to pursue his interest in the manner of his choosing.

With that plea, a not-so-distant memory, the government's rigorous and direct interventions in Vietnamese life to control the coronavirus is a reminder that they are in that special time where they need to suspend the otherwise individualistic and divisive drive for self-interest. In a hastily assembled meeting at the end of January 2021 following new infection cases of the third wave, Deputy Prime Minister Vu Duc Dam stopped halfway in his speech. "I always have confidence in Vietnamese, our people and our officials could be a little [...] (pause) [...] in normal times." Then he quickly resumed his talk, "but if anything happens, they will actively respond." He could have filled that split-second pause with "too distrustful of others" or a statement to that effect.

Public Consciousness among the Japanese

For the current generations of Japanese, the origins of the sense of *public* are not linked to a "national sentiment," a distant reminder of prewar militarism and the disasters of the 1940s. The sense of *public*, buried in the rhetoric of political leaders and individual narratives, has its seeds in a long history of self-seclusion in the Tokugawa era before its opening to the outside world in the mid-nineteenth century.

In pre- or early-modern Japan, Japanese farmers, accounting for over 90% of the population, experienced limited mobility. Their lives and livelihoods, much like those of the Vietnamese farmers, were limited to the small confines of their villages. However, there is one significant difference between Japanese and Vietnamese farmers. The former regularly had opportunities to observe, and even interact with, many non-villagers or *strangers*.

Sankin Kotai, the system of the alternate Edo (Tokyo) residence requirement for the *daimyō*s (feudal lords), introduced by the Tokugawa shogunate in 1635 and practiced throughout the Edo period until the 1860s, had the purpose of strengthening central control over the 250 plus *daimyō*s. It required these daimyōs to spend a year in Edo every two years as "proof" of their loyalty to the Shogun. Every one of the 250 daimyōs made a trip, on foot, every two years from his domain to Edo. The lack of change in the alternate residence requirement may be consistent with the rigid feudal system.

This durable requirement, however, blinds us to the impact of the presence of a mobile population. Each *daimyo*'s procession was accompanied by a sizable number of his retainers, ranging from a little over 100 to 5,000, depending on the size of the domain.

Each marched to Edo through any one of the five major routes with 214 post stations (or post towns). These travelers became "migrating messengers of change" (Rozman, 1974, p. 100) at places they passed, consuming local goods and services. The villagers, however immobile they might have been, regularly witnessed the traveling retinues. The *Sankin Kotai*

> revitalized the old imperial highway system, and led to the provision of facilities of a kind which could be used by all travelers, ... inns at which they could lodge, tea- houses at which they could rest, porters and horses whose services they could use.
>
> (Bolitho, 1990, p. 486)

The presence of this mobile population led to new local economies in these rural areas and more. Its impact may be slow in forming but is extensive, as a sociologist observes:

> [The villagers'] behavior and attitudes reflected the decreasing self-sufficiency and growing outside orientation. Changing family patterns resulting from popular aspirations for a higher living standard most likely closely corresponded to the commercialization of rural life. Marketing, probably more than migration, broadened the horizons of ordinary villagers.
>
> (Rozman, 1974, p. 105)

Efforts to place the interactions with the *strangers* in a stable perspective came as Japan's modernization began to pick up in the closing years of the nineteenth century. An increasing number of people migrated to Tokyo and other major cities. The number of white color workers in Tokyo was only 5.6% in 1908 but increased to 21.4% in 1920. Against this background, the Japanese Ministry of Education introduced a set of manners that people needed to observe in *public space* and *public time* in 1911 and 1913.

The keyword in these documents is *meiwaku* (nuisance or troublesome). The documents encouraged people not to become a nuisance to others, i.e., *strangers*, in public (space and time). From the 1920s on, the phrase *try-not-to-become-a-nuisance-to-others* began to appear more frequently to suggest the manners that were required of people *in public* (Enko, 2019). This *try-not-to-become-a-nuisance-to-others* rule is still dominant in public spaces.

Throughout the coronavirus pandemic, wearing masks or covering the mouth when coughing has never been mandatory in Japan. It is an etiquette that is expected of everyone *in public*. This emphasis on discretionary behavior is a promoter of what Lyn Lofland calls *cooperative motility* (Lofland, 1998, p. 29), the way "strangers work together to traverse space without incident."

This *cooperative motility* is rare among Vietnamese people. The *try-not-to-become-a-nuisance-to-others* principle does not make the Japanese patently collective-minded, as is often assumed by observers too eager to resort to cultural stereotyping. The *try-not-to-become-a-nuisance-to-others* principle is perfectly practical and rational because it is built on the calculation that *If I don't bother you, then you won't bother me* and the trust of others who would reciprocate this posture, which Goffman calls *deference ritual* (Goffman, 1956, p. 478). From this perspective, Abe's speech on April 7, 2020, cited above, to "protect other people's live," was less a call for action (even if he meant it to be so) and more an appeal to the Japanese sense of what one is to others.

The current coronavirus pandemic may have pushed many people to deviate from their much-accustomed everyday routines. College students may spend more time before their PCs, as schools offer online lectures and seminars. Office workers may find themselves more in their living rooms at home. Online shopping may have replaced weekend visits to supermarkets and other shops. All these alternatives to familiar routines appear to be no more than temporary, as the thought of "returning to the daily routine eventually" has never left the minds of many.

However, there is more to the daily routine.

Beyond the Pandemic

The restoration of everyday life may be in order in due time. That, however, should not blind us to the likelihood that the force working at a deeper layer of Vietnamese and Japanese consciousness has remained mostly undisturbed. The brief observations above make it clear that how people see themselves and behave among others, in the public, has gone through a long history. Besides, the opportunities are plenty where this force sways people's behavior. In public health, natural disaster prevention and relief, or even workplace human interactions, people expect constant and close interactions with others, mostly strangers, in their efforts to attain given goals. The people's perception of the public is likely to dictate their behavior, be it in Vietnam, Japan, or elsewhere.

Appendix

Differences between Directive No. 10 (2021 by Ho Chi Minh People Committee), Directive No. 15, and Directive No. 16 (Both 2020 by the Central Government)

	Directive 10	*Directive 15*	*Directive 16*
Public gatherings	People go out only when necessary No gathering of more than three people in public space, except office places, hospitals, and schools	Cancellation of events with more than 20 people per room Suspension of all cultural, sport, entertainment events Ban on the gathering of more than ten people outside offices, schools, and hospitals	Societal distancing. Everyone is required to stay home as much as possible and only go out under absolutely necessary circumstances Ban on gatherings of more than two people outside offices, schools, and hospitals
Minimum safe distance	1.5 meter	2 meter	2 meter
Service providers	Suspension of non-essential businesses and unorganized outdoor markets Service providers and production facilities of essential goods, factories, and production plants as such are allowed to operate if they implement required protection measures against the virus	Suspension of non-essential businesses and services Essential services are allowed to operate	Suspension of non-essential businesses and services Essential services are allowed to operate if they implement required protection measures against the virus
Public transportation	Suspension of public transportation Exceptions: transportation of food and essential goods, shuttle bus for factory workers, experts, and production goods if they implement required measures against the virus	Restrictions on traveling from coronavirus-hit localities to others Restrictions on transporting from Hanoi and Ho Chi Minh to other localities	Suspension of public transportation except for necessary circumstances Suspension of traveling from coronavirus-hit areas to other localities except for special cases

References

Abe, S. (2020, April 7). Press Conference. Asahi Shimbun Dejitaru. https://www.asahi.com/articles/ASN467JFGN46UTFK01R.html

Bolitho, H. (1990). Travelers' tales: Three eighteenth-century travel journals. *Harvard Journal of Asiatic Studies*, *50*(2), 485–504.

Directive No.10/CT-UBND on Enhancement of COVID-19 Prevention and Control Measures in Ho Chi Minh City. (2021, June 19). https://thuvienphapluat.vn/van-ban/The-thao-Y-te/Chi-thi-10-CT-UBND-2021-siet-chat-tang-cuong-bien-phap-phong-chong-dich-Covid19-Ho-Chi-Minh-478396.aspx

Directive No.15/CT-TTg on Climax Stage of COVID-19 Control Effort. (2020, March 27). https://thuvienphapluat.vn/van-ban/the-thao-y-te/chi-thi-15-ct-ttg-2020-quyet-liet-thuc-hien-dot-cao-diem-phong-chong-dich-covid-19-438342.aspx

Directive No.16/CT-TTg on Implementation of Urgent Measures for Prevention and Control of COVID-19. (2020, March 31). https://thuvienphapluat.vn/van-ban/The-thao-Y-te/Chi-thi-16-CT-TTg-2020-thuc-hien-bien-phap-cap-bach-phong-chong-dich-COVID-19-438648.aspx

Enko, M. (2019, February 2). Mijikana kotoba no rekishi o kanngaeru: 'meiwaku' to 'bunka' ni hisomu seijisei [Thoughts on familiar words' history: political character of 'nuisance' and culture)]. *Todai-shimbun Online*. https://www.todaishimbun.org/words_political_nature20190218/

General Department of Preventive Medicine (Cục Y tế Dự phòng). (2020, February 1). Công văn cục y tế dự phòng về việc tăng cường công tác kiểm dịch y tế phòng chống dịch bệnh lan truyền qua cửa khẩu [Document of Vietnam CDC on increased management on medical surveillance to prevent pandemic through border entries]. https://vncdc.gov.vn/cong-van-cuc-y-te-du-phong-ve-viec-tang-cuong-cong-tac-kiem-dich-y-te-phong-chong-dich-benh-lan-truyen-qua-cua-khau-nd14990.html.

Goffman, E. (1956). The nature of deference and demeanor. *American Anthropologist*. *58*(3), 473–502.

Goffman, E. (1971). *Relations in Public. Microstudies of the Public Order*. Routledge.

Government Decree 117/2020/ND-CP on Prescribing Penalties for Administrative Violations in the Medical Sector. (2020, September 28). https://thuvienphapluat.vn/van-ban/Vi-pham-hanh-chinh/Nghi-dinh-117-2020-ND-CP-quy-dinh-xu-phat-vi-pham-hanh-chinh-trong-linh-vuc-y-te-398159.aspx

Government Resolution 128/2021 NQ-CP on Provisional Regulations on Safety, Flexibility and Effective control of COVID-19. (2021, October 11). https://thuvienphapluat.vn/van-ban/The-thao-Y-te/Nghi-quyet-128-NQ-CP-2021-Quy-dinh-tam-thoi-thich-ung-an-toan-linh-hoat-dich-COVID19-490931.aspx?v=d

Hirata, T. (2020, April 9). 72% support the state of emergency over the virus in Japan, 70% say the Declaration came too late. *The Mainichi*. https://mainichi.jp/english/articles/20200409/p2a/00m/0na/013000c

Hoang Phuong & Viet Tuan. (2020, March 16). Cách ly quyết liệt sẽ giảm tổn thất do dịch bệnh [Aggressive Quarantine will reduce the costs of the Pandemic]. *VnEpress*. https://vnexpress.net/thoi-su/cach-ly-quyet-liet-se-giam-ton-that-do-dich-benh-4070024.html

Hoang Thuy. (2021, February 16). Quân đội kích hoạt trạng thái như thời chiến để phòng chống COVID-19 [The Military activated to war-mode in response to

the COVID-19]. *VnEpress*. https://vnexpress.net/quan-doi-kich-hoat-trang-thai
-nhu-thoi-chien-de-phong-chong-covid-19-4235789.html

Huu Cong, & Van Phu, Cong Khang (2021, November 4). Cuộc điều quân lớn
nhất sau chiến tranh [The largest deployment after the war]. *VnEpress*. https://
vnexpress.net/cuoc-dieu-quan-lon-nhat-sau-chien-tranh-4380801.html

Ito, N. (2021, January 18). Japan Cabinet's approval rating drops to 33%; Many
say coronavirus response 'too late'. *The Mainichi*. https://mainichi.jp/english/
articles/20210118/p2a/00m/0na/014000c

Johnston, E. (2021, February 4). Japan's new virus law: Fines for non-compliance
and support for hard-hit firms. *The Japan Times*. https://www.japantimes.co.jp/
news/2021/02/04/national/new-virus-law-explainer/

JTB Tourism Research & Consulting Co. (n.d.). Japan-bound statistics. Retrieved
2021, March 10 from https://www.tourism.jp/en/tourism-database/stats/
inbound/

Le Trai. (2021, July 15). Hồ Chí Minh phạt người vi phạm chỉ thị 16 hơn 8 tỷ đồng
[Ho Chi Minh city fined violators of Directive 16 with more than 8 billion vnd].
Zing News. https://zingnews.vn/tphcm-phat-nguoi-vi-pham-chi-thi-16-hon-8
-ty-dong-post1238439.html

Lofland, L. H. (1998). *The Public Realm. Exploring the City's Quintessential Territory*.
Routledge.

Maynes, M. J., Pierce, J. L., & Laslett, B. (2008). *Telling Stories: The Use of Personal
Narratives in the Social Sciences and History*. Cornell University Press.

Minh Cuong. (2021, January 30). Quảng Ninh truy vết được 23600 F1 đến F4
[Quang Ninh traced 23600 F1 ~ F4]. *VnEpress*. https://vnexpress.net/quang
-ninh-truy-vet-duoc-hon-23-600-f1-den-f4-4228967.html

Ministry of Health (Vietnam) (MOH). (2020a, January 27). *Thủ tướng: Chống
dịch như chống giặc* [Prime Minister: Fight the pandemic as if to fight a foreign
enemy].   https://moh.gov.vn/hoat-dong-cua-lanh-dao-bo/-/asset_publisher/
TW6LTp1ZtwaN/content/thu-tuong-chong-dich-nhu-chong-giac-

Ministry of Health (Vietnam) (MOH). (2020b, March 8). *"Cuộc chiến" chống
COVID-19: Bắt đầu chiến dịch mới* [The war against COVID-19: The new
operation   begins].   https://moh.gov.vn/tin-tong-hop/-/asset_publisher/
k206Q9qkZOqn/content/-cuoc-chien-chong-covid-19-bat-au-chien-dich-moi

Ministry of Health (Vietnam) (MOH). (2020c, May 22). *Phó thủ tướng: Chúng
ta vẫn chưa chiến thắng dịch bệnh* [Deputy Minister: We have not won the
pandemic]. https://moh.gov.vn/hoat-dong-cua-lanh-dao-bo/-/asset_publisher
/TW6LTp1ZtwaN/content/pho-thu-tuong-chung-ta-van-chua-chien-thang
-dich-benh

Ministry of Health, Labor and Welfare (Japan) (MHLW) (2020, March 31).
"Zenkoku kurasuta- mappu," [National Cluster Map]. https://www.mhlw.go.jp
/content/000657332.pdf

Nguyen, T. A. (2003). Village versus state: The evolution of state-local relations in
Vietnam until 1945. *Southeast Asian Studies*, *41*(1), 101–123.

NHK (Nippon Hoso Kyokai -Japan Broadcasting Corporation). (n.d.) "Tokubetsu
saito shingata korona uirus," [Special Site for Coronavirus]. https://www3.nhk.or
.jp/news/special/coronavirus/data-widget/#mokuji0

NHK. (2020a, April 21). "Sesshokusha no teigi henko: hasshou futsukamae 1 me-toru
inai 15 fun ijo," [Change in the definition of a close contact]. https://www3.nhk
.or.jp/news/html/20200421/k10012399231000.html

NHK (Nippon Hoso Kyokai). (2020b, December 24). "kazokunai kansen ha 'inshokunadokaishi kensenshita kekka' inshoku no taisaku wo," [Measures against the increased infections through family eating and drinking]. https://www3.nhk .or.jp/news/html/20201224/k10012781041000.html

Olson, M. (1971) [1965]. *The Logic of Collective Action: Public Goods and the Theory of Groups* (Revised ed.). Harvard University Press.

Quang Minh. (2021, July 11). *PM Demands Accelerated COVID-19 Vaccination Rollout*. Online Newspaper of the Government. http://news.chinhphu.vn/Home /PM-demands-accelerated-COVID19-vaccination-rollout/202111/46069.vgp

Rozman, G. (1974). Edo's importance in the changing Tokugawa society. *The Journal of Japanese Studies, 1*(1), 91–112.

Scott, J. C. (1976). *The Moral Economy of the Peasant: Rebellion and Subsistence in Southeast Asia*. Yale University Press.

Smith, M. (2020a, May 2). International COVID-19 tracker update: 2 May. *YouGov.* https://yougov.co.uk/topics/international/articles-reports/2020/05/02/ international-covid-19-tracker-update-2-may

Smith, M. (2020b, June 29). International COVID-19 tracker update: 29 June. *YouGov.* https://yougov.co.uk/topics/international/articles-reports/2020/06 /29/international-covid-19-tracker-update-29-june

Suga, Y. (2021, Jan 7). Press Conference. Prime Minister's Office of Japan. https:// www.kantei.go.jp/jp/99_suga/statement/2021/0107kaiken.html

Swift, R. (2021, Jan 22). Japan tourism push linked to surge in COVID-19 infections- study. *Reuters.* https://www.reuters.com/article/us-health-coronavirus-japan- travel-idUSKBN29R0J2

Tuan Kiet. (2021, June 18). Ngành Y tế TP Hồ Chí Minh: Hãy xem người đối diện mình như là một F0 [Medical Sector of Ho Chi Minh: Treat people in front of you as F0]. *Vietnamnet.* https://vietnamnet.vn/vn/suc-khoe/thong-diep-moi-cua -nganh-y-te-tp-hcm-hay-xem-nguoi-doi-dien-minh-nhu-la-mot-f0-746932.html

VnExpress. Covid-19 Data of Vietnam [Số liệu Covid-19 tại Việt Nam]. (n.d.). https://vnexpress.net/covid-19/covid-19-viet-nam. retrieved November 19, 2021.

Vu, L. T. C. (2020). *Agent Orange and Rural Development in Post-war Vietnam.* Routledge.

Vu, L. T. C. (2021). Surviving over Living: War generations' postwar narratives. *Rondo, III.* Global Studies Association, Doshisha University.

Worldometers.info. (n.d.). https://www.worldometers.info/. Accessed on November 19, 2021.

6 Psychological Responses, Health Literacy, and Information Behavior during the COVID-19 Pandemic in Japan and Korea

Jinah Lee

Introduction

While the COVID-19 pandemic continues worldwide, the way of dealing with the pandemic varies from country to country. This chapter explores how Japanese and Korean people have responded to the COVID-19 pandemic. In response to the global health crisis, Japan and Korea have taken strong measures at the border early in 2020 but did not impose mandatory domestic restrictions. Like many other countries, businesses were temporarily closed, schools offered online classes, and telecommuting was encouraged by the government in Japan and South Korea (hereafter, Korea). However, all these measures are requests from the government for "self-restraint" (Japan) or "social distancing" (Korea), sharply contrasted to forced lockdown measures taken in many other countries.

So-called the Japan model refers to the Japanese government's efforts to prevent the spread of infection and limit economic damage through a combination of declaration of a state of emergency which calls for stay home and follow-up investigations of individual cases, without resorting to legally enforceable measures to restrict behavior (Asia Pacific Initiative, 2020). The report pointed out that preparations for the threat of infectious diseases and the state of preparedness of the Japan model were insufficient even though Japan has suffered many disasters. However, the response of the Japanese people was entirely satisfactory (Asia Pacific Initiative, 2020). O'Shea (2020, December 18) pointed out that such Japanese government's response to COVID-19 was "national exceptionalism," and a Japanese politician even explained the success of Japan in a somewhat nationalistic manner while mentioning *Mindo* of the Japanese people, which means the quality of people.

Korea had the largest outbreak of Middle East respiratory syndrome (MERS) outside the Middle East in 2015, which led to stricter preventive measures against the infectious disease than Japan. However, rather than a forced lockdown, Korea also adopted a local quarantine strategy, the so-called K-Quarantine, to minimize economic damage and effectively prevent the spread of disease (Choi et al., 2020). Despite a temporary rise in infection rates during the first wave of the COVID-19 pandemic, the Korean government's response to the COVID-19 was evaluated as rapid and effective (Paek & Hove, 2021). Specifically, based

DOI: 10.4324/9781003286684-6

on the experience of the MERS outbreak, the Korean government enhanced crisis management and communication to promote citizens' preventive actions by using information communication technology, which raised public awareness of infectious diseases. The civic evaluation of the Korean government's preventive measures was generally positive. In addition, Cho and Kim (2021) indicated that political orientation affected the assessment of the Korean government's response to COVID-19: Those who were liberal in political orientation were more likely to support the government's response to COVID-19 positively. Even though the factors affecting government's evaluation in dealing with COVID-19 are not the focus of this study, it is worth noting that the government's response to COVID-19 would likely influence civic awareness and reaction toward the pandemic.

This chapter investigates how Japanese and Korean people responded to the COVID-19 pandemic in early 2021, as the third wave of COVID-19 infections hit hard in the two countries. Specifically, the study compares Japanese and Korean risk perception at various levels, psychological responses and preventive behavior, focusing on the social and cultural factors in response to COVID-19. The study also examines the extent to which people have acquired digital health literacy and self-efficacy on COVID-19 as of early 2021, at the one-year mark of the pandemic. Furthermore, this study explores how people seek and avoid information on COVID-19 and feel information overload amidst growing fatigue from the COVID-19 pandemic.

Social and Cultural Factors in Response to COVID-19

Previous studies highlighted social and cultural factors as predictors of preventive behavior, such as harmony seeking and avoidance of rejection, two aspects of interdependence (Hashimoto & Yamaguchi, 2013). In the context of self-construal theory, harmony seeking means interdependent self-construal (Hashimoto & Yamaguchi, 2013), and rejection avoidance refers to a tendency to avoid negative evaluations and rejection by others (Sakakibara & Ozono, 2020). These two factors present the reality that people must be in harmony with and be accepted by others in society (Hashimoto & Yamaguchi, 2013).

Studies have shown that Japanese people tend to seek harmony and avoid low ratings from others (Hashimoto & Yamaguchi, 2013, 2016). Regarding preventive measures against infectious diseases, in a survey conducted in early 2020, Sakakibara and Ozono (2020) found harmony seeking was positively associated with preventive behavior. On the other hand, rejection avoidance and social pressure factors did not affect preventive behavior. Based on the findings, Sakakibara and Ozono (2020) argued that the preventive behavior of Japanese people is not guided by social pressure but by individual awareness to prevent the spread of infection.

On the other hand, in the survey of early 2021, Lee (2021) showed the tendency to avoid rejection and the concerns that if infected, family and oneself could be criticized were significantly related to practicing self-restraint among the Japanese younger adults aged 20–29 years. Japanese media have often covered young adults who do not comply with the request to stay home, showing downtown areas full of young people (Siripala, 2021, January 2). In a survey conducted under Japan's first state of emergency, those concerned about COVID-19 infections showed negative feelings toward people who did not comply with the request for self-restraint (Motoyoshi, 2021). Media coverage has likely caused the public's negative feelings toward the younger adults who failed to take preventive behavior, leading to the concern for rejection avoidance and practicing self-constraint behavior among the young generation (Lee, 2021).

In the Korean context, Zhang and Lee (2021) revealed the role of subjective norms and interdependent self-construal in prevention behavior among Korean college students in the study conducted in 2020. Subjective norms such as "my family and friends tell me not to go to crowded places" and "my family and friends tell me to practice social distancing" positively affected the intention to continue the prevention behavior. In addition, the study showed that interdependent self-construal emphasizing relationships and groups was positively related to perceived severity and negative feelings about COVID-19, which affected the intention to continue COVID-19 prevention behavior.

Health Literacy, Self-Efficacy, and Information Behavior in the COVID-19 Pandemic

Citizens need to access reliable information and critically assess it to engage in health behaviors and make appropriate decisions during the pandemic and infodemic of COVID-19 (Dadaczynski et al., 2021). Health literates refer to "placing one's health and that of one's family and community into context, understanding which factors are influencing it and knowing how to address them" (Sørensen et al., 2012, p. 1). Studies have shown that people with limited or low health literacy are inundated with information from mass media and the Internet, making it difficult to evaluate information on COVD-19 (Okan et al., 2020).

In the same vein, self-efficacy on COVID-19 plays a significant role in coping with the COVID-19 pandemic. Zhang and Lee (2021) showed that self-efficacy positively affected the intention to continue COVID-19 prevention behavior among Korean citizens, based on the health belief model, which refers to how perceived susceptibility, severity, benefit, barrier, and self-efficacy are associated with engagement in health-promoting behavior. Ma et al. (2021) showed the role of health information efficacy in the relationship between health information search, trust on a social Q & A site, and prevention behavior in the context of COVID-19. The more search for information on COVID-19 on the Q & A site, the more active respondents were in preventive actions against COVID-19. The cognitive and emotional trust using the social Q & A site mediated this relationship, which was more significant for those with high health information efficacy.

Information avoidance is also a significant issue amid increasing concerns about the fatigue of the COVID-19 pandemic (Hornyak, 2020). Case et al. (2005) denoted that people often search for information actively but occasionally avoid it, leading to adverse outcomes. Unlike in the first phase of the pandemic, governments have become more difficult to engage citizens. People are fed up with the COVID-19 pandemic and its information. News from multiple sources is helpful during the pandemic, but it might also have detrimental consequences, such as information overload and negative psychological and behavioral responses (Soroya et al., 2021). Information overload might negatively affect coping intentions (Farooq et al., 2020) and even cause information avoidance.

Lee (2021) showed that the young Japanese generation relies on online media for COVID-19 information in the Japanese context. However, health literacy on COVID-19 among the young generations is not sufficient, and those who rely more on social networking sites and online news tend to feel overloaded with COVID-19 information. Although young adults with high personal risk perception managed not to avoid information about COVID-19, attitudes toward media coverage of COVID-19 and unreliability of COVID-19 information on the Internet and social media have led to information avoidance.

In a survey of Korean undergraduate students, Chun et al. (2021) revealed that digital health literacy had a positive effect on the use of health information or preventive behavior: For those with high digital health literacy, preventive health behaviors such as participation in quarantine and willingness to get vaccinated against COVID-19 tended to be increased. Although Korean undergraduate students use online media in everyday life, some have difficulty finding, understanding, and utilizing health information. Overall digital health literacy of Korean college students was relatively high, but almost half of the college students answered that they had difficulties evaluating the reliability of online information.

Research Questions

In response to COVID-19, there is little research to compare social and cultural factors such as interdependent self-construal between Japan and Korea. In addition, as previously mentioned above, studies have focused mainly on the relations between social and cultural factors and preventive behavior. Social and cultural factors might be related to the risk perception of COVID-19, which plays a significant role in psychological and behavioral responses to COVID-19. This study explores to what extent people perceived risk at various levels, such as the individual and societal levels, and the risk of infecting others with COVID-19 (RQ1). Also, the study looks at what factors are related to the risk perception of infecting others with COVID-19, focusing on the interdependent culture of the two countries (RQ2).

RQ1: What are the levels of risk perception of COVID-19 at the individual and societal levels, and what risk perception of infecting others with COVID-19 in Japan and Korea?

RQ2: What factors are related to the risk perception of infecting others with COIVID-19 in Japan and Korea?

People need to continue their health prevention behaviors, and it is important to examine factors associated with health literacy and information behavior. This study focuses on digital health literacy, given the growing importance of online information during the pandemic. This study explores the extent to which people have acquired digital health literacy and self-efficacy on COVID-19 at the one-year mark of the pandemic (RQ3) and what factors are related to digital health literacy on COVID-19 (RQ4).

RQ3: What are the levels of digital health literacy and self-efficacy on COVID-19 in Japan and Korea?
RQ4: What factors are related to digital health literacy on COVID-19 in Japan and Korea?

In addition, considering the growing fatigue of the COVID-19 pandemic, this study examines the extent to which people seek and avoid information on COVID-19 and feel overloaded and fatigued with COVID-19 information (RQ5). Also, the study investigates what factors are associated with information seeking and avoidance of COVID-19 (RQ6), focusing on risk perception, information overload and fatigue.

RQ5: What are the levels of information seeking, avoidance, and feeling of overload and fatigue of COVID-19 in Japan and Korea?
RQ6: What factors are related to information seeking and avoidance on COVID-19 in Japan and Korea?

Furthermore, this study examines factors related to preventive behavior, such as self-restraint in Japan and social distancing in Korea, emphasizing information behavior, including information seeking and avoidance (RQ7).

RQ7: What factors are related to the practice of self-restraint in Japan and social distancing in Korea in the context of COVID-19?

Study 1

Sample

Study 1 is based on online surveys conducted in Japan and Korea. The study focuses on the responses to COVID-19, including risk perception, health literacy, and self-efficacy on COVID-19 in Japan and Korea (RQ1 to RQ4). The online survey was conducted among a panel of Internet research companies in Japan and Korea, and the sample size was assigned by age and gender. Considering the areas with a high number of infected people, the survey was conducted on 1,500 residents of the main regions in Kanto and Kinki aged 18–69 in Japan, from February 10 to 11, 2021 (Male: $N = 750$, Female: $N = 750$, Age: $M = 41.84$, $SD = 14.436$). Nine hundred fifty-five residents of main metropolitan areas aged

18–69 completed the online survey for a Korean sample between March 12 and March 16, 2021 (Male: $N = 476$, Female: $N = 479$, Age: $M = 39.66$, $SD = 13.733$).

Measurement

The study assessed the degree of risk perception of COVID-19 at the individual and societal levels and risk perception of infecting others with COVID-19 on a five-point scale ranging from 1 (not at all) to 5 (absolutely), using a self-developed risk perception scale. This study combined four individual risks of infection items into a scale ($\alpha = .928$), and details of the risk perception items are shown in Appendix.

Regarding social and cultural factors, harmony seeking was adopted from Hashimoto and Yamagishi (2016): "I value maintaining harmony with others." The study adopted one item from Hashimoto and Yamagishi (2016) to assess avoidance of rejection: "I sometimes get so anxious about what other people might think that I am prevented from doing what I really want to do." The following two items of sensitivity to criticism were rated on a five-point scale from 1 (not at all) to 5 (absolutely): "I am concerned that people criticize my family and myself if infected" and "I am concerned that people criticize my family and myself if not practicing self-restraint (Japan) / social distancing (Korea)."

The digital health literacy scale was adapted from Dadaczynski et al. (2021). Respondents assessed digital health literacy on COVID-19, such as evaluating and understanding COVID-19 information and determining how to respond based on COVID-19 information (see Appendix). The study combined these 11 items into a scale ($\alpha = .940$). The study also measured self-efficacy on COVID-19, focusing on the prevention of COVID-19 and affecting government measures to COVID-19 on a five-point scale: "If everyone thoroughly takes measures to prevent infection, COVID-19 can be prevented" and "People can reflect their opinions on the government's COVID-19 measures." Willingness to get vaccinated against COVID-19 was also measured (see Appendix).

Findings

Risk Perception and Psychological Responses to COVID-19

The first research question addressed the risk perception of COVID-19 at the individual and societal levels and the risk perception of infecting others with COVID-19 among Japanese and Korean respondents.

Table 6.1 shows respondents' risk perception of COVID-19, as well as the risk perception of infecting others with COVID-19 in Japan and Korea. Overall, the level of risk perception was high in both countries. Japanese respondents perceived higher individual risk (Japan: $M = 3.87$, $SD = .948$, Korea: $M = 3.79$, $SD = .892$, $t\,(2,121.197) = -2.052$, $p < .05$, 95% $CI[-0.152, -0.003]$) and risk of infecting others with COVID-19 than Korean respondents did (Japan: $M =$

Table 6.1 Means and Standard Deviations for Risk Perception of COVID-19

	Japan M (SD)	Korea M (SD)	t (df)	Cohen's d
Individual risk	3.87 (.948)	3.79 (.892)	−2.052 (2,121.197)*	0.927
Risk of infecting other people	3.78 (1.038)	3.64 (1.075)	−3.210 (2,453)**	1.053
Societal risk	3.86 (1.034)	3.91 (.894)	1.104 (2,237.834)	0.982

*p < .05; **p < .01.

Table 6.2 Multiple Regression Analyses Predicting for Risk Perception of Infecting Others with COVID-19

	Japan β	Korea β
Gender [a]	−.155**	−.037
Age	.079*	−.086*
Harmony seeking	.219**	.086*
Avoidance of rejection	.049†	.239**
Adjusted R^2	.093**	.086**

†$p < .1$; *$p < .01$; **$p < .001$.

[a]Gender was coded: female = 0, male = 1.

3.78, $SD = 1.038$, Korea: $M = 3.64$, $SD = 1.075$, $t(2,453) = -3.210$, $p < .01$, 95% CL [−0.225, −0.054]). The effect size using Cohen's d was 0.927 and 1.503, respectively, a large effect by Cohen's standards. On the other hand, there was no significant difference in the societal risk in both countries, showing the public's great social concern for the unprecedented global health crisis.

The second research question looked at factors related to the risk perception of infecting others with COVID-19 in Japan and Korea, focusing on both countries' interdependent cultures and relations. Table 6.2 summarizes the results of the multiple regression analyses for risk perception of infecting others with COVID-19 as a dependent variable among Japanese and Korean respondents.

The results showed that harmony seeking was positively related to the risk of infecting others with COVID-19 in both countries (Japan: $\beta = .219$, $p < .001$, Korea: $\beta = .086$, $p < .01$). Avoidance of rejection was also positively associated with the risk of infecting others with COVID-19 among Japanese ($\beta = .049$, $p = .059$) and Korean respondents ($\beta = .239$, $p < .001$). Among Japanese respondents, harmony seeking was a more significant factor, whereas avoidance of rejection was the main factor in the risk perception of infecting

Table 6.3 Means and Standard Deviations for Sensitivity to Criticism in the Context of COVID-19

	Japan M (SD)	Korea M (SD)	t (df)	Cohen's d
Criticism due to infection	3.42 (1.032)	3.77 (.995)	8.349 (2,085.075)*	1.017
Criticism due to failing to practice self-restraint / social distancing	3.29 (1.057)	3.69 (.997)	9.478 (2,117.343)*	1.034

*p < .001.

others with COVID-19 among Korean respondents. These results may be due to concerns about social criticisms among Korean respondents from the vivid experience of the MERS in 2015. As presented in Table 6.3, Korean respondents were more sensitive to criticism of the infection (Korea: $M = 3.77$, $SD = .995$, Japan: $M = 3.42$, $SD = 1.032$, $t (2,085.075) = 8.349$, $p < .001$, 95% $CL [0.267, 0.431]$) and the lack of social distancing (Korea: $M = 3.69$, $SD = .997$, Japan: $M = 3.29$, $SD = 1.057$, $t (2,117.343) = 9.478$, $p < .001$, 95% $CL [0.318, 0.484]$). The effect size using Cohen's *d* was 1.017 and 1.034, respectively, a large effect by Cohen's standards.

Digital Health Literacy and Self-Efficacy on COVID-19

The third research question examined to what extent people acquired digital health literacy and self-efficacy on COVID-19 among Japanese and Korean respondents. As shown in Table 6.4, Korean respondents indicated a higher level of digital health literacy (Korea: $M = 3.72$, $SD = .582$, Japan: $M = 3.10$, $SD = .678$, $t (2,453) = 23.144$, $p < .001$, 95% $CL [0.563, 0.668]$). Cohen's *d* was 0.643, a medium effect by Cohen's standards.

Table 6.4 Means and Standard Deviations for Self-efficacy on COVID-19

	Japan M (SD)	Korea M (SD)	t (df)	Cohen's d
Digital health literacy	3.10 (.678)	3.72 (.582)	23.144 (2,453)*	0.643
Self-efficacy preventing COVID-19	3.57 (.990)	4.20 (.869)	16.422 (2,217.551)*	0.945
affecting government measures	2.87 (.942)	3.29 (.959)	10.723 (2,005.503)*	0.949

*p < .001.

In addition, Korean respondents tended to perceive a high level of self-efficacy about preventing COVID-19 (Korea: $M = 4.20$, $SD = .869$, Japan: $M = 3.57$, $SD = .990$, $t(2,217.551) = 16.422$, $p < .001$, 95% $CL[0.550, 0.699]$), and affecting government measures to COVID-19 compared to Japanese respondents (Korea: $M = 3.29$, $SD = .959$, Japan: $M = 2.87$, $SD = .942$, $t(2,005.503) = 10.723$, $p < .001$, 95% $CL[0.345, 0.500]$). The effect size using Cohen's d was 0.945 and 0.949, respectively, a large effect by Cohen's standards.

Another set of multiple regression analyses was conducted to examine the relationship between the risk perception, harmony seeking, and rejection of avoidance, and the self-assessed digital health literacy on COVID-19 (R4). As presented in Table 6.5, the results showed that younger respondents showed a higher level of digital health literacy in Japan ($\beta = -.054$, $p < .05$) and Korea ($\beta = -.060$, $p = .054$), most likely as a result of the media usage patterns of the young generation. Those who perceive a higher societal risk of COVID-19 showed a higher level of digital health literacy in Japan ($\beta = .081$, $p = .053$) and Korea ($\beta = .148$, $p < .001$). Harmony-seeking was also positively associated with digital health literacy (Japan: $\beta = .163$, $p < .001$, Korea: $\beta = .255$, $p < .001$).

In addition, the perceived risk of infecting others with COVID-19 was positively related to digital health literacy among Japanese respondents ($\beta = .104$, $p < .05$). Avoidance of rejection was negatively associated with digital health literacy among Japanese respondents ($\beta = -.061$, $p < .05$). In contrast, there were no such significant relations among Korean respondents.

To sum, both countries' perceptions of societal risk and harmony seeking were predictors of digital health literacy, indicating the significance of interdependent culture and social relation factors.

Regarding the willingness to get vaccinated against COVID-19, Korean respondents ($M = 3.48$, $SD = 1.131$) were more likely to be willing to get vaccinated than Japanese respondents ($M = 3.24$, $SD = 1.104$, $t(1,995.606) = 5.182$,

Table 6.5 Multiple Regression Analyses Predicting for Digital Health Literacy

	Japan β	Korea β
Gender[a]	.058*	.018
Age	-.054*	-.060†
Individual risk	.029	.048
Risk of infecting others	.104*	-.023
Societal risk	.081†	.148**
Harmony seeking	.163**	.255**
Avoidance of rejection	-.061*	-.048
Adjusted R^2	.073**	.108**

†$p < .1$; *$p < .05$; **$p < .001$.

[a]Gender was coded: female = 0, male = 1.

$p < .001$, 95% CL [0.149, 0.331]). The effect size using Cohen's d was large (d = 1.115). Although it is not the main research focus to examine factors related to the willingness to get vaccinated, it is worth noting that digital health literacy was slightly correlated with the willingness to get vaccinated against COVID-19 in both countries (Japan: $r = .239$ $p < .001$, 95% CL [.149, .270], Korea: $r = .210$, $p < .001$, 95% CL [.190, .286]), indicating that digital health literacy is a significant factor in adopting preventive health behavior.

Study 2

Sample

Study 2 examined to what extent people seek or avoid information on COVID-19, considering the growing fatigue from COVID-19 (RQ 5 and 6). The online survey was conducted among a panel of Internet research companies in Japan and Korea, and the sample size was assigned by age and gender. In Japan, considering the areas with a high number of infected people, the survey was conducted on residents of the main regions in Kanto, Chubu, and Kinki aged 20–69, on February 26, 2021 (Male: $N = 400$, Female: $n = 400$, Age: $M = 44.65$, $SD = 14.035$). For a Korean sample, the study analyzed the same sample as Study 1 ($N = 955$).

Measurement

For information seeking and avoidance of COVID-19 and a feeling of overload with COVID-19 information, participants answered to what extent they seek and avoid information about COVID-19 (information seeking scale: $\alpha = .843$, information avoidance scale: $\alpha = .813$) and to what extent they experience information overload on a five-point scale from 1 (not at all) to 5 (absolutely). The scale items were modified from Soroya et al. (2021), considering the Japanese and Korean contexts and expressions. The study also measured fatigue of COVID-19 information on a five-point scale (see Appendix 1 for the scale). The following two items of concerns about COVID-19 information were also assessed using self-developed scales: "I am concerned that I am missing important information about COVID-19" and "I am concerned that the information I got about COVID-19 might be wrong."

Furthermore, the study assessed the degree of risk perception of COVID-19 at the individual and societal levels (hereafter referred to as individual and societal risk) and the perceived risk of infecting others with COVID-19 using the same scales as Study 1 (see Appendix). The study combined four items of individual risk of infection into a scale ($\alpha = .929$). To assess the degree of preventive behavior, participants rated the item on a five-point scale from 1 (not at all) to 5 (absolutely) (Japan: "I am refraining from going out unnecessarily under the emergency declaration," Korea: "I am practicing social distancing").

Findings

Seeking and Avoiding COVID-19 Information, and Overload and Fatigue of COVID-19 Information

Table 6.6 presented to what extent people seek, avoid COVID-19 information, and feel overload and fatigue of COVID-19 information among Japanese and Korean respondents (RQ5). There was no significant difference between Japanese and Korean respondents in information avoidance, which means that citizens in both countries are attentive to the COVID-19 information amid the continuing pandemic.

On the other hand, the study showed contrasting results regarding seeking and fatigue of COVID-19 information. Concerning the degree of information seeking, Korean respondents searched for more information about COVID-19 (Korea: $M = 3.31$, $SD = .804$), Japan: $M = 3.01$, $SD = .991$), t (1,532.376) $= 6.820$, $p < .001$, 95% CL [0.212, 0.383]). Although fatigue of COVID-19 information was not strong in both countries, Japanese respondents showed a stronger feeling of fatigue of COVID-19 information (Japan: $M = 2.95$, $SD = 1.110$, Korea: $M = 2.69$, $SD = 1.098$, $M = t$ (1,693.058) $= -4.858$, $p < .001$, 95% CL [−0.361, −0.153]). It is also interesting to note that Japanese respondents were more concerned about the correctness of the information (Japan: $M = 3.08$, $SD = .979$, Korea: $M = 2.98$, $SD = .924$, t(1,753) $= -2.112$, $p < .05$, 95% CL [−0.185, −0.007]), while Korean respondents were more concerned about whether missing important information (Korea: $M = 3.03$, $SD = .941$, Japan: $M = 2.85$, $SD = 1.004$, t(1,656.660) $= 3.762$, $p < .001$, 95% CL [0.084, 0.268]). The effect size using Cohen's d was between 0.894 and 1.104, a large effect by Cohen's standards.

Table 6.6 Means and Standard Deviations for Information Behavior in the Context of COVID-19

	Japan M (SD)	Korea M (SD)	t (df)	Cohen's d
Information seeking	3.01 (.991)	3.31 (.804)	6.820 (1,532.376)**	0.894
Information avoidance	2.50 (1.007)	2.56 (.868)	1.245 (1,587.523)	0.934
Information overload	3.48 (1.015)	3.48 (.810)	.005 (1,517.317)	0.910
Information fatigue	2.95 (1.110)	2.69 (1.098)	−4.858 (1,693.058)**	1.104
Concerns about				
correctness of information	3.08 (.979)	2.98 (.924)	−2.112 (1,753)*	0.950
whether missing important information	2.85 (1.004)	3.03 (.941)	3.762 (1,656.660)**	0.970

*$p < .05$; **$p < .001$.

Table 6.7 Multiple Regression Analyses Predicting for Information Seeking and Avoidance

	Information seeking		Information avoidance	
	Japan β	Korea β	Japan β	Korea β
Gender[a]	.109***	.071*	.014	−.035
Age	.049	−.018	−.088**	−.012
Individual risk	.075	.053	−.159**	.093*
Risk of infecting others	.115*	.066	.133**	.058
Societal risk	.110*	.144***	−.010	−.160***
Information overload	.308***	.315***	.071 †	.043
Information fatigue	−.085*	−.156***	.468***	.539***
Adjusted R^2	.232***	.194***	.268***	.324***

† $p < .1$; * $p < .05$; ** $p < .01$; *** $p < .001$.

[a]Gender was coded: female = 0, male = 1.

The sixth research question investigated factors related to seeking and avoiding COVID-19 information in Japan and Korea. Table 6.7 summarizes the results of the multiple regression analyses for seeking and avoidance of COVID-19 information in both countries.

In terms of perceptions of individual risk and risk of infecting others with COVID-19, the results exhibited different patterns among Japanese and Korean respondents. While the perception of individual risk was negatively associated with avoidance of COVID-19 information in Japan ($\beta = -.159$, $p < .01$), perception of individual risk was positively related to avoidance of COVID-19 information in Korea ($\beta = .093$, $p < .05$). Although there was no significant relationship between the perceived risk of infecting others with COVID-19 and information seeking or avoidance in Korea, the perceived risk of infecting others with COVID-19 was positively related to information seeking ($\beta = .115$, $p < .05$) and information avoidance ($\beta = .133$, $p < .01$) in Japan. Perception of societal risk was positively associated with information seeking of COVID-19 in both countries (Japan: $\beta = .110$, $p < .05$, Korea: $\beta = .144$, $p < .001$), and those with a higher societal risk were less likely to avoid information in Korea ($\beta = -.160$, $p < .001$). Overall, the results showed that societal risk resulted in a high level of information seeking about COVID-19 in both countries, indicating it is essential to provide adequate risk information.

Regarding information fatigue, those who felt fatigued with COVID-19 information were less likely to seek information (Japan: $\beta = -.085$, $p < .05$, Korea: $\beta = -.156$, $p < .001$) and more likely to avoid COVID-19 information (Japan: $\beta = .468$, $p < .001$, Korea: $\beta = .539$, $p < .001$), as expected. Among Japanese respondents, the relation between information overload and information avoidance was marginally significant ($\beta = .071$, $p = .050$), but the feeling of overload with COVID-19 information was positively associated with seeking COVID-19 information in both countries (Japan: β = .308, p < .001, Korea: β = .315, p < .001), contrary to the expectation. Taken together, these results showed that the fatigue of COVID-19 information was related to a high level of information avoidance or a low level of seeking information. However, the feeling of overload with COVID-19 information rather led to information seeking in both countries.

The seventh research question investigated what factors predict taking preventive behavior, such as self-restraint in Japan and social distancing in Korea in the context of COVID-19. As shown in Table 6.8, Japanese and Korean respondents indicated a high performance of preventive behavior, and Korean respondents were more likely to practice preventive behavior than Japanese respondents (Korea: M = 4.10, SD = .812, Japan: M = 3.62, SD = 1.049, t (1,487.538) = 10.374, p < .001, 95% CL [0.382, 0.561]). Cohen's d was 0.928, a large effect by Cohen's standards.

Table 6.9 shows the results of the multiple regression analyses with practicing preventive behavior as the dependent variable. Regarding the perceived risk of COVID-19, perception of societal risk was positively related to practicing preventive behavior in Japan (β = .249, p < .001) and Korea (β = .204, p < .001), and those who searched for more information were more likely to practice preventive behavior in both countries (β = .145, p < .001, β = .171, p < .001). The individual risk was positively associated with self-restraint in Japan (β = .216, p < .001),

Table 6.8 Means and Standard Deviations for Preventing Behavior in the Context of COVID-19

	Japan M (SD)	Korea M (SD)	t (df)	Cohen's d
Preventing behavior	3.62 (1.049)	4.10 (.812)	10.374 (1,487.538)*	0.928

*p < .001.

Table 6.9 Multiple Regression Analyses Predicting for the Practice of Preventive Behavior in the Context of COVID-19

	Japan β	Korea β
Gender[a]	.007	−.051†
Age	.097*	.090*
Individual risk	.216**	.039
Risk of infecting others	.031	−.058
Societal risk	.249**	.204**
Information seeking	.145**	.171**
Information avoidance	−.007	−.194**
Adjusted R^2	.310**	.154**

†p < .1; *p < .01; **p < .001.

[a] Gender was coded: female = 0, male = 1.

whereas there was no significant relation to social distancing in Korea. Besides, avoidance of COVID-19 information was negatively related to the practice of social distancing among Korean respondents ($\beta = -.194$, $p < .001$), but there was no significant relation among Japanese respondents.

To summarize, societal risk and information seeking are the main factors in preventive behavior, emphasizing the importance of recognizing societal risks and promoting information-seeking behavior.

Discussion

The COVID-19 pandemic approach in Japan and Korea contrasted with those that adopted strict lockdown measures. Whether or not practicing self-restraint in Japan and social distancing in Korea effectively suppresses the spread of COVID-19 largely depends on individual responses and voluntary cooperation of the citizens. Japan and Korea have successfully contained COVID-19 in the early stage of the pandemic, showing very low infection and mortality rates. However, as the COVID-19 pandemic continues, it is becoming difficult for the government to appeal to people. This study compared the risk perception and preventive behavior among Japanese and Korean respondents, focusing on the social and cultural factors in response to COVID-19. Also, this study looked at factors related to digital health literacy and information behavior, as people need to continue to practice preventive health measures.

Overall, people in both countries perceived a high level of risk at the individual and societal levels, resulting in a high level of taking preventive behavior, such as self-restraint in Japan and social distancing in Korea. Japanese respondents were more likely to perceive individual-level risk and risk of infecting others with COVID-19 than Korean respondents. Korean respondents were more likely to experience social pressure in responding to COVID-19. Also, those seeking to avoid rejection perceived a higher risk of infecting others with COVID-19 among Korean respondents. The recent Korean experience of MERS might have led to sensitivity to social pressure.

The study also investigated to what extent people gained digital health literacy and self-efficacy to cope with COVID-19. Both Japanese and Korean respondents showed a high level of digital health literacy on COVID-19, with Korean respondents demonstrating a higher digital health literacy. Regarding self-efficacy in preventing COVID-19 and influencing government action against COVID-19, Korean respondents showed a higher level of self-efficacy than Japanese respondents. Furthermore, social relation factors such as societal risk and harmony seeking were related to digital health literacy in both countries.

The level of avoidance of COVID-19 information was relatively low in both countries, and there was no difference between Japanese and Korean respondents. Korean respondents tended to search for more details about COVID-19, and Japanese respondents felt more fatigued with COVID-19 information than Korean respondents. Interestingly, regarding the COVID-19 information,

Japanese respondents cared more about the correctness, while Korean respondents were more concerned about whether important information was missing.

The overall results of the analysis of factors relating to seeking and avoiding COVID-19 information showed that societal risk, overload, and fatigue of COVID-19 information were the main factors. The societal risk was associated with a high level of information seeking and a low level of avoidance of COVID-19 information in both countries, which means it is essential to provide adequate risk information. Fatigue of COVID-19 information was negatively associated with information seeking of COVID-19 in both countries.

It was predicted that the feeling overloaded with COVID-19 information would be inversely related to information seeking, but the findings of study 2 showed that the feeling of overload with COVID-19 information was positively related to information seeking in both countries. Although study 2 has not measured digital health literacy in both countries, it is likely that the feeling overloaded with COVID-19 information may not hinder information-seeking behavior, based on the result showing a high level of digital health literacy in Study 1. The high level of the risk perception of unprecedented health crisis may also be a reason for the result. Among Japanese respondents, the feeling overloaded with COVID-19 information was positively related to avoiding COVID-19 information in Japan, which is a concern amid the ongoing pandemic.

Perception of societal risk was associated with preventive behavior in Korea and Japan, and individual risk was related to self-restraint in Japan. Those who looked for more information took preventive behaviors in both countries, and those who were low in the level of information avoidance of COVID-19 tended to practice social distancing in Korea. These results show the significance of civic awareness of risk at the societal level and promoting information-seeking behavior in risk communication.

As the global health crisis continues at the time of writing this chapter, citizens should continue to engage in health prevention behaviors. Digital media has become an indispensable medium for preventing and managing infectious diseases during the COVID-19 pandemic. Overall, the results of this study indicate that it is essential to provide and access accurate risk information, improve digital health literacy and self-efficacy on COVID-19 and deal with information avoidance presumably resulting from fatigue in the COVID-19 pandemic. Considering the sociocultural background and COVID-19 fatigue in Japanese and Korean contexts, further study into the response to COVID-19 from the perspective of health literacy and information behavior is necessary for the long-term battle against COVID-19.

Note

This study assessed multicollinearity in the multiple regression model (Tables 6.2, 6.5, 6.7, and 6.9) using variance inflation factor (VIF, less than 4), and there was no multicollinearity between independent variables in the model.

Acknowledgments

This study was funded by Keio University Global Research Institute (Korean survey for Study 1 and 2, and Japanese survey for Study 1). The two online surveys were conducted with the study of Chapter 7: Media Cynicism, Risk Perception of COVID-19, and the Civil Values in Japan and Korea, and the data related to risk perception was shared with Chapter 7. Japanese survey for Study 2 was supported by the Institute for Journalism, Media & Communication Studies, Keio University. The content is solely the author's responsibility and does not represent the official views of the granting organization.

Appendix

Measures of Study (five-point scale)

Items

STUDY 1 and 2

  Risk Perception of COVID-19

  Individual Risk (Self-developed scale, Study 1: α=.928 and Study 2: α= .929)

  I am worried that my family and I will get infected with COVID-19.

  I am worried if my family and I have symptoms like COVID-19.

  I am worried that my family and I might get worse because of COVID-19.

  I am worried that my family and I might get infected with COVID-19 and die.

  Risk of Infecting Others

  I am worried that I might infect people close to me with COVID-19.

  Societal risk

  I am worried that the number of people infected with COVID-19 will increase throughout Japan/ Korea.

STUDY 1

  Harmony Seeking (Adopted from Hashimoto & Yamagishi, 2016)

  I value maintaining harmony with others.

  Avoidance of Rejection (Adopted from Hashimoto &Yamagishi, 2016)

  I sometimes get so anxious about what other people might think that I am prevented from doing what I really want to do.

  Sensitivity to criticism (Self-developed scale)

  I am concerned that people criticize my family and myself if infected.

  Japan: I am concerned that people criticize my family and myself if not practicing self-restraint.

  Korea: I am concerned that people criticize my family and myself if not practicing social distancing.

  Digital Health Literacy on COVID-19 (Adapted from Dadaczynski et al., 2021, α = .940)

  I can easily find information about COVID-19 on the Internet.

  I can easily find the information I am looking for regarding COVID-19 on the Internet.

(Continued)

Items

I can understand well the information about COVID-19 that I got from the Internet.

I can determine which information about COVID-19 I got from the Internet is important to me.

I can judge whether the information about COVID-19 I got from the Internet is correct or not.

I can easily determine how to act from the information about COVID-19 I got from the Internet.

It is easy to determine how you can use the COVID-19 related information you find on the Internet on your own

I can get reliable information about COVID-19 on the Internet.

I can tell which information on the Internet about COVID-19 is written to sell products or for commercial purposes

If I were to ask a question about COVID-19 on social media or an Internet forum, I would be able to ask it appropriately.

If I were to express my thoughts about COVID-19 on social media or Internet forums, I would describe them appropriately.

Self-Efficacy (Self-developed scale)

Preventing COVID-19

If everyone thoroughly takes measures to prevent infection, COVID-19 can be prevented.

Affecting Government measures to COVID-19

People can reflect their opinions on the government's COVID-19 measures.

Willingness to Get Vaccinated Against COVID-19 (Self-developed scale)

I want to get vaccinated against COVID-19.

STUDY 2

Information-Seeking on COVID-19 (Adopted and modified from Soroya et al., 2021, $\alpha = .843$)

I am checking out various sources for COVID-19-related information.

I am searching for COVID-19-related information.

Avoidance of COVID-19 Information (Adopted and modified from Soroya et al., 2021, $\alpha = .813$)

I try not to look at COVID-19-related information.

I intentionally avoid COVID-19-related information.

Overload of COVID-19 Information (Adopted and modified from Soroya et al., 2021)

The media I usually use is full of COVID-19-related information.

Fatigue of COVID-19 Information (Self-developed scale)

I got tired of COVID-19 information.

Concerns about COVID-19 Information (Self-developed scale)

I am concerned that I am missing important information about COVID-19.

I am concerned that the information I got about COVID-19 might be wrong.

Degree of Preventive Behavior (Self-developed scale)

Japan: I am refraining from going out unnecessarily under the emergency declaration.

Korea: I am practicing social distancing.

References

Asian Pacific Initiative. (2020). *Shingata korona taio minkan rinji chosa-kai chosa kensho hokokusho [The Independent investigation commission on the Japanese government's response to COVID-19: Report on best practices and lessons learned]*. Discover 21.

Case, D. O., Andrews, J. E., Johnson, J. D., & Allard, S. L. (2005). Avoiding versus seeking: The relationship of information seeking to avoidance, blunting, coping, dissonance, and related concepts. *Journal of the Medical Library Association, 93*(3), 353–362. https://www.ncbi.nlm.nih.gov/pmc/articles/PMC1175801/

Cho, Y. L., & Kim, S.-Y. (2021). Gongjung-ui yeonlyeong-gwa jeongchi seonghyang-kolona19 wiheom insig, wiheom jeongboui tamsaeg cheoli, jeongbuui jaenan daeeung pyeong-ga-e michineun yeonghyang [How public's age and political orientation affect COVID-19 risk perceptions, risk information seeking and processing, and evaluation of government's response to COVID-19]. *Korean Journal of Journalism & Communication Studies, 65*(4), 106–147. https://doi .org/10.20879/kjjcs.2021.65.4.003

Choi, K., Choi, H., & Kahng, B. (2020). Covid-19 epidemic under the K-quarantine model: Network approach. arXiv:2010.07157

Chun, H., Yoon, H-R, Choe, S. K., & Park, E. J. (2021). Daehagsaeng-ui dijiteol geongangliteoleosiwa yebangjeog geonganghaengdong: kolona19 baegsinjeobjong uihyang mich bang-yeog cham-yeoleul jungsim-eulo [COVID-19 related digital health literacy and preventive health behaviors among college students: Intention to vaccinate and adherence to preventive measures]. *Korea Journal of Population Studies, 44*(2), 121–141. https://doi.org/10.31693/KJPS.2021.06.44.2.121

Dadaczynski, K., Okan, O., Messer, M., Leung, A. Y. M., Rosário, R., Darlington, E., & Rathmann, K. (2021). Digital health literacy and web-based information-seeking behaviors of university students in Germany during the COVID-19 pandemic: Cross-sectional survey study. *Journal of Medical Internet Research, 23*(1), e24097, 1–17. https://doi.org/10.2196/24097

Farooq, A., Laato, S., & Islam, A. N. (2020). Impact of online information on self-isolation intention during the COVID-19 pandemic: Cross-sectional study. *Journal of Medical Internet Research, 22*(5), e19128, 1–15. https://doi.org/10 .2196/19128

Hashimoto, H., & Yamagishi, T. (2013). Two faces of interdependence: Harmony seeking and rejection avoidance. *Asian Journal of Social Psychology, 16*(2), 142–151. https://doi.org/10.1111/ajsp.12022

Hashimoto, H., & Yamagishi, T. (2016). Duality of independence and interdependence: An adaptationist perspective. *Asian Journal of Social Psychology, 19*(4), 286–297. https://doi.org/10.1111/ajsp.12145

Hornyak, T. (2020, December 18). Why Japan, once a COVID-19 success story, faces the prospect of a dark, deadly winter. https://time.com/5922918/japan -covid-19-cases-fatigue/

Lee, J. (2021). Responses to media coverage of the Covid-19 pandemic and information behaviour in the Japanese Context. *SEARCH The Journal of Media and Communication Research, 13*(1), 111–126. https://fslmjournals.taylors.edu .my/responses-to-media-coverage-of-the-covid-19-pandemic-and-information -behaviour-in-the-japanese-context/

Ma, J. Park, H-R., & Choi, J. (2021). Sosyeol Q&A saiteueseoui geongangjeongbogeomsaeggwa yebanghaengdongui gwangyee daehan yeongu: kolonabaileoseugam-yeomjeung-19leul jungsimeulo [Health information seeking on social Q&A sites and preventive behavior: Focusing on coronavirus infection-19]. *Journal of Digital Contents and Society, 22*(6), 959–967. https://doi.org/10.9728/dcs.2021.22.6.959

Motoyoshi, T. (2021). Shingata korona uirusu kansensho ni yoru hitobito e no shinriteki eikyo[Psychological impact of the COVID-19 on Japanese people]. *Journal of Societal Safety Sciences, 11*, 97–108. https://www.kansai-u.ac.jp/Fc_ss/center/study/pdf/bulletin011_2.pdf

Okan, O., Bollweg, T. M., Berens, E.-M., Hurrelmann, K., Bauer, U., & Schaeffer, D. (2020). Coronavirus-related health literacy: A cross-sectional study in adults during the COVID-19 Infodemic in Germany. *International Journal of Environmental Research and Public Health, 17*(15), 5503. https://doi.org/10.3390/ijerph17155503

O'Shea, P. (2020, December 18). Sweden and Japan are paying the price for COVID exceptionalism. *THE CONVERSATION.* https://theconversation.com/sweden-and-japan-are-paying-the-price-for-covid-exceptionalism-151974

Paek, H. J., & Hove, T. (2021). Information communication technologies (ICTs), crisis communication principles and the COVID-19 response in South Korea. *Journal of Creative Communications, 16*(2), 213–221. https://doi.org/10.1177/0973258620981170

Sakakibara, R., & Ozono, H. (2020, July 13). Nihon ni okeru shingata koronauirusukansensho o meguru shinri kodo ni kansuru chosa: Yobokodo shorai no mitoshi joho kakusan ni shoten o ateta kento [A survey on psychology and behavior regarding new coronavirus infections in Japan: Focusing on preventive behavior, prospects, and information dissemination]. https://doi.org/10.31234/osf.io/635zk

Siripala, T. (2021, January 2). Japan faces its worst COVID-19 outbreak yet: Record breaking infections in Tokyo have sparked a sense of impending crisis in the capital's battle against the coronavirus. THE DIPLOMATE. https://thediplomat.com/2021/01/japan-faces-its-worst-covid-19-outbreak-yet/

Sørensen, K., Van den Broucke, S., Fullam, J., Doyle, G., Pelikan, J., Slonska, Z., Brand, H., & (HLS-EU) Consortium Health Literacy Project European (2012). Health literacy and public health: A systematic review and integration of definitions and models. *BMC Public Health, 12*, 80. https://doi.org/10.1186/1471-2458-12-80

Soroya, S. H., Farooq, A., Mahmood, K., Isoaho, J., & Zara, S-e. (2021). From information seeking to information avoidance: Understanding the health information behaviour during a global health crisis. *Information Processing & Management, 58*(2), 102440, 1–16. https://doi.org/10.1016/j.ipm.2020.102440

Zhang, Y, & Lee, S. Y. (2021). Kolona19 yebanghaengdong jisog-uido-e yeonghyang-eul michineun yoin yeongu: geongangsinnyeommodel(HBM),midieo/daeinj eongbonochul, bujeongjeog gamjeong, jagihaeseogseonghyang-eul jungsim-eulo [A study on the factors influencing the intention to continue COVID-19 preventive behavior: Focusing on the health belief model (HBM), media/interpersonal information exposure, negative emotions, and interdependent self-construal]. *Journal of Speech, Media & Communication Research, 20*(4), 315–348. https://www.earticle.net/Article/A403272

7 Media Cynicism, Risk Perception of COVID-19, and the Civil Values in Japan and Korea

Kwangho Lee

Introduction

In many democracies, it is widely observable that there is a tendency among citizens to have a skeptical and cynical attitude toward conventional journalism and the news media. The tendency is obvious on the Internet. There are particular disdainful expressions toward journalism commonly known in many languages; "Le journalisme des ordures" in French, "Müll Journalismus" in German, "periodismo basura" in Spanish, and of course "garbage journalism" in English. According to Al-Rawi (2020)'s analysis, "garbage journalism" was the 12th most used expression in tweets with the #fakenews hashtag on Twitter.

East Asian countries are not exceptional. In Japan, there is the slang word "masugomi." The sound of this word is very similar to "masukomi," which is an abbreviation of "mass communication," and has the meaning of "mass media" in the Japanese language. "Masugomi" is a term coined by changing the "komi" of "masukomi" to "gomi," which means garbage; therefore, "masugomi" implies expressing a strong feeling of disdain or distrust for the mass media, especially for the nature of news reporting. This expression can often be detected on the Internet or social media, although it is not common usage in everyday life.

In South Korea (hereafter, Korea), the term "giregi" is widely used as a derogatory term for reporters. It is a combination of "gi" from the Korean word "gija" (meaning "reporter") and "regi" from the Korean word "suregi" (meaning "garbage"). It indicates "reporters who write garbage articles." Unlike in Japan, this expression is relatively broadly used not only on the Internet but also in daily life. Kim Eo-jun, a famous personality of the radio program titled "the News Factory of Kim Eo-jun," often uses this term even on live broadcasting in criticizing conservative news media. A recent and typical example demonstrates how "giregi" is accepted in Korean society. In March 2021, Korea's Supreme Court overturned the convictions of the first and second instance courts (insult, fine of 300,000 won) and acquitted a person accused of insulting a reporter by writing a comment, "This is called 'giregi,' isn't it?" to the reporter's article on a website. The reason for the acquittal is as follows: The word "giregi" is a relatively common word used to criticize the content of an article or the actions of a reporter, and it is not significantly malicious compared to other comments on the article

DOI: 10.4324/9781003286684-7

in question (Jang, 2021). This case illustrates the fact that derogatory remarks about journalists and news media have become so commonplace that they no longer have the nuance of being an outright attack on character.

Despite the fact that such a strong disdainful attitude toward journalists and the news media is widespread, few studies have taken seriously this issue as a subject in audience studies. To shed new light on the subject, I have utilized and developed the concept of "media cynicism" to describe this negative attitude toward journalists and the news media and conducted some research in Korean society to show that it is widespread to a considerable extent (Lee, 2019, 2020a, b). Lee (2020a) illuminates that the "hostile media perception" is one of the factors that give rise to media cynicism and that media cynicism can affect the audience's use of political information sources, including selective exposure. By analyzing the case in Japan, Lee (2021) has found that hostile media perception reached a certain level and that the higher levels of it led to stronger media cynicism.

Built on my previous studies, this chapter examines whether media cynicism can also affect the reception process of risk-related information, which is not ostensibly political issue. Further, it explores how the reception process is related to the level of various risk perceptions about COVID-19 and how the risk perception leads to the acceptance of preventive measures that limit individual freedom and human rights. In doing so, this chapter demonstrates that media cynicism may hinder the formation of new civic values demanded in the pandemic era through its influences on the use of information sources and the resulting risk perceptions.

Media Cynicism and Hostile Media Perception

Cappella and Jamieson (1996) in their article titled "News frames, political cynicism, and media cynicism" have introduced the concept of media cynicism that explains an audience's negative reaction to news media. Cappella and Jamieson (1996, 1997) demonstrate that political coverage could directly influence people's cynicism toward governments, policy debates, and political campaigns depending on the news frame. They argue that the "strategic frame," which focuses on politicians' selfish motives and strategic actions, increases voters' distrust of politics, which in turn leads to reduced involvement and low participation in politics. Then they proposed the idea of "media cynicism" in pointing out that such political reporting can lead not only to cynicism about politics but also to cynicism about the media themselves.

> The public's trust in this institution is falling; in part, this may be due to the media's own sowing of the seeds of public cynicism. Public distrust of political institutions and processes may have attached itself to the bearers of information about those institutions—the news media themselves ... Media cynicism may result from political cynicism or vice versa.
>
> (Cappella and Jamieson, 1996, p. 83)

Their concept of media cynicism seems to have similar components to the operational definition of political cynicism. In their book *The Spiral of Cynicism* (1997), Cappella and Jamieson have introduced measurement scales of media cynicism used in their survey, which tap on evaluations of journalistic performances and commercial motives of news media. Besides that, the scale includes favorable and unfavorable attitudes toward news reporting in general and an evaluation of the media's contribution to solving social problems. Based on the composition of the scale, it seems clear that with the concept of media cynicism, they try to indicate a negative attitude toward journalists and news organizations formed on the perceptions and evaluations about their journalistic performances and selfish motives. However, their notion of media cynicism has received little attention compared to political cynicism, and they do not seem to have developed it in their subsequent studies. Some researchers have even used the term in a completely different meaning to describe the "cynical media" (e.g., Poletti & Brants, 2010).

In defining the concept of media cynicism more clearly, Dekker and Meijerink's (2012) review of the concept of political cynicism offers numerous clues. They point out that cynicism is different from distrust, skepticism, and indifference. According to them, mistrust is an attitude that includes unpredictability about the future actions of the other party, and skepticism is an attitude of questioning and seeking information. However, cynicism is more of an attitude that comes from anticipating future actions and thinking that one knows everything about the other party. They also argue that if you are indifferent, you don't think much about the other party and do not act, but if you are cynical, you take active action against the other party.

Furthermore, according to the *Oxford English Dictionary*, the word "cynical" contains a more specific and limited nuance of disposition to find faults and disbelieve the sincerity or goodness of the other party (OED, n.d.) rather than just a general meaning of negative. Therefore, by combining Cappella and Jamieson's original notion with Dekker and Meijerink's review and dictionary meaning, this chapter defines media cynicism as an attitude that is formed from the belief that the journalist and news organizations lack competence and morality and that demeans and ridicules them out of the confidence of knowing well about them.

Although many possible factors leading to media cynicism, one of the factors that this study will focus on in this chapter is hostile media perception, which Vallone et al. (1985) have discovered in an experiment. The hostile media perception is a cognitive distortion experienced by partisan audiences and refers to perceiving news content as hostile to one's own camp. In the early years, studies on such phenomena have tended to focus on "biased information processing for specific political coverage" caused by group affiliation such as ethnicity (e.g., Israel vs. Arab). Subsequent studies have revealed that the same phenomenon occurs in social issues such as abortion and sports coverage (Giner-Sorolla & Chaiken, 1994; Arpan & Raney, 2003; Hansen & Kim, 2011).

While the conventional concept of hostile media perception has focused on perceptions of a specific or a series of news content (Gunther and Schmit, 2004; Gunther et al., 2009; Perloff, 2015), Lee (2019) has broadened the scope and reframed it as the perception that could be established against "certain news organizations" as well. It proposes the assumption that if a particular news organization persistently reports (or is perceived to report) in support of a position that is opposed to one's own camp across multiple issues, then hostile media perceptions can be formed not only for the content of a particular report but also for the news organization itself. To understand the reality and dynamics of despising reactions of audiences to the news media in today's political situation, it is necessary and efficient to expand this concept.

Here, the cognitive dissonance theory (Festinger, 1957) helps explain the process by which such hostile media perceptions degrade news organizations' performance and morality evaluations. The perception that a news organization "hostile" to one's own camp provides "accurate, objective, and neutral" news coverage is dissonant with the self-cognition that one's own camp is correct. To suppress or eliminate the occurrence of such dissonance, the evaluations of hostile media's performance and morality must be lowered.

Hostile media perception itself is thought to be influenced by the strength of one's attitude toward various issues. The stronger the attitude toward an issue, the greater the probability and degree to which a particular news report on that issue differs from one's attitude. Furthermore, it can be inferred that hostile media perceptions are strongest when an individual has strong attitudes across multiple issues and when a particular news organization's coverage of those multiple issues is consistently different from one's own. If partisanship means consistent attitudes toward multiple issues, then the strength of such partisanship can be a major factor in generating hostile media perceptions. As I have verified by analyzing survey data in Japan and Korea (Lee, 2020a, 2021), there exists a clear relationship between these three variables, i.e., the strength of partisanship → hostile media perception → media cynicism.

Perception of the media partisanship may also influence hostile media perception. It can be predicted that highly partisan individuals will experience the strongest hostile media perceptions toward the media that are (perceived to be) highly partisan in the opposite direction. This is a matter of cognition of what one believes a particular media outlet to be like, apart from its actual argument on multiple issues. There is clear media partisanship in Japan and Korea where this chapter conducted survey research. In Japan, the *Yomiuri Shimbun*, the *Sankei Shimbun*, and the *Nihon Keizai Shimbun* are seen as conservative, while the *Asahi Shimbun*, the *Mainichi Shimbun*, and the *Tokyo Shimbun* are regarded as liberal. In Korea, the *Chosun Ilbo*, *The Dong-A Ilbo*, and *JoongAng Ilbo* are considered conservative, while the *Kyunghyang Shinmun* and *Hankyoreh* are seen as liberal. The mere acceptance of these "reputations" of partisanship can lead to hostile media perceptions, even among people who are not actual readers of the respective newspapers.

Media and Risk Perception

The media coverage of risk sources and measures to deal with these risks may influence risk perception. There is some existing literature that deserves to be referred to. Based on their content analysis of newspapers and a telephone survey of the residents, Flynn et al. (1998) have examined the issue of risk perception and stigma toward nuclear detonator production facilities. The results have shown that media coverage affects "social amplification of risk." By examining the impact of the media on the April 2009 H1N1 virus pandemic, Lin and Lagoe (2013) have found that higher reliance on news media, including television, newspapers, and the Internet is associated with higher risk perceptions. Chang (2012) has demonstrated that exposure to television news about the H1N1 flu in Taiwan is associated with higher perceived severity and vulnerability levels. It has also analyzed the impact of how risk stories were framed. It illustrates that news about H1N1 flu in Taiwan used the "alarm frame" more than the "coping frame" and found through experiments that alarm frame stories evoke greater fear and enhance perceptions of severity and vulnerability. Several other studies have also confirmed the relationship between news media and risk perception (Culbertson & Stempel, 1985, Coleman, 1993, Morton & Duck, 2001, Dudo et al., 2007).

In Japan and Korea, news reports on the new coronavirus began to appear in January 2020, with daily reports on the symptoms of COVID-19, the risk of severe illness and death, the domestic and overseas' number of the infected, the details of quarantine measures, and the development of vaccines and medicines. The number of reports containing the keyword "corona" was 66,615 in the Asahi Shimbun, 60,961 in the *Yomiuri Shimbun* throughout the two years of 2020 and 2021 (Tokyo morning edition only). During the same period, the Korean news media reported 40,051 articles in *The Dong-A Ilbo*, 66,460 in *The JoongAng Ilbo*, and 63,580 in the public broadcaster KBS.[1] Thus, the enormous amount of COVID-19 news reports seemed to put the people of both countries into high-risk perceptions and at the same time in a situation of information overload, as explained in Chapter 6 of this book.

With the growing presence as a source of information, the role of social media cannot be underestimated. In particular, health and medical issues have received scholarly attention in understanding, reacting to, and sharing information about various risk events (Chew & Eysenbach, 2010; Signorini et al., 2011; Song et al., 2016). Among others, Choi et al. (2017) have disclosed that during the 2015 Middle East respiratory syndrome (MERS) outbreak in Korea, social media use enhanced risk perception by interacting with information processing modes. Song et al. (2017) have analyzed big data (8,671,695) of postings collected from 171 online sources, including Twitter, blogs, message boards, and 149 news sites during the MERS outbreak in Korea. The results revealed that 82.3% of postings on Twitter and 74.8% of online groups were more related to negative emotions such as worry and fear. In comparison, 65.3% of postings on news sites were more associated with positive emotions such as calm and composed. Besides, Song et al. (2017) have revealed that 171 online sources contained 174,589 false information such as "general hospitals were closed because of MERS," "eating chicken can prevent MERS," "taking antipyretics can cure MERS," and fake lists of hospitals that were claimed to have confirmed MERS patients.

Risk Perception and Civic Value

Risk perception influences our coping behavior toward risk sources. When risk perception is high, a stronger motivation to avoid risk sources and more support for measures to prevent risk are expected (Brewer et al., 2007). It can be inferred that as the risk perception of COVID-19 increases, the support for various preventive measures becomes stronger. Most preventive measures for infectious diseases limit personal freedom or protection of personal information. Supporting these restrictive measures means that democratic values must be temporarily reserved. Therefore, changes in civic values can occur depending on how risk perception is formed.

Based on the previous research and discussion above, this study poses and tests four research questions.

RQ 1: To what extent does media cynicism relate to negative attitudes toward mass media coverage of COVID-19?

RQ 2: To what extent do the negative attitudes toward mass media coverage relate to using information sources regarding COVID-19?

RQ 3: How are the use of information sources related to the risk perception of COVID-19?

RQ 4: What is the relationship between risk perception of COVID-19 and support for restrictive preventive measures?

Method

Sample

The survey in Japan was conducted over two days, from February 10 to February 11, 2021, using the panel members of the i-Bridge Corporation. The survey was completed when the number of respondents reached 1,500. Respondents were recruited from the Tokyo metropolitan area (*Tokyo, Saitama, Chiba*, and *Kanagawa*), the Kanto region (*Ibaraki, Tochigi*, and *Gunma*), and the Kinki region (*Osaka, Kyoto, Mie, Shiga, Hyogo, Nara*, and *Wakayama*). The Korean survey was conducted over five days from March 12 to March 16, 2021, using the panel members of Macromill Embrain, and ended when 955 respondents were reached. Respondents were recruited from the metropolitan area (*Seoul, Inchon*, and *Kyoengkido*) and the four major regional municipalities (*Daejeon, Daegu, Busan*, and *Gwangju*). In both countries, equal numbers of men and women were assigned. The age range (18–69) was the same in both samples. The average age was 41.8 years in Japan and 39.7 years in Korea. The respondents living in the metropolitan area were 67.1% in Japan and 42.4% in Korea.

Measurement

The variables measured in this survey are as follows. The details of measurement items are listed in the tables and figures showing the survey results.

- *Hostile media perception* (HMP). Five items developed by Lee (2021) (Japan: α = .870, Korea: α = .919).
- *Media cynicism.* Eighteen items developed by Lee (2021) (Japan: α = .910, Korea: α = .928). This measurement consists of nine items measuring evaluations of journalistic performances, four items measuring perceptions of selfish motives, and five items measuring derogatory attitudes against journalists and news organizations.
- *Negative attitudes toward COVID-19 reporting* (NAC). Thirteen items developed for this study (Japan: α = .923, Korea: α = .865). The items measure the quantity, appropriateness of content, accuracy, neutrality, sensationalism, diversity, and professionalism of COVID-19 news coverage by newspapers and broadcasters.
- *Use of information sources on COVID-19.* Fourteen sources, including public and private broadcasters' news programs, social media, government and local government websites, and health and medical information websites.
- *Risk perception of COVID-19.* Four items measuring risk perception at the individual level, one item at the interpersonal level, and two items at the societal level (Japan: α = .937, Korea: α = .918).
- *Acceptance of restrictive measures to prevent virus-induced infection in the future* (ARM). Ten items developed for this survey (Japan: α = .859, Korea: α = .795).
- *Attribution of causes for the COVID-19 spread in the home country.* Twelve items developed for this study (Japan: α = .853, Korea: α = .800).

All variables were measured on a five-point scale except the HMP and ARM which were measured with a four-point scale. In addition to the above variables, sex and age were also measured for control purposes. Statistical program HAD developed by Shimizu (2016) was used for the data analysis.

Findings

Media Cynicism and Its Relationship with Hostile Media Perception

Figure 7.1 shows the means of the 18 items to measure media cynicism in Japan and Korea. Overall, Korean respondents showed a lower evaluation of performances and higher ratings of selfish motives of journalists and news organizations than their Japanese counterparts.

First, regarding the evaluations of journalists, Korean respondents indicate significantly lower ratings for the political neutrality and the fact-reporting efforts of their country's journalists than their Japanese counterparts. There was no significant difference between the two countries in the evaluations of journalists' professionalism, truth-revealing efforts, and contribution to the people's right to know, with means below the midpoint of three overall. Regarding the intention to use the position of journalists to pursue personal gain and to cozy up with the political and business elites, both countries' respondents estimated that these highly, with Korean respondents being much stronger in their views.

What do you think of the following evaluations of journalists and news organizations?

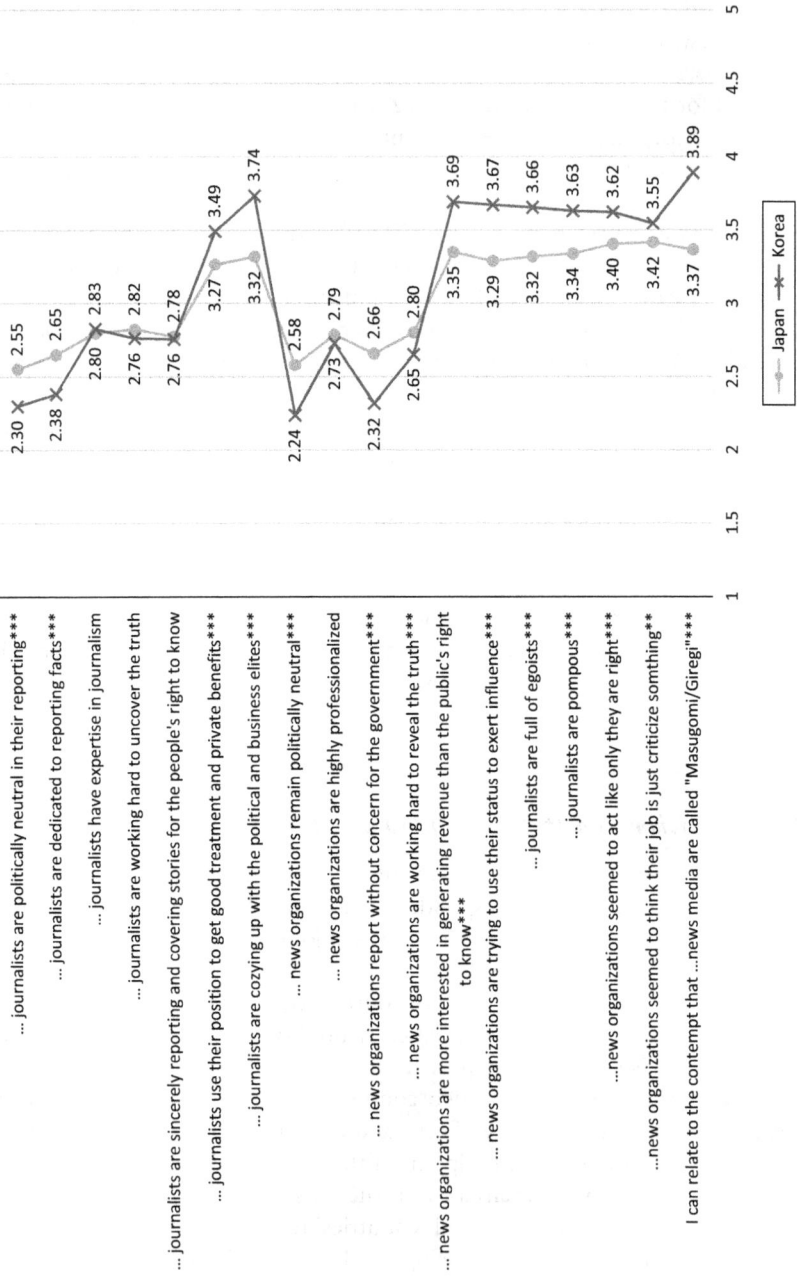

Figure 7.1 Japan–Korea differences in evaluations of journalists and news organizations. Note: Means of those items marked with asterisk(s) in all figures are significantly different at the corresponding significance levels of *p < .05, **p < .01, and ***p < .001

The evaluation of the news media as an organization was also severe. The scores for political neutrality, professionalism, independence from political power, and efforts to clarify the truth were all below the midpoint of 3. Concerning political neutrality and independence, the rating among Korean respondents was significantly lower than Japan's, and its average score is approaching 2. On the other hand, estimates of the selfish motives of news organizations are high overall as the means for the pursuit of commercial interests and the intention to exert influence are above the midpoint. Again, Korean respondents viewed their news organizations as more selfish than their Japanese counterparts.

In addition, derogatory attitudes toward journalists and news organizations are evident, given these low-performance ratings and high estimates of selfish motives. The negative attitude that journalists are egotists and pompous was stronger in both countries, particularly Korea. There was also a strongly negative assessment that "the news organizations always seemed to act like only they are right," and "they seemed to think their job is just criticize something." Moreover, the average score for empathy with the insult of "Masugomi" and "Giregi" was 3.37 in Japan and a whopping 3.89 in Korea. In terms of the percentage of respondents, 40.9% in Japan and 69.6% in Korea showed their consent to the despising attitude.

As mentioned earlier, it can be inferred that such media cynicism is related to HMP. First, the degree of media cynicism, calculated by summing the scores of the 18 items (*range* = 18–90), was 59.6 (*SD* = 11.02) for Japan and 64.0 (*SD* = 11.92) for Korea. Although the score among Korean respondents was significantly higher (t = −4.348, $p < .001$, d = −0.382), the difference was not as large as expected. The HMP score (*range* = 4–20) was 13.7 (*SD* = 3.27) among Japanese respondents and 14.5 (*SD* = 3.44) among Korean respondents. Although Korean respondents expressed a significantly higher HMP (t = −0.83, $p < .001$, d = −0.249), the difference was relatively small, indicating that HMP is quite widespread in both countries. As shown in Table 7.1, the mean values of the individual items of HMP do not differ much between the two countries, except for the item "Some of the media report against the politicians and parties

Table 7.1 Japan–Korea Differences in Hostile Media Perceptions

Some of [the Japanese|Korean] News Media...	Japan	Korea	t	d
are at odds with my views	2.70	2.76	−1.757	−0.072
report against the politicians and parties I support	2.53	2.93	−11.749***	−0.480
defend people and countries that I don't like	2.76	2.97	−6.620***	−0.271
are very angry to watch.	2.92	3.02	−3.121**	−0.129
are hostile to watch	2.70	2.76	−1.900	−0.079

$*p < .05$; $**p < .01$; $***p < .001$.

I support." And as expected, there was a moderate correlation between HMP and media cynicism, $r = .549$ ($p < .001$) in Japan and $r = .538$ ($p < .001$) in Korea.

Negative Attitude toward COVID-19 Reporting

Figure 7.2 shows the means of each item developed to access NAC. Japanese respondents have more NAC overall, while media cynicism tends to be significantly higher among Korean respondents, as indicated in the previous section. Japanese respondents were more likely than Korean respondents to think that mass media's COVID-19 reporting is useless because it repeats the same information every day, neither providing the necessary information nor adequately communicating the problem. They also appeared to think that the COVID-19 coverage was more sensational than Korean respondents. They were significantly more dissatisfied than Korean respondents that non-specialists, celebrities, and entertainers expressed their opinions on COVID-19 and that some experts appeared on TV repeatedly and became famous like celebrities. Predictably, respondents in both countries evaluated that there was too much news about COVID-19.

As media cynicism increases, this study predicts that NAC will become stronger. As expected, there was a moderate positive correlation between media cynicism and NAC in Japan ($r = .575$, $p < .001$) and Korea ($r = .371$, $p < .001$).

Use of Information Sources and Risk Perceptions

This study found differences between the two countries regarding the media used to obtain information about COVID-19. The most used information source in Japan was the news service provided by portal sites such as Yahoo! Japan, Google News, and Line News (62.1%), followed by news (55.7%) and information programs (46.3%) of commercial broadcasters. The public broadcaster NHK's news was used by 40.3% of the Japanese respondents. Social networking sites (34.9%) and YouTube (36.9%) were also used to some extent, while government and local government websites, healthcare-related websites, and websites of medical institutions such as hospitals were consulted by around 20% of the respondents.

In Korea, news from the public broadcaster KBS was used by the largest proportion of people (47.9%) even though not a significant lead over other sources. News from other TV stations also was selected as a frequent source for COVID-19 information by around 45% of respondents (MBC 45.6%, SBS 43.5%). In Korea, people often read news provided by various newspapers on portal sites such as *NAVER*, but the usage rate for news from the preferred newspaper was 27.3%, which was not as high as expected. In Korea, government (28.9%) and local government (27.9%) websites were used more than in Japan, while SNS (37.2%) and YouTube (35.4%) were accessed almost as much as in Japan. The healthcare-related websites were viewed by 27.2% of respondents, a little higher than in Japan, but hospitals and other medical institutions' websites were consulted about the same as in Japan, at around 20%.

What do you think of the following evaluations of COVID-19 coverage in newspapers and broadcasts?

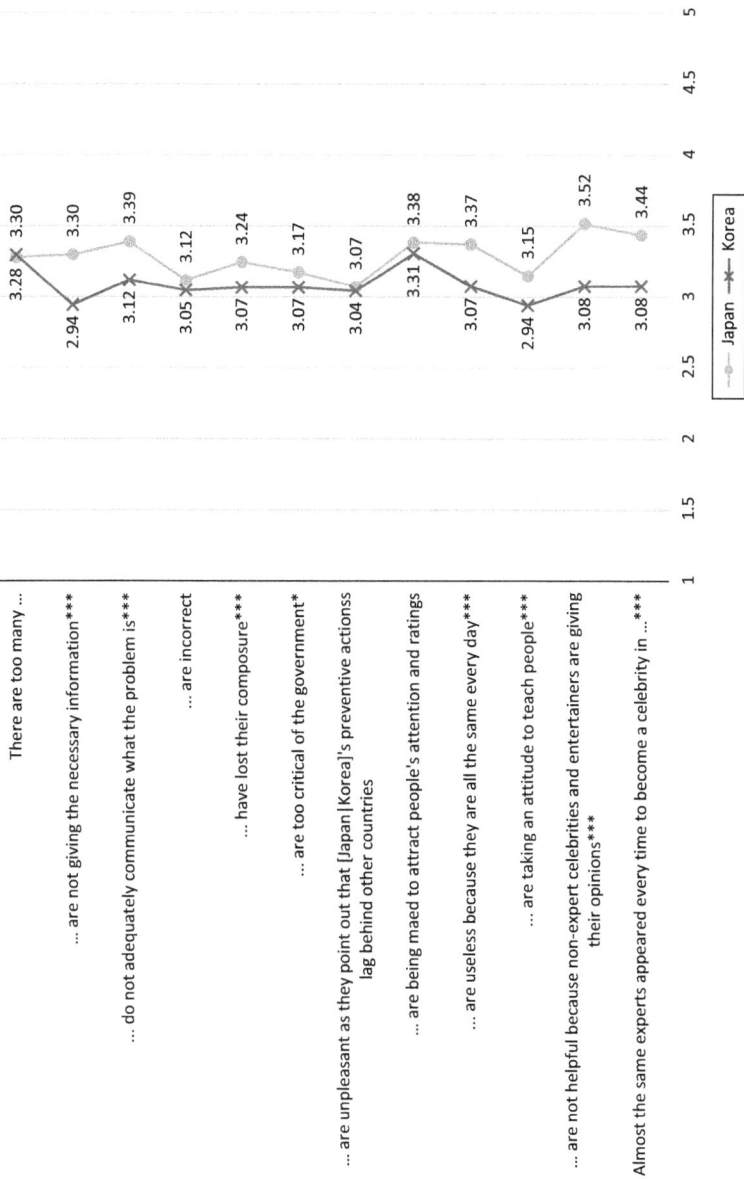

There are too many ...

... are not giving the necessary information***

... do not adequately communicate what the problem is***

... are incorrect

... have lost their composure***

... are too critical of the government*

... are unpleasant as they point out that [Japan|Korea]'s preventive actionss lag behind other countries

... are being maed to attract people's attention and ratings

... are useless because they are all the same every day***

... are taking an attitude to teach people***

... are not helpful because non-expert celebrities and entertainers are giving their opinions***

Almost the same experts appeared every time to become a celebrity in ...***

	Japan	Korea
There are too many	3.28	3.30
... are not giving the necessary information***	2.94	3.30
... do not adequately communicate what the problem is***	3.12	3.39
... are incorrect	3.05	3.12
... have lost their composure***	3.07	3.24
... are too critical of the government*	3.07	3.17
... lag behind other countries	3.04	3.07
... are being maed to attract people's attention and ratings	3.31	3.38
... are useless because they are all the same every day***	3.07	3.37
... are taking an attitude to teach people***	2.94	3.15
... their opinions***	3.08	3.52
Almost the same experts... ***	3.08	3.44

Figure 7.2 Japan–Korea differences in negative attitudes toward mass media's COVID-19 reporting

Table 7.2 Japan–Korea Differences in Risk Perceptions

I am worried that...	Japan	Korea	t	d
I or my family might be infected with the new coronavirus	3.85	3.95	−2.524*	−0.102
I or my family might have symptoms similar to the new coronavirus	3.91	3.87	0.997	0.041
I or my family might get the new coronavirus and become very sick	3.89	3.83	1.417	0.058
I or my family might die from the new coronavirus	3.82	3.51	6.747***	0.283
I might infect someone close to me with the new coronavirus	3.78	3.64	3.186**	0.133
the number of people infected will increase throughout the country	3.86	3.91	−1.104	−0.044
the whole of the country will suffer economically from the new coronavirus	3.92	4.01	−2.457*	−0.098

$*p < .05; **p < .01; ***p < .001.$

Risk perception was quite high in both countries. As shown in Table 7.2, most of the individual risks, i.e., the risk of infection, severe illness, and death of oneself and one's family members, were perceived highly to the degree exceeding the mean value of 3.8. Even though some of the *t*-test results were significant, there was little difference in individual risk perception between the two countries.

The risk of infecting other people was also high, especially among Japanese respondents. In contrast, Korean respondents were more worried about the risks of increasing infection on a societal scale and worsening the country's economic situation, although the differences were not large. The last two items were combined into the societal risk for the subsequent analysis.

One of the main research questions of this chapter is how NAC, which may be enhanced by media cynicism, relates to the risk perceptions of COVID-19. To confirm this, a correlation coefficient was calculated between NAC and risk perceptions, but there were no noticeable associations between them. The risk perception is expected to decrease as NAC increases, but the Japanese data showed a weak positive correlation, and the Korean data had no significant correlation. This unexpected result is presumably due to the high level of risk perceptions, which might produce ceiling effects.

This study conducted multiple regression analyses to examine the relationships between the use of information sources and risk perceptions. Gender and age were included in the analysis as control variables. The results showed that portal sites news ($\beta = .218, p < .001$), commercial broadcast news ($\beta = .137, p < .001$), and SNS ($\beta = .107, p < .01$) were the predictors for the risk perceptions in Japan.

In Korea, government websites (β = .099, p < .05) were slightly associated with the risk perception, but none of the other sources predicted the risk perception.

Risk Perception and Acceptance of Restrictive Measures

It is expected that increased risk perception will strengthen the intention to take preventive actions against risks. Particularly in the case of infectious diseases, which are spread through interpersonal contacts, restrictive measures against individual freedom to move and privacy of locations are central to preventive actions. In the case of the COVID-19 pandemic, the quarantine authorities in many countries have taken various restrictive measures such as mandatory mask-wearing, restrictions on going out, travel, and meetings, shortening of business hours, and identifying personal information of infected people and close contacts, even though the severity varies from country to country. It is also true that many citizens, especially in western countries, expressed their opposition to the restrictive measures and confronted it sometimes violently.

In Japan, especially in the first half of 2020 before the Tokyo Olympics and Paralympics, there was a reluctance to heighten the risk perception of COVID-19 and to take restrictive measures, as the catchphrase "fear correctly" well illustrates. On the other hand, Korea seems more willing to take restrictive measures. One reason is its experience with the 2015 MERS epidemic. Another reason is the outbreak of a large cluster in the first stages of the COVID-19 epidemic. In fact, in the first half of 2020, there was a noticeable tone in which Japan viewed Korea's proactive preventive measures as "disrespect for individual freedom and human rights," while Korea criticized Japan's lax response as "a cover-up of infection status for hosting the Tokyo Olympics" (e.g., Park & Kim, 2020).

After that, Japan eventually decided to postpone the Tokyo Olympics and Paralympics, and a relatively large spread of infection (the third wave in Japan) occurred at the end of 2020, resulting in a sharp increase in severe injuries and deaths. Risk perception of COVID-19 also has increased dramatically. The data used in this chapter were obtained in February 2021 when Japan was in the middle of the third wave.

On the other hand, Korea has been so confident in its quarantine measures after the initial spread of COVID-19 to name their preventive system "K-Quarantine." Because no significant spread of the COVID-19 has occurred since the first outbreak, except a cluster in a Christian church in the metropolitan area at the end of August 2020, Korea was confident of the effectiveness of its restrictive measures. However, with the arrival of a major wave of infection at the end of 2020 (the third wave in Korea), the risk perception seems to have increased even more than before. The survey in Korea was conducted when the peak of the third wave had just passed, but the number of cases had stopped falling, and infection was still spreading to a certain extent.

Since Korea faced a large spread of infection despite its "proud" K-quarantine in place, it might be possible that doubts about the effectiveness of restrictive measures have grown at the point of data collection. In Japan, on the other hand, there may have been a change in the optimistic belief that strong restrictive measures were unnecessary because citizens would take preventive actions voluntarily.

Figure 7.3 shows the results of ARM, which was measured by listing 12 typical restrictive measures and asking respondents whether they could accept them or not with a four-point scale. The results show that Korean respondents are significantly more receptive than Japanese to most measures except lockdown and restriction of going out. Japan respondents also have a positive attitude toward restrictive measures, scoring above the midpoint 2.5 in all measures. School closures ($M = 2.55$) may be frowned upon because of the ripple effect on the work of parents, but the result seems to be influenced by the memory of the sudden closure of schools implemented by then Prime Minister Abe in the spring of 2020 when COVID-19 had not yet spread, did more to deprive children of educational opportunities than to help prevent infection. Next, there were relatively large gaps between Japan and Korea, attitudes toward privacy infringement, such as collecting location information of infected people by GPS (Japan: $M = 2.61$, Korea: $M = 3.12$) and leaving personal information when entering facilities (Japan: $M = 2.67$, Korea: $M = 3.16$). On the other hand, there was a relatively high acceptance of mandatory mask-wearing in Japan ($M = 3.15$).

Korean respondents are particularly positive toward mandatory mask-wearing ($M = 3.64$) and seems to have a lesser feeling of rejection toward collecting personal information. They are also more willing to accept government control of medical supplies and PCR testing of all residents in the area where the infection spreads, as is done in China. The bottom two items in Figure 7.3, which were only included in the Korean survey, represent a high level of support for temporarily restricting religious meetings and political gatherings and demonstrations. This result seems to be related to the perception that the spread of COVID-19 in Korea in 2020 occurred mainly through worship services at Christian churches and was exacerbated by rallies and marches organized by conservative political groups. This explanation is immediately confirmed by the results on causal attribution of the spread of infection (Figure 7.4).

Causal Attribution of the Spread of Infection

Figure 7.4 shows the results of the causal attribution of the spread of COVID-19 in Japan and Korea. The major difference between the two countries in this figure can be found in the attribution to the government response and quarantine system. The Japanese respondents believe that the spread of COVID-19 was due to the government's priority on the economy ($M = 3.65$) and inadequate testing system ($M = 3.64$), isolation of infected people ($M = 3.61$), and public health system ($M = 3.18$), while the Korean respondents, as mentioned in the previous section, regard the meetings, rallies, and demonstrations of religious ($M = 4.16$) and political ($M = 3.99$) groups as the cause of the spread of the infection, and not so much the government's quarantine measures and system. They believe that the government's quarantine measures and systems

What do you think of taking the following measures next time a new virus-induced infection occurs?

Measure	Japan	Korea
Locating infected people through GPS*	2.61	3.12
Imposing a lockdown to prohibit movement between regions	2.76	2.81
Mandatory mask-wearing in public places*	3.15	3.64
Ordering shorter hours for restaurants*	2.75	2.94
Temporary restriction on everyone's going out	2.78	2.83
Leaving personal information when entering facilities*	2.67	3.16
PCR testing of all residents of the area where the infection is spreading*	2.92	3.11
Mandatory vaccination*	2.75	2.98
Closing schools, including elementary, middle, and high schools*	2.55	3.01
Government control over the procurement and distribution of medical supplies*	2.87	3.14
Temporarily restricting meetings or worship services of religious organizations		3.53
Temporarily restricting freedom of assembly and demonstration		3.46

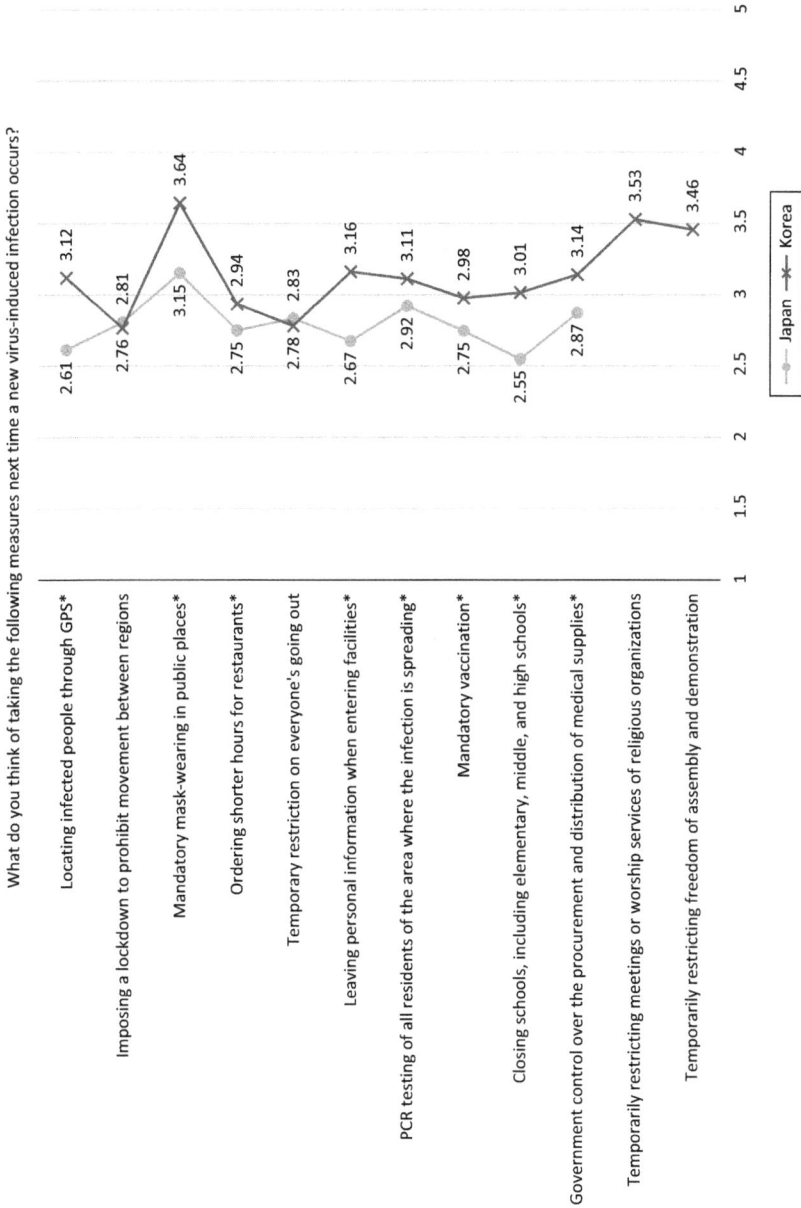

Figure 7.3 Japan–Korea differences in acceptance of restrictive measures

What do you think of the following causes of the COVID-19 spread? (It's because ...)

Cause	Japan	Korea
... the government did not strictly restrict the entry of foreigners**	3.73	3.85
...Japan/Korea values individual freedom	3.10	3.17
...Japan/Korea is an advanced democratic society	2.94	2.87
...Japan/Korea values the protection of personal information	3.01	2.99
... the government has given priority to the economy***	3.65	2.95
... the inspection system was inadequate.***	3.64	2.79
... the system for isolating the infected was inadequate***	3.61	2.97
... the public health and sanitation system is inadequate***	3.18	2.63
... young people spread the infection	3.28	3.30
... individual's public awareness is low	3.45	3.37
... the information from Japanese government did not resonate with the people***	3.53	2.89
... the information from local governments did not resonate with the residents***	3.38	2.93
... religious people worshiped in violation of the ban	4.16	—
... political groups held rallies in violation of the ban	3.99	—

Japan —— Korea —*—

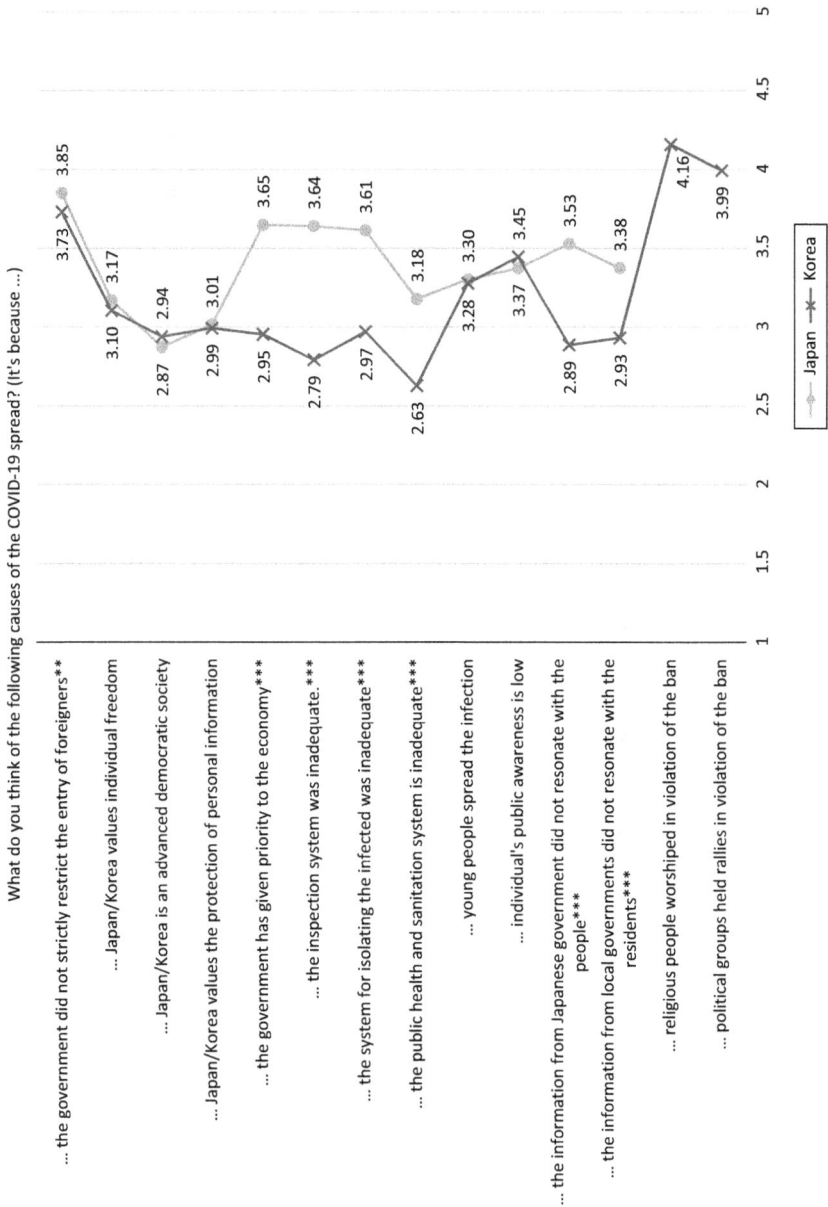

Figure 7.4 Japan–Korea differences in attributing the cause of the COVID-19 spread

are not responsible for the increase of infected people. Taken together, Japanese respondents tried to find the reason for the spread of the disease in "the failure of government policies and quarantine systems," while Korean respondents attributed it to "the exercise of freedom by some selfish people who ignored the public interest."

Both countries' respondents were very similar in their tendency to seek the cause of the spread of infection in the permission of foreigners to enter the country (Japan: M = 3.85, Korea: M = 3.73), the protection of personal freedom (Japan: M = 3.17, Korea: M = 3.10) and personal information (Japan: M = 3.01, Korea: M = 2.99), and the respect of democratic values (Japan: M = 2.87, Korea: M = 2.94). The perception that young people are spreading the disease (Japan: M = 3.30, Korea: M = 3.28) and that the lack of public awareness (Japan: M = 3.37, Korea: M = 3.45) is one of the reasons for the infection showed a similar pattern in both countries.

Along with the risk perception, this pattern of causal attribution of the COVID-19 spread may be linked to the ARM discussed in the previous section. To confirm this link, a multiple regression analysis was conducted with the ARM as the target variable and the three kinds of risk perceptions (i.e., individual, interpersonal, and societal risk perception), and causal attributions as explanatory variables. The patterns of causal attributions were summarized into three types of attribution: attribution to policy and system failure, attribution to protecting democratic values, and attribution to disregarding public interests.

Table 7.3 presents the results of the multiple regression analysis. First, concerning risk perceptions, only individual risk perception (β = .195, p < .001) was a significant predictor variable in Japan, whereas in Korea, societal risk perception (β = .121, p < .05) was more strongly associated with ARM than individual risk perception. That means that Korean respondents were more willing to accept

Table 7.3 Results of Multiple Regression Analysis for the Acceptance of Restrictive Measures

Dependent Variable: Acceptance of Restrictive Measures	Japan	Korea
Male	−.036	−.058*
Age	.048*	.105***
Individual risk	.195***	.096
Risk of infecting other people	.045	−.023
Societal risk	.050	.121*
Attribution to protecting democratic values	.137***	.152***
Attribution to policy and system failure	.240***	−.099**
Attribution to exercise of freedom without regarding public interests	–	.279***
Adjusted R²	.260***	.183***

*p < .05; **p < .01; ***p < .001.

stricter quarantine measures, as society would be forced into a difficult situation, rather than the concern that they or their family members would be infected with COVID-19 and suffer health problems.

In terms of causal attribution for the spread of infection, attribution to policy and quarantine system failures was the most important explanatory variable in Japan (β = .240, p < .001). In contrast, the most significant predictor in Korea was attribution to the religious and political groups ignoring the public interest (β = .279, p < .001). It can be said that Japanese respondents are tired of the government's inaction and lack of preparedness and have come to accept stricter quarantine measures, while Korean respondents have questioned the selfish and blind demands for freedom without regard to social responsibility and came to want more restrictive measures. The perception that attempts to protect demo-cratic values provided the cause for the spread of infection was also associated with the ARM with approximately the same strength in both countries.

Conclusion

This chapter has identified the prevalence of media cynicism in Japanese and Korean societies, which may also affect the acceptance of crucial infection-related information during a pandemic. The more media cynicism people had, the more negative their attitudes toward COVID-19-related mass media reporting. It can be thought that such attitudes might encourage people to approach alternative sources of information that are less reliable and vulnerable to rumors, miscommu-nications, and fake news, thus preventing them from forming appropriate risk per-ceptions. However, the survey results uncovered that both Japanese and Korean respondents, while critical of COVID-19 reporting, basically received the infor-mation provided by the mass media and formed a high level of risk perception.

Media cynicism, which is thought to be formed mainly by HMP to the news media in the era of political polarization among citizens and the media, may not be influential enough to overcome the growing dependence on the news media during a pandemic health crisis. While expressing dissatisfaction with the quality of information conveyed by the news media and sometimes disdain for the anx-iety-provoking manner it was delivered, most people in Japan and Korea appear to have received more than enough information to feed their preventive actions.

However, it is also true that media cynicism is negatively correlated with the use of public and commercial broadcast news. It is also interesting to note that although the association was weak, there was a negative association between media cynicism and overall media use, including online media. Therefore, media cynicism may interfere with obtaining appropriate risk-related information by bringing about a general decline in media use.

In addition, since media cynicism is primarily formed from HMP, selective exposure to preferred media outlets likely occurs. In the Korean study, we found that a negative correlation exists between media cynicism and unfavorable broad-cast news use (r = −.321, p < .001) and between media cynicism and unfavorable newspaper use (r = −.317, p < .001). Particularly in Korea, it is likely that selective exposure affects the level of risk perception because the government's reaction to COVID-19 mostly becomes a political issue and has been treated differently by conservative and liberal media.

Although risk perception was formed quite high in both countries, the level of ARM was significantly higher in Korea than in Japan overall. This difference seems to be strongly influenced by Korea's experience of the MERS epidemic in 2015 and Japan's trust in the peoples' voluntary cooperation.

Japan and Korea also differed in their perceptions of the causes of the COVID-19 spread. Japan attributed the cause to government policies and inadequate public health care systems. In contrast, Korea was more favorable to the performance of the quarantine authorities and saw religious and political groups that disobeyed their instructions as the "culprits" of the spread. In both countries, the protection of democratic values was also perceived to accelerate the spread. Such attributions can be susceptible to media framing, but that is beyond the scope of this chapter and requires further study.

The heightened risk perception and causal attribution patterns increased the ARM in both countries. This seems to be a manifestation of civic values in the pandemic era, in which democratic values should be temporarily reserved and social crisis prevention should be prioritized while preserving one's own and others' lives.

Note

1 Japanese data were searched in the respective newspaper article databases, while Korean data were obtained at the Big Kinds news database of Korea Press Foundation.

References

Al-Rawi, A. (2020). *News 2.0: Journalists, Audiences, and News on Social Media.* Wiley-Blackwell.

Arpan, L. M., & Raney, A. A. (2003). An experimental investigation of news source and the hostile media effect. *Journalism & Mass Communication Quarterly, 80*(2), 265–281. https://doi.org/10.1177%2F107769900308000203

Brewer, N. T., Chapman, G. B., Gibbons, F. X., Gerrard, M., McCaul, K. D., & Weinstein, N. D. (2007). Meta-analysis of the relationship between risk perception and health behavior: The example of vaccination. *Health Psychology, 26*(2), 136–145. https://doi.org/10.1037/0278-6133.26.2.136

Cappella, J. N., & Jamieson, K. H. 1996. News frames, political cynicism, and media cynicism. *The Annals of the American Academy of Political and Social Science, 546*(1), 71–84. https://doi.org/10.1177/0002716296546001007

Cappella, J. N., & Jamieson, K. H. (1997). *Spiral of Cynicism: The Press and the Public Good.* Oxford University Press.

Chang, C. (2012). News coverage of health-related issues and its impacts on perceptions: Taiwan as an example. *Health Communication, 27*(2), 111–123. https://doi.org/10.1080/10410236.2011.569004

Chew, C., & Eysenbach, G. (2010). Pandemics in the age of twitter: Content analysis of tweets during the 2009 H1N1 outbreak. *PLoS ONE, 5*(11), e14118. https://doi.org/10.1371/journal.pone.0014118

Choi, D. H., Yoo, W., Noh, G. Y., & Park, K. (2017). The impact of social media on risk perceptions during the MERS outbreak in South Korea. *Computers in Human Behavior*, *72*, 422–431. https://doi.org/10.1016/j.chb.2017.03.004

Coleman, C. L. (1993). The influence of mass media and interpersonal communication on societal and personal risk judgments. *Communication Research*, *20*(4), 611–628. https://doi.org/10.1177/009365093020004006

Culbertson, H. M., & Stempel, G. H. (1985). "Media malaise": Explaining personal optimism and societal pessimism about health care. *Journal of Communication*, *35*(2), 180–190. https://psycnet.apa.org/doi/10.1111/j.1460-2466.1985.tb02242.x

Dekker, H., & Meijerink, E. (2012). Political cynicism: Conceptualization, operationalization, and explanation. *Politics, Culture and Socialization*, *3*(1–2), 33–48.

Dudo, A. D., Dahlstrom, M. F., & Brossard, D. (2007). Reporting a potential pandemic: A risk-related assessment of avian influenza coverage in US newspapers. *Science Communication*, *28*(4), 429–454. https://doi.org/10.1177/1075547007302211

Festinger, L. (1957). *A Theory of Cognitive Dissonance*. Stanford University Press.

Flynn, J., Peters, E., Mertz, C. K., & Slovid, P. (1998). Risk, media, and stigma at Rocky Flats. *Risk Analysis*, *18*(6), 715–725. https://doi.org/10.1111/j.1539-6924.1998.tb01115.x

Giner-Sorolla, R., & Chaiken, S. (1994). The causes of hostile media judgments. *Journal of Experimental Social Psychology*, *30*(2), 165–180. https://doi.org/10.1006/jesp.1994.1008

Gunther, A. C., & Schmitt, K. (2004). Mapping boundaries of the hostile media effect. *Journal of Communication*, *54*(1), 55–70. https://doi.org/10.1111/j.1460-2466.2004.tb02613.x

Gunther, A. C., Miller, N., & Liebhart, J. L. (2009). Assimilation and contrast in a test of the hostile media effect. *Communication Research*, *36*(6), 747–764. https://doi.org/10.1177/0093650209346804

Hansen, G. J., & Kim, H. (2011). Is the media biased against me? A meta-analysis of the hostile media effect research. *Communication Research Reports*, *28*(2), 169–179. https://doi.org/10.1080/08824096.2011.565280

Jang, Y. (2021). Giregineun jwegaoptta daebop giregi daetkkeure modokjjweanya [The expression of 'Giregi' is innocent. The Supreme Court said, 'Giregi' Isn't a crime of blasphemy]. *The Hankyoreh* Internet edition, 2021/3/25 https://www.hani.co.kr/arti/society/society_general/988176.html retrieved 2021/4/20.

Lee, K. (2019). Tekitaiteki media ninchi to media shinishizumu: Kankoku shakai ni okeru sono jittai no haaku [Current State of Hostile Media Perception and Media Cynicism in Korean Society]. *Media Communication*, *69*, 85–95. https://koara.lib.keio.ac.jp/xoonips/modules/xoonips/download.php/AA1121824X-20190300-0085.pdf?file_id=142869

Lee, K. (2020a). Media shinishizumu to seiji jōhōgen no riyō : Kankoku shakai ni okeru seijiteki kyokuseika o haikei ni [Media cynicism and the use of political information sources in the context of political polarization in Korean society]. *Media Communication*, *70*, 19–27. https://koara.lib.keio.ac.jp/xoonips/modules/xoonips/download.php/AA1121824X-20200300-0019.pdf?file_id=151669

Lee, K. (2020b). Kankoku ni okeru media shinishizumu to seiji nyūsu no "shōhi," sentakuteki sesshoku [Media cynicism, political news consumption and selective exposure in South Korea]. *Hōgaku kenkyū [Journal of Law, Politics and Sociology]*, *93*(12), 71–94. https://koara.lib.keio.ac.jp/xoonips/modules/xoonips/download.php/AN00224504-20201228-0343.pdf?file_id=159465

Lee, K. (2021). Media shinishizumu no yōin to kekka: tekitaiteki media ninchi oyobi "posuto shinjitsu shugiteki taido" tono kanren [Media Cynicism in Japan: An Analysis on the Relations with Hostile Media Perception and Post-truth Attitude]. *Media Communication*, *71*, 103–116. https://koara.lib.keio.ac.jp/xoonips/modules/xoonips/download.php/AA1121824X-20210300-0103.pdf?file_id=156696

Lin, C. A., & Lagoe, C. (2013). Effects of news media and interpersonal interactions on H1N1 risk perception and vaccination intent. *Communication Research Reports*, *30*(2), 127–136. https://doi.org/10.1080/08824096.2012.762907

Morton, T. A., & Duck, J. M. (2001). Communication and health beliefs: Mass and interpersonal influences on perceptions of risk to self and others. *Communication Research*, *28*(5), 602–626. https://doi.org/10.1177/009365001028005002

OED (n.d.). Cynical. In *Oxford English Dictionary*. Retrieved February 14, 2022, from https://www.oed.com/view/Entry/46639

Park, H., & Kim, B. (2020). il jungjeungman korona gomsa hwakjjinja chuksso uihok [Only severe COVID-19 test... Suspicion of reducing the number of confirmed cases] *The Donga Ilbo*, 2020/2/26 https://www.bigkinds.or.kr/v2/news/search.do;Bigkinds=38C5299345E54B62BDD0335956CABB67# retrieved 2022/2/14

Perloff, R. M. (2015). A three-decade retrospective on the hostile media effect. *Mass Communication and Society*, *18*(6), 701–729. https://doi.org/10.1080/15205436.2015.1051234

Poletti, M., & Brants, K. (2010). Between partisanship and cynicism: Italian journalism in a state of flux. *Journalism*, *11*(3), 329–346. https://doi.org/10.1177/1464884909360923

Shimizu Y. (2016). Furī no tōkei bunseki sofuto HAD: Kinō no shōkai to tōkei gakushū kyōiku, kenkyū jissen ni okeru riyō hōhō no teian [An introduction to the statistical free software HAD: Suggestions to improve teaching, learning, and practice data analysis]. *Journal of Media, Information and Communication*, *1*, 59–73. https://repository.tku.ac.jp/dspace/bitstream/11150/10815/1/JMIC01-05.pdf

Signorini, A., Segre, A. M., & Polgreen, P. M. (2011). The use of twitter to track levels of disease activity and public concern in the U.S. during the influenza A H1N1 pandemic. *PLoS ONE*, *6*(5), e19467. https://doi.org/10.1371/journal.pone.0019467

Song, J., Song, T. M., Seo, D.-C., Jin, D.-L., & Kim, J. S. (2017). Social big data analysis of information spread and perceived infection risk during the 2015 middle east respiratory syndrome outbreak in South Korea. *Cyberpsychology, Behavior, and Social Networking*, *20*(1), 22–29. https://doi.org/10.1089/cyber.2016.0126

Song, H., Omori, K., Kim, J., Tenzek, K. E., Hawkins, J. M., Lin, W.-Y., Kim, Y.-C., & Jung, J.-Y. (2016). Trusting social media as a source of health information: Online surveys comparing the United States, Korea, and Hong Kong. *Journal of Medical Internet Research*, *18*(3), e25. https://doi.org/10.2196/jmir.4193

Vallone, R. P., Ross, L., & Lepper, M. R. (1985). The hostile media phenomenon: biased perception and perceptions of media bias in coverage of the Beirut massacre. *Journal of Personality and Social Psychology*, *49*(3), 577. https://doi.org/10.1037//0022-3514.49.3.577

8 Mediated Experience of the COVID-19 Pandemic and the Politics of Emotion in Japan

Shuzo Yamakoshi and Fumie Mitani

Introduction

Ever since emerged in late 2019, the COVID-19 pandemic has influenced our everyday life. We have seen and learned how horrible the pandemic has been through the media. Many lost their family members, too. The fear of death has become more familiar and closer than ever. Under unprecedented and unexpected circumstances, every government on the globe, regardless of democratic or authoritarian regimes, introduced various kinds of measurements to contain and control the pandemic. Such measurements restricted and changed how we enjoyed our daily life, and yet we have managed to adjust to the new way of life. One major reason is that mediated experience has a great impact on our perception and understanding of the pandemic. Then the question becomes how we have accepted governmental control in our everyday life.

An emotion like fear and anxiety, as this chapter suggests, is one element that helps us accept its severe control and situation. The chapter attempts to understand the COVID-19 pandemic as a risk from the perspective of people's mediated experience. For regarding the pandemic in contemporary society as a mediated experience, two points need to be considered. First is the nature of today's media environment, which is a "hybrid media system." Andrew Chadwick (2017, p. xi) argues that

> (t)he hybrid media system is built upon interactions among older and newer media logics—where logics are defined as bundles of technologies, genres, norms, behaviors, and organizational forms—in the reflexively connected social fields of media and politics. Actors in this system are articulated by complex ever-evolving relationships based upon adaptation and interdependence and concentrations and diffusions of power.

Our mediated experience can be understood as a complex of diverse media practices by various actors through mainstream and social media. Then it helps to construct "reality" for each one of us.

Second, in the hybrid media system, these mediated experiences and "realities" are politically constructed. In many democratic nations, digital media

DOI: 10.4324/9781003286684-8

technologies have created filter bubbles and echo chambers. But importantly, the divided media ecosystem is driven by ideological struggles and has evolved into a political and social divide. People tend to use only the media they want to believe in and try to exclude the other media. Thus, the media system and the public sphere become divided and disrupted (Bennett & Livingston, 2018; Dahlgren, 2018).

In these media environments, our mediated experience in modern society is constructed by "the political" that facilitates we/they discrimination (Mouffe, 2005, p. 9). Each individual and group construct their version of "reality." Japan is not a unique case. From the outset of the pandemic, the "struggle over meaning"—how and what people see the pandemic—is activated through a conflict of each reality. For example, the meaning of the COVID-19 pandemic has become a symbol of struggling between "crisis" and "everyday life." Not only do politicians politicize the pandemic, but also do the ordinary citizens who exclusively listen to the voice that they like to hear. Thus, wearing a face mask has become a political symbol, although the Japanese have used to wearing it in ordinary times. Supporters and opponents of vaccination have experienced and understood their "reality" respectively.

How then is "the political" activated in the mediated experience of the COVID-19 pandemic? To understand how "the political" works in democratic societies such as Japan, this chapter introduces the idea and role of "emotions" and regards that the pandemic has an aspect of "politics of emotions." Karin Wahl-Jorgensen (2019) sheds new light on the role of emotions in mediated politics. She defines emotions as "the relational interpretation of affect experienced in individual bodies" (Wahl-Jorgensen, 2019, p. 8). People's "anxiety," "anger," and "sadness" form a collective identity and influence the political process and social order. Such emotions are constructed, circulated, and shared through the media. The mediated experience of the pandemic contributes to constructing emotions.

In analyzing the mediated experience of COVID-19 and its risk from the perspective of the "politics of emotion," it is important to note that this experience has related to the "politics of post-truth" where "alternative facts" replace facts, and feelings have more weight than evidence (McIntyre, 2018). We have come to understand that "post-truth politics" has been developing not only in Trump's populism in the United States but also in the era of the pandemic in many parts of the globe. The "anxiety," "anger," and "fear" surrounding COVID-19 amplify the "distrust" of governments, experts, science, and the media, and people come to believe in what they want to believe in their filter bubbles. People's mediated experiences and emotions thus become an impediment to effective risk communication.

Against this backdrop, we need to critically analyze the function of the media in the pandemic of COVID-19. What kind of emotions does the media construct? How have those emotions been distributed and shared in a hybrid media system? And what risks and obstructions do contemporary media environments and mediated experiences pose for pandemic solutions?

This chapter draws a case study from Japan's experience of encountering COVID-19 from March through May 2020. It was the time that the first wave of COVID-19 hit Japan. It is significant to analyze the first wave because how people went through mediated experiences in their first contact with COVID-19 determined their understanding and behavior. The chapter will first outline Japan's COVID-19 control measures until December 2021 and the media environment. It then analyzes the resonance of television and social media during the first wave of the pandemic and the moral panic of "quarantine vigilantes" caused by its resonance. Finally, it will discuss the findings of the "politics of emotion" and the "politics of post-truth."

Japan's COVID-19 Control Measures and Media Environment

The COVID-19 Pandemic in Japan

Japan experienced the outbreak of the COVID-19 pandemic five times till December 2021. However, there was no forcible lockdown. Besides, the number of patients and deaths is much lower than in Europe and the United States.

On January 5, 2020, the Japanese government announced a new type of viral pneumonia in China. The first case of the coronavirus patient in Japan was confirmed on January 15. However, concern about the disease in Japan was not high at first.

Public concern about the coronavirus increased when the Chinese government announced on January 21 that the disease was transmitted on a "human-to-human" basis, and Wuhan was locked down on January 23. The Japanese government decided to support the return of Japanese citizens from Wuhan. The arrival of a charter flight to Japan was broadcast live on TV and became a media event.

A series of events that occurred in February heightened public concern and fear of COVID-19. First, a cruise ship with infected passengers, the Diamond Princess, was anchored at the Port of Yokohama in Tokyo Bay. The infection spread and infection clusters were caused on board. Second, infection clusters were confirmed in Tokyo and other areas. This meant that the novel coronavirus had been spreading in Japan. Amidst the growing social unrest, the government suddenly announced on February 27 to close schools temporarily for about two weeks from March 2. This decision caused social confusion and made people understand that COVID-19 was a "crisis."

Japan had experienced the first wave of the COVID-19 pandemic by mid-March 2020 (Figure 8.1). The news about the spread of the disease and the lockdown in Europe and the United States made people anxious. The Japanese citizens wondered if Tokyo would have an explosive outbreak like New York and London in a few weeks.

Amid such growing anxiety, Tokyo Governor Yuriko Koike, who was known as a populist politician, called for future vigilance from the citizens of Tokyo by

Newly comfirmed cases in Japan, Daily, in 2020 and 2021

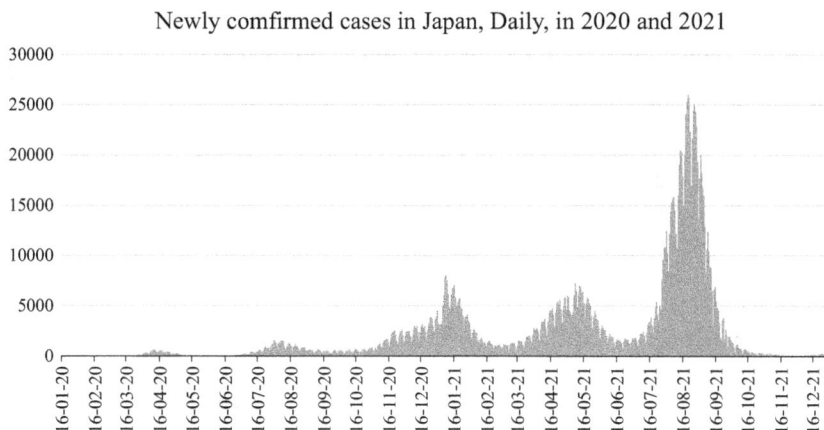

Figure 8.1 Newly confirmed cases in Japan, daily, in 2020 and 2021 [Source: Ministry of Health, Labour and Welfare (2022)]

referring to the "lockdown" that was taking place in cities of Western countries at that time in the conference. She also said, "there is a possibility that we will have to take strong measures such as a blockade of the city, a so-called lockdown, depending on the future development in the situation" on March 23 (Tokyo Metropolitan Government, 2020a). Her media conference had a great impact on people's behavioral change. Her strong words such as "city blockade" and "lockdown" raised tensions in weakening the self-restraint mood (Asia Pacific Initiative, 2020, p. 140).

On March 24, Prime Minister Shinzo Abe announced that the Tokyo Olympic and Paralympic Games would be postponed. The next day of its announcement, Governor Koike held up a signboard with the message "Spread of infection in a serious phase" (Tokyo Metropolitan Government, 2020b). This message of the explosive outbreak of infection and serious phase was widely reported with a remark of "lockdown" and inflated public sense of crisis (Asia Pacific Initiative, 2020, p. 140). People were also terrified by the death of a celebrity in March due to the coronavirus. The fact that Japan's control measures were different from those of other countries also made them more suspicious. Besides Governor Koike agitated the fear.

On April 7, the government declared a state of emergency and asked people to stay home. This containment did not apply any penalties, but the number of infected people began to decline. The state of emergency was lifted on May 25. The government then adopted a policy of promoting travel and eating at a restaurant. This resulted in an increased number of confirmed cases. The second wave of the pandemic came in July and August, and the third wave came in December 2020 and January 2021. On January 7, the government declared a state of emergency for the second time. Following the declaration, the number of people going out decreased, which in turn decreased the number of positive cases. The state of emergency was lifted on March 21. During the third wave, the Japanese government began to vaccinate healthcare workers. The number of people who received the second vaccination by the end of March is about 125,000 (Ministry of Health, Labour and Welfare, 2021). The number was still low, and people needed to stay-at-home.

However, the number of confirmed cases increased again due to a week-holiday called "Golden Week" starting at the end of April, and began the fourth wave. As a result, a state of emergency was declared for the third time on April 26. The Japanese government lifted it on June 20 except for Okinawa Prefecture—in Okinawa where the number of patients is relatively high, healthcare delivery system was strained by scarcity of medical resources. The point here is that lifting the declaration of a state of emergency did not mean removing the restrictions on people's actions. Although the declaration of the state of emergency was lifted, semi-state emergency COVID-19 measures, which lowered the level of activity restrictions, continued. However, the semi-state measures were not sufficiently effective in promoting behavioral change.

The fifth wave had come due to the increased flow of people for the Tokyo Olympic and Paralympic Games, and a state of emergency was declared on July 12—less than one month after the third declaration was lifted. During this period, the declaration of a state of emergency had little effect. One reason for this was the growing distrust of the government, which had decided to hold the Olympics despite the declaration of a state of emergency.[1] A message from the government to stay home was not widely heeded. In addition, as the characteristics of the novel coronavirus infection became clearer, the emotions of fear and anxiety faded away. The fourth declaration was lifted on October 1.

In Japan, there were five waves of a pandemic, and the government issued a state of emergency four times by December 2021. It was during the fifth wave that the number of confirmed cases was the highest. However, at this time, the pandemic situation had become familiar due to the multiple waves experienced, many people had been vaccinated twice,[2] and thus social anxiety and fear were reduced. In December 2021, a variant of COVID-19 called "Omicron" began spreading in Japan. The Omicron variant infection has easily and quickly spread more than the other variants such as the Delta variant and caused less severe illness, while the vaccines seem to be not effective enough to block the Omicron variant. Even under these circumstances, the movement of people during the year-end and New Year holidays of 2021 to 2022 was higher than the last year.

Social anxiety and fear caused by unknown viruses were inflated the most during the first wave. For that reason, this chapter will focus its analysis on the period of the first wave.

The "Japanese Model" for the COVID-19 Control Measures

This section will discuss the strategy of Japan's countermeasures against the COVID-19 pandemic. Japan's initial measure of this pandemic was different from that of Europe and the United States. The Japanese government called it the "Japanese model" (Asia Pacific Initiative, 2020). This chapter will focus on the fact that this model failed to control social emotions while succeeding in controlling the number of infections and deaths.

Japan has adopted a national health insurance system, which is mandatory for residents in Japan and has the highest number of hospital beds per population in the world. Thus, it is inherently able to obtain full medical services at a low cost. However, there were few resources for COVID-19 control. First, Japan performed fewer PCR tests for the virus in the early stage of the pandemic. Its test has focused on high-risk groups and people associated with suspected clusters. Second, as a result of neoliberal reforms, local government budgets for public health were reduced and the system of the public health center was weakened. Third, public medical facilities that deal with diseases had also been forced to undergo neoliberal reforms. Fourth, there were no legal systems that would allow for strong regulations that would be able to restrict human rights during a pandemic.

Under these circumstances, the government's expert panel was established in February 2020. The expert panel sought a pragmatic response with limited resources. First, the expert group propounded the "*San mitsu* [Three Cs]," a strategy to encourage behavioral change to avoid closed spaces, crowded places, and close-contact settings (Asia Pacific Initiative, 2020, p. 33). This strategy was widely promoted in combination with ensuring social distance and wearing a face mask. Second, resources were invested in measures for infection clusters in collaboration with public health centers. This involved conducting an active epidemiological investigation to capture the source of cluster outbreaks and take immediate action to slow down or minimize the spread of future infections (Omi & Oshitani, 2020; Asia Pacific Initiative, 2020, p. 39, see also Figure 8.2). Third, a state of emergency, which requested restaurants to refrain from business and people to stay home, was declared by the government. The experts of the panel presented the need for a simulation of an 80% reduction in human contact and succeeded in persuading people.

With these measures, the first wave of the pandemic in March 2020 was brought under control. Prime Minister Abe said on May 25, when the state of emergency was lifted, "We have shown the excellence of the Japanese model" (Asia Pacific Initiative, 2020, p. 458).

However, Japan's initial response to COVID-19 was not appreciated by people, especially due to the "dysfunction of risk communication"—insufficient strategy to send out the message of how to respond to this crisis and share it with broad audiences in Japan (Asia Pacific Initiative, 2020, pp. 350–352). First, the Japanese model did not adequately explain why and how different it is from the responses of other countries and why the number of PCR tests was lower than others. Second, the Prime Minister did not adequately send information about their measures. In addition to the small number of press conferences, he did not sufficiently answer reporters' questions. Third, the heads of local governments spoke out aggressively in the media individually. Some of them deployed populistic discursive strategies. And fourth, the mass media and

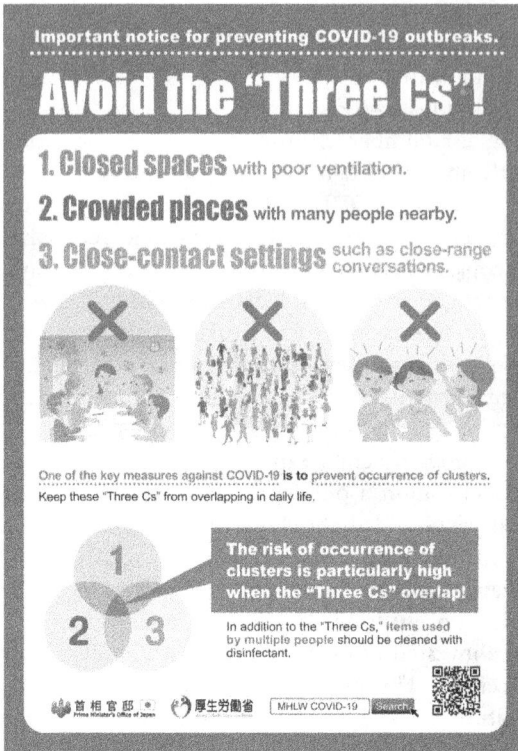

Figure 8.2 Avoid the "Three Cs"! [Source: Prime Minister's Office in Japan (2020)]

social media activated a discourse of criticism and distrust of the government and experts. As a result, emotions such as anxiety, fear, and anger have inflated widely in society.

Hybrid Media System in Japan

In Japan, the influence of traditional media, such as television and newspapers, remains relatively strong. Many Japanese citizens regularly watch television news, carried by the public broadcaster NHK and/or the five major commercial news networks. For the sake of the analysis, this study focuses on an infotainment program called "*waido-shō* [wide-show]" in Japanese instead of news programs. It picks wide-shows partly because they provide intriguing cases to observe a Japanese style of hybrid media system, and partly because more audiences spend time watching wide-shows because the stay-home policy prevailed under the state of emergency.

Wide-shows have a uniquely Japanese style of programming and are typically composed of two genres: infotainment and talk-show. They are initially targeted at housewives, with celebrity gossip and health information being the main topics. On weekdays, five commercial news networks broadcast live wide-shows for two to three hours from morning to around noon. Since wide-shows see topicality important, the topics they cover are similar regardless of networks. With the trend of news becoming more entertaining, they become more integrated with news programs. As a result, they tend to cover topics such as politics and social issues.

However, wide-shows do not have their news-gathering system. Their style is to introduce issues covered by other news programs on their networks, or information that has become a hot topic in newspapers, magazines, or social media, and later the guests make comments on the issues. Wide-shows focus more on the talk between hosts and commentators in the studio than on finding out the new aspects of the issues. The guest commentators are celebrities, critics, journalists, and experts and provide comments on topics even though they are not familiar with them. The talk focuses on gaining the sympathy of the audience rather than analyzing issues. This style results in the content often including speculation, rumors, disinformation, and sensationalism. Since spring 2020, the COVID-19 pandemic has been a major topic on the wide-shows. Ratings for many wide-shows increased because of a state of emergency (Takahashi & Hara, 2020).

Under the pandemic, social media also became a major source of people's mediated experience. Twitter was used by 38.7% of the Internet users, making it the second most used social media after the messenger app Line (Institute for Information and Communications Policy, 2020, p. 15). Twitter is used for sharing and spreading the news or for criticism and comment. During the pandemic, the audience of wide-shows made comments on Twitter and spread them, while wide-shows introduced tweets that have become a hot topic. Thus, this resonance between social media and television, especially wide-shows, was widely seen in the first wave (Takahashi & Hara, 2020; Nanasawa et al., 2021).

Both wide-shows and Twitter have a great impact on the representation, evocation, and sharing of emotions. In this way, an emotional regime surrounding the pandemic is constructed from the resonance between wide-shows and Twitter. An emotional regime allows for the expression of emotions that are specific to a certain time or a certain political order (Reddy, 2001, pp. 124–125; Wahl-Jorgensen, 2019). It is also constructed through media practices, and at the same time, it defines the normative expression of emotions through media practices. Therefore, it is important to analyze the figurations of media discourses and practices in clarifying the emotional regime of the pandemic.

Resonance of Emotions

The Discursive Practice of "Criticism" in Wide-Shows and Constructing Emotions

This section analyzes the process by which the mediated experience of the pandemic constructed the emotional regime of "anxiety," "fear," and "anger" by focusing on wide-shows and Twitter during the first wave.

It draws examples from the "Morning Show," which is a popular morning wide-show broadcasted on the TV Asashi News Networks (ANN). In April 2020, its average monthly rating was 12.3%, up from 9.2% of the previous year. It also had a higher rating than other wide-shows in the same time slot (Takahashi & Hara, 2020, p. 7). Also, the Morning Show became a hot topic on Twitter during the first wave.

Like other wide-shows, this program introduces information from the news of ANN, newspaper articles, magazine articles, and the commentators respond to the introduced information. Two commentators caught people's attention. One was Toru Tamagawa, who is also a corporate journalist for ANN. He has long been known for his critical stance toward the government. The other was Harue Okada, a professor of infectious diseases and public health and a former researcher at the National Institute of Infectious Diseases. The discursive practices of these two commentators strongly criticized the government's measures against the COVID-19 pandemic and constructed "anxiety," "fear," and "anger" in the audience.

The logic of their discursive practices has the following three characteristics. First, they formed the discourse that the government's measures against the COVID-19 pandemic are wrong. For example, Okada talked about the government's measures against infections cluster and said, "I think it is a big mistake" in the show on April 23. This criticism is based on the fact that Japan has a lower number of PCR tests than in Europe and the United States and on the fact that it has taken a unique control measure. By pointing out the insufficient measures of the government, the commentators provoked "anxiety" and "anger" in the program.

The second is the discourse that there must be many more infected people, especially those in Tokyo. For example, Tamagawa said, "(The actual number of infections is) probably at the level of one in a thousand to one in a hundred" on April 13. However, at that time, the total number of PCR test-positive cases in Tokyo was 2,124 (April 12), and this is 0.015% or 1 in 7,000–10,000. In addition, Okada made comments as follows.

We cannot detect an explosive outbreak on the current testing system.
(Okada, April 21, 2020)

I think that Tokyo has already experienced community spread very fast right now.
(Okada, April 21, 2020)

These quotations imply that the government's PCR testing is inadequate and that the current number of confirmed cases is only a fraction of the total. This criticism raises questions about the low number of confirmed cases in Japan. In other words, they formed the discourse that the number of hidden confirmed cases that have not been subjected to PCR testing is much larger than one might imagine. It is a discursive practice suggesting that there are far more infected people than the government and local governments grasp and that an explosive outbreak is invisibly underway. Thus, the commentators showed "anger" in the program by criticizing the government's measures.

The third is the discourse that Tokyo will eventually become in the same situation as New York. The "Morning Show" introduced how bad the situation of New York and Bergamo was, and then, they made comments on the situation in Tokyo as follows.

> That's why I have talked again and again to hurry up (to declare a state of emergency). Don't let it become like Bergamo or New York.
>
> (Okada, April 6, 2020)

> Tokyo will be hell in a few weeks.
>
> (Okada, April 13, 2020)

> The number of cases for severely ill and dead will possibly surge after the Golden-Week holidays.
>
> (Tamagawa, April 27, 2020)

As mentioned in the quote above, the devastation in New York was frequently referred to during March and April. The first confirmed case in New York was on March 1, 2020. Since then, the number of confirmed cases has increased dramatically. Because of the pandemic, the mayor of New York City declared a state of emergency on March 7 and a lockdown on March 22. Moreover, a Japanese doctor treating novel coronavirus patients in New York issued a strong warning over the virus situation in Tokyo, saying that Tokyo now "looks like" New York two to three weeks ago on April 4 (Jiji Press News, April 5, 2020). The "Morning Show" reported how patients were being forced to rest in the corridors at a hospital because there were not enough beds for them, and how the streets in New York were deserted almost every day. Thus, the program formed a discourse that Tokyo will be like New York.

These discursive practices suggest that the number of severe symptoms and deaths in Japan will surge dramatically as a result of the failure of the government's COVID-19 control measures. Thus, this logic that provoked "fear" and "anger" suggests to the audience of "Morning Show" that the COVID-19 pandemic cannot be prevented by the measures taken by the Japanese government, the pandemic is invisibly underway, and the government is covering it up.

The logics of these discursive practices in the "Morning Show" show that it constructed "anxiety," "fear," by sending the message that the number of confirmed cases is higher than what the government is offering and that the situation in Tokyo would get worse. It also provoked "anger" by criticizing the insufficient government's measures.

Resonance of Emotions through Twitter

The above discursive formation of "anxiety," "fear," and "anger" on TV was amplified, shared, and spread by Twitter. This section analyzes the tweets of reactions to the "Morning Show" during this period. The analysis is based on tweets tagged with *#mōningshō* [#morningshow]. These tweets were categorized as follows.

1) Expression of "fear" and "anxiety"

First, some tweets represent the fears and anxieties of the audience that are evoked by watching the show.

> I was really anxious so that I couldn't sleep last night. And I'm still anxious very much.
>
> (@o8GcKuuTLrfj6JG, March 27, 2020)

> My fears are becoming more and more real. Tokyo will become like New York City in a week in the worst scenario … Tokyo in 10 days is terrifying.
>
> (@ucchi_ucchi, April 1, 2020)

2) Sympathy with the commentators

Tweets were agreeing with Tamagawa and Okada's comments. Many of them took the stance that Tamagawa and Okada, unlike the government, were telling the "right thing" and the "truth."

> Tamagawa, he is very good! I feel exactly the same! I think you're right.
>
> (@Ctada2, April 6, 2020)

> It's happening just like Ms. Okada said it would. That's why I can imagine what will happen next by watching this show and listening to her, I'm very terrified that the government won't do anything about it.
>
> (@onmaau, April 10, 2020)

> Ms. Okada said we might be experiencing an explosive outbreak … I'm really scared! Abe's administration is the worst.
>
> (@WYbZer5EQK5R9nv, April 6, 2020)

These tweets expressed sympathy with the commentators, expressing that they are the ones who understand "our" emotions. The sympathy with the commentators evolved into not only fear and anxiety but also distrust and anger towards the government.

3) Antipathy toward the Morning Show

In contrast to sympathy with the commentators, some of the tweets expressed frustration, anger, and antipathy towards the program. Often, they were also associated with distrust and dissatisfaction with the mainstream media.

Even if the government declares a state of emergency, these guys will just complain again.

(@bLV7NW2YIQ2A4Ds, April 6, 2020)

Trying to stir things up by edit, edit, edit. Tamagawa has been exposed as A SCUM who only needs to be able to criticize as he doesn't understand anything. His critics make no sense. Get rid of Tamagawa.

(@Zafonic9, April 9, 2020)

Ms. Okada, please stop stirring up public anxiety without presenting any plan to combat coronavirus infection. It's disgusting.

(@oshiguchi, April 1, 2020)

As described above, the tweets expressed sympathy and antipathy for the program. It is important to note that even in the case of criticism of the program, the emotions of anger and distrust are expressed. In other words, emotions such as anxiety, fear, and anger were activated by this program as the nexus. These emotions are also related to and activated by the three logics seen in the discourse on the pandemic in the "Morning Show," as described in the previous section. The discourse of the "Morning Show" was organized on the logic of criticism of the government's measures against the novel coronavirus infection, distrust of the data presented by the government, and the idea that the situation would become more critical. This discourse resonated with Twitter, allowing for the expression of negative emotions such as anxiety, fear, and anger on social media. In other words, this is how the emotional regime surrounding COVID-19 was formed.

Media Practice as Quarantine Vigilantes and Emotional Regime

The emotional regime, once formed, conditions media practices. The resonance between the wide-show and social media was developed through the emotional regime. One of the examples is the media practice called "*jishuku keisatsu* [quarantine vigilantes]" in Japanese. The quarantine vigilantes are the media and general people who criticize people for breaking quarantine requests and make a public spectacle of them. This is a kind of moral panic. It is not only an act driven by emotions such as "anxiety," "fear," and "anger," but also a practice that seeks empathy for such emotions.

The wide-shows in Japan acted as quarantine vigilantes. On April 13, the "Morning Show" focused on people who did not refrain from their normal life and reported on crowded shopping streets, people going out for drinks, and people playing on beaches and rivers.

On social media, the audience's emotion of anger, which resonated with the program, was inflated.

I'm pretty pissed off that people are making excuses and not staying at home while we are trying to put an end to Coronavirus.

(@manami_719, April 13, 2020)

Are you only thinking about yourself!? Take it seriously! Shit.

(@VvenLBES15zrb3x, April 13, 2020)

Interestingly, some social media users practiced their "quarantine vigilantes" on Twitter. For example, a tweet by @VRG_Ray compared two photos of shopping streets on April 4. One shows Harajuku, popular among the young, and the other shows Sugamo, popular among the old. Harajuku was less crowded while Sugamo was more crowded in the photos. The poster of the tweet then wrote, "The difference between the old people who don't understand the seriousness of the situation and the young people with a sense of crisis." This tweet accuses the old people of not staying at home and was retweeted more than 17,000 and 43,000 liked. At that time, there was strong criticism of the youth on TV which showed many young people walking around shopping streets. His media practice could be thought to criticize such mainstream media discourse.

The media practice as quarantine vigilantes was shared between wide audiences and Twitter users. This was enabled by the emotional regime of anxiety, fear, and anger. During the first wave of the pandemic, the act of quarantine vigilantes escalated. Later, it developed to social media bashing and flaming of the infected people. It is impossible to verify who first started these acts of quarantine vigilantes. This is because the contents of wide-shows are often influenced by social media information. However, this resonance between wide-shows and social media shows that the emotional regime of anxiety, fear, and anger was widely shared in Japanese society in the analyzed period.

Media as Risk and "Politics of Emotion"

As shown above, the "Morning Show" contributed to constructing the emotional regime and sharing it with broad audiences, and the audiences such as the Twitter users responded to the program with emotions such as "anxiety," "fear," and "anger." The emotional regime, which is composed of "anxiety," "fear," and "anger," subsequently conditioned media practices. Moreover, it also helped to condition people's political process. For example, around March 2020 when the pandemic approached and threatened daily life, criticism of the administration became more salient on social media. From April to May 2020, there was a spin-off development of emotions of "anxiety," "fear," and "anger" evolved into hashtag activism on Twitter; it developed into the other social movement on social media against the bill to amend the Public Prosecutor's Office Act.[3]

This emotional regime not only conditioned media practices and the political process but also restricted people's understanding and interpretation of the COVID-19 pandemic. It led to affect the government's countermeasures as well as activate media and political distrust among people. In a sense, the emotional regime constructed amid a risk gave rise to new risk.

The chapter has also suggested that social media users do not distinguish between wide-shows and news broadcasting. This implies that the category of "news" has become ambiguous. Social media users do not pay attention to the significant difference between the information and the professionally edited news reporting; they do not care if there is any. In other words, there is no distinction between commentators' comments, social media tweets, and news produced by professional journalists. Responses to the program suggested that some showed sympathy with the commentators and fully accepted the ideas and thoughts shown in the program, while some showed antipathy against the "Morning Show" and strongly rejected it. It implies that the audiences believed in what they wanted to believe. This situation had the potential to develop into a risk of increasing media distrust and making the politics of emotions more difficult to control.

This risk could promote a "post-truth" situation, as McIntyre (2018) describes. Although Japan does not see any particular kind of system of disinformation as it has in the US, it has experienced a "post-truth" situation in its way. The professional journalism of the mainstream media has lost the influence that they enjoyed in the past. There is a growing tendency that people regard information from wide-shows and the Internet as "news." A hybrid media system contributes to the construction of an emotional regime of anxiety, anger, and fear in society. Thus, in the post-COVID-19 society, the politics of emotion in a hybrid media system would be more important than before.

Conclusion

This chapter has demonstrated that the emotional regime, which consists of "anxiety," "anger," and "fear," was constructed by the complex practices of mainstream media and social media in the hybrid media system during the pandemic of COVID-19. Our analysis has demonstrated that emotions promoted behavioral change and contributed to the suppression of the first wave of the pandemic in Japan. At the same time, however, these emotions could contribute to causing social division and discrimination, which in turn stimulate political dissent. Political dissent they have stimulated turned into dissatisfaction with how the government handled the pandemic and other issues and led to the resignation of two cabinets. In this way, the pandemic as a risk activated the "politics of emotion" in Japan.

This chapter has also illuminated that the media is deeply involved in the politics of emotions, and the contemporary hybrid media environment has activated the interaction between mainstream media and social media. The function of the media in the politics of emotions is ambivalent to the solution to the pandemic. The media amplified emotions generally played a significant role in suppressing the first wave of COVID-19, while those emotions also promoted distrust of politics and the mainstream media. As a result, risk communication messages—how people should behave during the pandemic and deal with the novel coronavirus—have become increasingly difficult to convey; once being set their mind to COVID-19 during the first wave, it got increasingly difficult for them to change it afterward. This is exactly the hidden power of the "politics of emotions" which is uncontrollable and undecidable.

Notes

1 There was no significant bias in the age group of those who don't stay at home. Although the vaccination coverage as of July was more than 30% of the total population, most of them were the elderly.
2 The percentage of people who have completed their second vaccination in Japan is 77.8% on December 24, 2021 (Prime Minister's Office in Japan, 2021).
3 In April 2020, the Abe administration introduced the amendment to the parliament aiming at allowing prosecutors to extend their retirement age. This amendment was seen as an unjustified intervention in the judiciary by the administration but failed to be realized in the end.

References

Asia Pacific Initiatives. (2020). *Shingata korona taiou minkanrinji chousakai: chousa kenkyu houkokusho [The Independent Investigation Commission on the Japanese Government's Response to COVID-19: Report on Best Practices and Lessons Learned]*. Discover.

Bennett, W. L., & Livingston, S. (2018). The disinformation order: Disruptivecommunication and the decline of democratic institutions. *European Journal of Communication, 33*(2), 122–139. https://doi.org/10.1177/0267323118760317

Chadwick, A. (2017). *The hybrid media system: Politics and power (Second edition)*. Oxford University Press.

Dahlgren, P. (2018). Media knowledge and trust: The deepening epistemic crisis ofdemocracy. *Javnost-the Public, 25*(1–2), 20–27. https://doi.org/10.1080/13183222.2018.1418819

Institute for Information and Communications Policy. (2020). *Reiwa gannen do joho tsushin media no riyou jikan to joho kodo ni kansuru chousa houkoku sho [FY2020 Survey Report on Usage Time of Communication Media and Information Behavior]*. Ministry of Internal Affairs and Communications, Institute for Information and Communications Policy. https://www.soumu.go.jp/main_content/000708015.pdf

Jiji Press News. (2020, April 5). *N.Y. doctor alarmed by virus situation in Tokyo*. https://sp.m.jiji.com/english/show/4054

McIntyre, L. (2018). *Post-truth*. MIT Press.

Ministry of Health, Labour and Welfare. (2021). Shingata korona wakuchin no sesshu jisseki ni tsuite (4 gatsu 9 noka made) [Results of the novel coronavirus vaccination (till April 9, 2021)]. https://www.mhlw.go.jp/stf/seisakunitsuite/bunya/vaccine_sesshujisseki.html

Ministry of Health, Labour and Welfare. (2022). Opun data, shinki yousei sha suu no suii (nichi betsu) [Open data, newly confirmed cases (Daily)]. UpToDate. Retrieved January 1, 2022, from https://www.mhlw.go.jp/stf/covid-19/open-data.html

Mouffe, C. (2005). *On the Political*. Routledge.

Nanasawa, K., Higashiyama, K., & Takahashi, K. (2021). Shingata korona uirusu ha donoyou ni tsutae raretaka: terebi to social media no renkan no naka de [dai 2 bu] PCR kensa terebi no "gidai settei" to Twitter no hannou [How television reported COVID-19: Looking at the correlation between television and social media [Part II] PCR testing: 'agenda setting' by broadcasters and reaction on twitter]. *The NHK Monthly Report on Broadcast Research, 71*(1), 24–61.

Omi, S., & Oshitani, H. (2020, June 1). Japan's COVID-19 response [English version of press conference presentation slide on May 29, 2020]. Press Conference of Government Advisory Panel on COVID-19. Ministry of Health, Labour and Welfare. https://www.mhlw.go.jp/content/10900000/000635891.pdf

Prime Minister's Office in Japan. (2020). Avoid the "three Cs"! https://www.kantei.go.jp/jp/content/000061935.pdf

Prime Minister's Office in Japan. (2021). Shingata korona wakuchin ni tsuite [On vaccination of the novel coronavirus]. UpToDate. Retrieved December 28, 2021 from https://www.kantei.go.jp/jp/headline/kansensho/vaccine.html

Reddy, W. (2001). *The Navigation of Feeling: A Framework for the History of Emotions*. Cambridge University Press.

Takahashi, K., & Hara, Y. (2020). "Shingata korona uirusu" ha donoyou ni tsutaeraretaka—terebi to social media no renkan no nakade—[dai 1 bu] data de souransuru houdou to toukou no 200 nichi [How television reported COVID-19: Looking at the correlation between television and social media [Part I] Summarizing the 200 days of reports and posts through data]. *The NHK Monthly Report on Broadcast Research*, *70*(12), 2–35.

Tokyo Metropolitan Government. (2020a). Koike chiji "chiji no heya"/ kisha kaiken (reiwa 2 nen 3 gatsu 23 nichi) [Governor Koike "governor's office" /press conference (March 23, 2020)]. https://www.metro.tokyo.lg.jp/tosei/governor/governor/kishakaiken/2020/03/23.html

Tokyo Metropolitan Government. (2020b). Koike chiji "chiji no heya"/ kisha kaiken (reiwa 2 nen 3 gatsu 25 nichi) [Governor Koike "governor's office"/ press conference (March 25, 2020)]. https://www.metro.tokyo.lg.jp/tosei/governor/governor/kishakaiken/2020/03/25.html

Wahl-Jorgensen, K. (2019). *Emotions, Media and Politics*. Polity.

9 Coronationalism in the Risk Society

The Nationalist Discourses of Taiwanese Professional Baseball during the Outbreak of COVID-19

Chang-de Liu

Introduction: COVID-19, Nationalism, and Baseball in Taiwan

Coronavirus disease 2019 (COVID-19), which outbroke in Wuhan (China) in mid-January 2020, has impacted all aspects of daily human lives globally. Within only three months, confirmed cases worldwide had increased to more than 118,000 in 114 countries, and on March 11, 2020, the World Health Organization (WHO) announced that the disease was characterized as a pandemic (WHO, 2020). Most people around the world had experienced the threat of COVID-19, including rising deaths and health risks, lockdown and disrupted routines, economic hardship and pressures, etc. As the result, racial attacks and discrimination against Chinese and Asians break out in many countries around the world during the pandemic era (BBC News Chinese, 2020).

As the pandemic got worse in 2020, racism and nationalism had been spurred by the outbreak around the world. Combining the two words—coronavirus and nationalism—into a compound word "coronationalism" in his commentary, Colijn (2020), a senior research fellow of international relations think tank in the Netherlands, described how the US and the European countries in early 2020 taking protectionism policies for national sovereignty rather than multilateralism for global cooperation. Later, a Belgian politician, Cindy Franssen, also referred to the term, coronationalism, in a commentary to criticize the far-right parties for spreading misinformation about the pandemic (Ozkirimli, 2020).

Pandemic often triggers the rise of exclusionary nationalism, the rise of racism, and the emergence of authoritarian politics. COVID-19 is highly relevant to issues of race and international politics, including naming the disease as "Chinese virus" by politicians in many countries, the controversy over whether the origin of the virus is China or the US, and the extremely inequality in vaccine distribution between the Global North and Global South (Rogers et al., 2020; Oxfam, 2021). Prevent policies of COVID-19, such as lockdowns and mandatory vaccinations, have greatly affected the daily lives of ordinary people in many countries. Fear and aversion to viruses "from other countries" reinforced biases and stereotypes about migrants and minorities. Moreover, restrictions on human rights, such as freedom of movement and temporarily closing the national border, have

DOI: 10.4324/9781003286684-9

resulted in politics of fear, which have become breeding grounds for far-right political parties and authoritarian regimes (Bieber, 2020).

In Taiwan, the pandemic has intensified political and military tensions with China and worsened the conflicts of national and political identities. Different political camps—mainly depending on different attitudes toward China—opposed each other in many controversies, for instance, the official mandarin name for the disease is still "Wuhan Pneumonia" (武漢肺炎) in Taiwan; the "Xiaoming controversy" (小明事件) over whether the children of Taiwanese businessmen who lived in China could return at the beginning of the outbreak; the debate about changing the name of China Airlines, which was responsible for delivering masks to allied countries in order to implement the government's "epidemic prevention diplomacy" (Tsai et al., 2020).

While lockdown and border control had become routine around the world, Taiwan was comparatively "successful" in controlling the virus transmission by the early response—such as tightly regulating travel, rigorous contact tracing, technology-enforced quarantine, and universal mask-wearing—and thus achieved a record of more than 250 days without a locally transmitted case from April 12 to December 22 (Bloomberg, 2020). The relatively effective disease prevention by the public health authority in 2020 had led to a sense of "national pride" in Taiwan. The government's strategy to enhance national identity and facilitate nation-building through pandemic prevention has ignited nationalism during the COVID-19 period (Tsai, 2020).

Many important sports events were canceled or postponed due to the COVID-19 pandemic at the beginning of 2020. However, Taiwanese professional sports—the Chinese Professional Baseball League (CPBL)—started on April 12 and became the first and the "only" professional baseball season in the world till Korean professional baseball resumed on May 5. Less than one month later—before the opening of Japanese and American professional baseball on June 19 and July 24, respectively—CPBL opened ballparks to spectators on May 8, the world's first sporting games with live attendances at that time. While the COVID-19 pandemic "lockdown" sporting events around the world, Taiwan's success in containing the COVID-19 pandemic provided the local baseball a rare opportunity for international exposure. The CPBL launched its first-time English-language online streaming via Twitter, and the broadcasting of each game attracted more than one million viewers worldwide, especially those from the US where the Major League Baseball (MLB) games were postponed. Taiwanese baseball, therefore, has become a national pride that represents the achievement of preventing the pandemic.

Therefore, coronationalism in Taiwan during the era of the pandemic is different from its counterparts in European and North American societies. Coronavirus nationalism in Western countries is characterized by racial discrimination, xenophobia, and deglobalization. However, because of the history of diplomatic isolation and the need to seek international recognition, Taiwan's coronationalism represented a certain degree of national anxiety to be recognized and accepted by international society, especially by developed countries like the US and Japan, as well as seeking to integrate into globalization.

Through examining the international promotion of Taiwanese professional baseball (the Chinese Professional Baseball) during the COVID-19 era, this research is aimed at exploring the characteristics of sport nationalism in the world risk society. The "Coro-nationalism" in Taiwan baseball could be regarded as a nexus to understand the relationship between international conflicts and nationalism in the globalization age, as well as to further explore the sociological understanding of the pandemic in the world risk society.

Literature Review

Diseases, Nationalism, and the World Risk Society

There is a strong correlation between disasters or diseases and ethnic or national conflicts. For example, racist theories of black biological inferiority were prevailing during the 1918 pandemic (often referred to as the Spanish flu) as African Americans had a higher proportion of the cases and deaths, which in fact resulted from their low income and the lack of medicine and sustainable public health system (Gamble, 2010; Brooks, 2020).

Beck et al. (1994: vii) emphasize, "what is 'natural' is now so thoroughly entangled with what is 'social' that there can be nothing taken for granted about it anymore." The development of natural science is highly influenced and shaped by political and economic power. The risk society, which has been formed by modernity, is full of crises and disasters, such as ecological or financial risks, beyond human control. Furthermore, nationalist sentiments and xenophobia have been aroused as global crises were uncontrollable by international governmental bodies (Beck, 1996; Zhou, 2021).

The issues of diseases and pandemics such as COVID-19 are a socially constructed process rather than merely scientific or public health debates. In East Asian developing countries, the development of biotechnology has related to nation-building and identity. For example, Gottweis and Kim (2010) argue that the South Korean government mobilized the public to support the stem cell study project and constructed an emerging "bionationalism" that exceeded traditional ethnic nationalism in reshaping Korean identity and national economic prospects. The governments of developing countries usually attempted to form a consensus among citizens, namely "communities of fate," to overcome the national crisis of epidemics or diseases (Ong & Chen, 2010).

Coronationalism or "Covid nationalism" has emerged in European and North American societies, as evidenced by the anti-restriction and anti-vaccination protests that blend viral conspiracy theories with patriotism. In the global political economy context of the US–China conflict in recent years, the coronavirus, China, the United Nations, the WHO, and transnational technology corporations, have become the enemies of right-wing groups, and "deglobalization" has also become the target of far-right politics and exclusionary nationalism (Juergensmeyer, 2020).

In the pandemic prevention policy in the UK, for example, Fitzgerald (2022) points out that the discourse formed by public health experts and scholars focused on border control and framed the issues centered on national conflict and nationalism. What he called "viral nationalism" regards national border controls as the primary battleground for controlling COVID infections; therefore, it ignored the need for involuntary international traffic of migrants and refugees. In order to ensure domestic safety, viral nationalism is "at least occasional recourse to forms of rhetoric, metaphor, and imagery that are violent, militaristic, or dehumanizing."

In early 2021, high-income countries, which account for 16% of the global population, purchased up to 60% of the world's vaccines. Vaccination rates in the high-income and upper-middle-income countries had reached 85%, while those in low-income countries were only 1%. Inequalities in the distribution of vaccines between rich and poor countries represented the transition of globalization. In the open market of vaccines, the rich countries of the Global North control the vaccine. High-income countries monopolized limited-production doses of vaccines in order to ensure domestic need. The race to acquire and reserve as more amount of new vaccines as possible for domestic use constitutes "vaccine nationalism" (Zhou, 2021). Paradoxically, vaccine (or viral) nationalism and protectionism in rich countries resulted in the globalization of the virus because most people of the Global South have been excluded from the protection of full vaccination. Global conflicts between the rich and poor countries, thus, have become worse during the pandemic period (Zhou, 2021; Mittelman, 2021).

The unequal distribution of COVID-19 vaccines has deepened the contradictions and conflicts between countries and the trend of deglobalization. Global public health governmental bodies such as the United Nations and the WHO are unable to control the crisis due to geopolitical conflicts, insufficient financial resources, and lack of enforcement power. People in poor countries have been put into the dilemma of insufficient vaccine prevention; therefore, the threat of COVID-19 has been continuing on a global scale.

Moreover, vaccine and virus nationalism have also been influenced by geopolitics, that is, the political and economic confrontations between the US and China since the 2010s. China was the epicenter of the outbreak at the end of 2019, while later the US had most infections and deaths caused by pandemic 2020. Therefore, the R&D and distribution of vaccines have become a battleground between the two world powers and reinforcing protectionism, populism, authoritarianism, and racism around the world, rather than a "world village" or multilateralism for cooperation and mutual interests (Zhou, 2021).

National identity, on the one hand, is often formed and reproduced or invented by formal social institutions, rituals, symbols, and traditions. On the other hand, nationalism is also constructed and mobilized through discourses among elites and ordinary people (Anderson, 1983; Hobsbawm, 1983). In the process of national building, mass media have played an important role. News coverage and commentaries on national newspapers, for example, draw cultural and political boundaries between us and others for the imagined community. Under the threats of risks such as disasters and diseases, media discourse has also become an important field for reproducing collective identity and the so-called "coronationalism" or viral nationalism.

For example, following the European Union banned British beef imports to prevent "mad cow disease" (CJD/BSE: Creutzfeldt-Jakob Disease and Bovine Spongiform Encephalopathy) in 1996, xenophobia and nationalist sentiments permeated the UK mass media, especially in tabloid newspapers. In the coverages of the final four of the Euro '96 football championships, in which England played against Germany, the British popular press portrayed the opponent football team as the Nazi German militaries in World War II, provoking historical war hatred. The anti-European discourse on mass media drew the line between "us" (the UK) and "other" (European Union) and reproduced the stereotype of Germany. The tabloids emphasized conflicts between British society and European countries and escalated the public health crisis into risk and threat to the local beef industry and national economy (Brookes, 1999).

During the COVID-19 era, media in the US and Korea have also represented and mutually shaped national identity in the two countries, respectively. A comparative study found that liberal and conservative news media in both countries used a similar strategy to construct the image of the major "other," China, during the pandemic. Both liberal and conservative media in the US identify "Us" as a powerful nation-state. In the context of political and economic confrontation with China in recent years, both liberal and conservative media regard China as the racial "Other," who is "secretive, corrupt, and insidious." Meanwhile, conservative media in the US are more inclined to depict China as "an evil communist regime that is hyper-ambitious." The threat of COVID-19 evoked a sentiment of national pride and crisis in South Korea. Conservative media criticized China, a "rogue state," for manipulating information about the coronavirus in the outbreak, which is the main reason for the global spread of COVID-19, and denounced the liberal government for hesitating to blame China's cover-up of the disease. Nevertheless, liberal media were inclined to praise the government's effective prevention policies and depict South Korea as a "model state" outperforming China and Western countries in handling the pandemic crisis. For liberal newspapers, Korean people are proud of controlling the spread of the virus without lockdown or travel restrictions, as well as the ability to help other countries with mask donation and medical support (Chung et al., 2021).

As the international governing bodies are unable to respond to cross-border global risks, such as diseases and disasters, racism and exclusionary nationalism have prevailed around the world, which led to the unequal distribution of vaccines and intensified geopolitical conflicts between superpower states, China and the US. During the pandemic era, the media played a critical role in the cultural construction of imagined communities by distinguishing "others" from "us." On the one hand, coronationalism creates a positive self-image that contributed to national identity; on the other hand, nationalist discourses and sentiments are inclined to regard the "enemy" or "other" as another nation, immigrants, minority groups, etc., rather than virus or diseases.

Sports, National Identity, and Globalization

Since the nineteenth century, the sport has become an effective vehicle for molding collective national identity. International sports events or contests manifest national pride and glory, constituting an ideal propaganda showcase of official nationalism whereby patriotism is mobilized. As a society facing a splitting identity crisis, such as Northern Ireland and Catalonia, sport's nationalistic linkage has become a two-edged sword. It carries the cultural mission of consolidating a unified national identity constructed by the central government. Yet political separationists also seek to nationalize a local team to claim political independence. Scotland and the Northern Ireland football players hardly fight for their British nationality. A Catalonian team and its Spanish compatriot can become adversaries (Bariner, 2001; Maguire, Jarvie, Mansfield & Bardley, 2002). National glory, in these cases, is played out at odds with the ascribed nationalities. In the globalizing landscape of the cultural economy, sports join a number of centrifugal cultural forces contributing to the disjuncture of the nation from the state.

The discursive struggle of sporting nationalism also reflects the changing role of the nation-state in the globalizing flow of transnational capital. Hardt and Negri (2000) argue for the emergence of a global media empire, whose existence no longer relies on territorial annexation or colonization. A new global empire wins over the government and its people in consensus, fine-tuning, and micromanaging to the appeal of national or cultural identities of diverse regions, yet in general in keeping with the requirement of the globalizing logic of capital.

The phenomenon of the so-called "new international division of cultural labor" (NICL) characterizes this new model of imperial expansion. By recruiting talented, but underpaid athletes from various parts of the world, professional sports leagues such as those in the US have effectively reduced costs on labor output. Furthermore, trans-border recruitment helped expand the US sport's international market as the already broad national fanbase of the migrant athletes was also taken over (Miller et al., 2003).

National identity was appropriated as a segmentation strategy of commodification by the transnational sports capital, a spinoff product promoting "corporate nationalism" (Silk, Andrews, & Cole, 2005), such as the collaboration of New Zealand yachting clubs with local and multinational corporations (John & Jackson, 2010), or Nike's promotional finesse by articulating its product image with traditional Japanese sports (Kobayashi, 2011). In these cases, patriotism finds the perfect avatar in national sports teams through the magic hand of commercial branding. National identity is brought under the sway of transnational capital.

To those nations exporting players overseas, transnational capital also impacted the way baseball's national tradition is constructed. With Korean players being enrolled in the MLB, the media's sports coverage in South Korea began emphasizing such aspects as individual performance, global competition, and the responsibility of mercenary players to their mother nation. The commoditization logic of neo-liberal globalization also dictates that Korea's colonization past be conscripted to the increment of the lure of the game. In MLB's World Baseball Classic, the Korean/Japanese matchup tends to be underlined with an overtone of anti-colonial rivalry. The commercialization of historic colonial violence ultimately serves the interests of MLB and its corporate sponsors. Yet the provoked anti-Japanese sentiment amounts to a re-colonization of the collective consciousness (Cho, 2008; Lee, 2012). As many elite Taiwanese baseball players attempted to pursue their career in the MLB, the American professional baseball has successfully expanded its labor pool and market in Taiwan since the mid-2000s. Meanwhile, the perspective of global capitalism that defines "self" and "others" by the MLB—the core of global baseball—has dominated the Taiwanese sports field. The nationalist discourse of Taiwanese baseball regards MLB as the center or the highest arena and praises all the efforts of local elite athletes to migrate into the transnational baseball industry, including MLB and NPB (Liu, 2008).

While dominated by political power in the past, discursive struggles in the field of national sports have usually been characterized by the conflicts between official and civic nationalist discourses or between the different political identities. Nowadays sports nationalism in the age of global capitalism has also become a tool for transnational corporations to increase their markets on a global scale. Meanwhile, the worldview of local sports fans has gradually been impacted by global sports industries as a cultural consequence of globalization.

Nationalist Discourse about the CPBL Games during the Pandemic

COVID-19 as a global crisis has intensified nationalism and racism in the media around the world. Sports events during the pandemic have become a center for the cultural construction of imagined community—that is, the nation-state. In order to understand the characteristics of Taiwanese nationalism in the pandemic era, this study examines the media representations of the international exposure of CPBL in the outbreak of COVID-19. A total of 285 news articles in three mainstream newspapers between April 12 and May 12 are collected through online databases—180 reports from *The Liberty Times* (自由時報), 72 from *The United Daily News* (聯合報), and 33 from *The Apple Daily* (蘋果日報), respectively. Through discourse analysis, this study illustrates how the nationalist news coverage of the global risk shape local identity, as well as the public understanding of disease and sport.

The Whole World Is Watching: Pandemic Prevention and Baseball as the National Glory

In the early days of the 2020 pandemic, both pandemic prevention and professional baseball emerged as the national glory identified collectively throughout Taiwan primarily through two interrelated discourse strategies. First, acceptance and recognition from the US, Japan, and European countries have always been the long-term need of the Taiwanese government and society. Due to China's oppression, Taiwan has encountered diplomatic isolation—that is, being unable to be recognized as a country for many years—and by 2021 less than 15 countries have diplomatic relations with Taiwan. Therefore, foreign media reports on Taiwan's pandemic prevention and CPBL games have become a symbol of "the whole world is watching Taiwan."

Second, by associating professional baseball with the nation's success and international reputation in containing the COVID-19 pandemic, the nationalist discourses during the pandemic have formed the CPBL games as "a national pride" and Taiwan as "a community against the viral threat." Local media tended to connect the success of virus prevention with the achievement of being "the first nation to open its professional baseball season amid global lockdowns."

Because of the relatively successful control of the pandemic, the opening season of CPBL in April 2020 highlighted Taiwan as "the first country to start a professional baseball season during the global lockdown," attracting the attention of the international press. Local media translated the dispatch from foreign news agencies or foreign media reports, as well as collected and edited Tweets from US and Japanese baseball writers, commentators, and fans, "The whole world is watching our games." The media reports emphasized that the media of various countries were keeping eyes on Taiwan (Apple Daily, 2020a), and even the negative images and events, such as the bench-clearing clash between the two teams due to a hit-by-pitch, were also stressed to be "seen by the world" (Lo, 2020b).

In this topic of coverage, attention from well-known foreign media often became the focus. For example, the reports from US or Japanese news organizations:

> Taiwan is the only country where professional baseball events are still being held under the COVID-19 pandemic. CPBL games attracted more and more international media's attention. CNN has joined the ranks, with its coverage pointing out that Taiwan's successful containment of the pandemic has enabled the opening season of CPBL to be commenced. CPBL seize this opportunity to strengthen its broadcast capacity to enable the whole world to watch the game simultaneously.
>
> (Wu, M., 2020b)

> The Japanese baseball columnist Hideyoshi Komada, who is based in Taiwan, gave an in-depth introduction of Taiwan's successful containment of the pandemic, the professional baseball operation model, and the players' aspirations in his article, detailing CPBL's successful experience of holding its season-opening under a global public health crisis, which made headlines on Japan's Yahoo baseball page.
>
> (Wang & Wang, 2020)

As the only professional baseball continuing "play-ball" around the world at that time, CPBL became the focus of the international media and was magnified into a symbol of Taiwan's international recognition. For example, the former general manager of the MLB's LA Dodgers expressed "being happy" about the exposure that CPBL and Taiwan received. The news report quoted his post in which he regarded Taiwan as a "country."

> Dan Evans, the former Dodgers general manager, retweeted the news on Liberty Times Sports that CPBL games had reached 5.25 million overseas views, and wrote: "Taiwan is such a great nation, and baseball is vibrant there […] The nation is beautiful, and I love its culture."
>
> (Liberty Times, 2020i)

A report in *The New York Times* was translated by Taiwanese media and featured Taiwanese professional baseball as a "national pride":

> The Taiwanese government's successful containment of the pandemic has allowed CPBL to take the lead in the world to start its season. As a result, CPBL was featured in *The New York Times*, in which its article mentioned that CPBL has become the pride of the Taiwanese and a symbol of success in the fight against the pandemic.
>
> (Liberty Times, 2020n)

Taiwan's long-term predicament about not being "recognized" by other countries diplomatically has been compensated by the "recognition" of various national symbols by the international media during the pandemic:

> Bloomberg Taipei Bureau Chief, Samson Ellis, posted a short clip at Xinzhuang Baseball Stadium (新莊球場) on Twitter, sharing with the world the precious experience such as the bat hitting the baseball and the cheers of the audience. Ellis said: "That sound baseball fans all over the world have been missing. Life in Taiwan slowly gets back to normal with the first pro baseball game with fans back in the stadium." […] The website of the South China Morning Post, an English-language newspaper in Hong Kong, used a video provided by Reuters to present the live broadcast of a Taiwanese baseball game, with a huge national flag unfurled in the outfield by the Republic of China Armed Forces.
>
> (Central News Agency, 2020; see Chang, 2020; Ellis, 2020)

The English-language anchor who broadcasts the CPBL game also noted that "This is also a way for Taiwan to show itself to the world." Therefore, the significance of CPBL's game broadcast to Taiwan is not limited to baseball; instead, it is an opportunity for the international promotion of Taiwan's culture and country:

> I hope that after watching the CPBL game, foreign audiences can have a better picture and understand Taiwan bit by bit," Richard Wang added […]

Wayne McNeil said, "[…] everything is a great exposure opportunity for Taiwan, which is bigger than baseball itself.

(Liberty Times, 2020o)

After the first step of "Taiwan-being-seen," the next step is to emphasize Taiwan's "world number one" status both in pandemic prevention and in professional baseball. The success of pandemic containment was the "pride" of Taiwanese society at the time. For example, the Canadian media reported that foreign players lauded the effectiveness of local pandemic prevention (Liberty Times, 2020h), and Reuters was "amazed" by Taiwan's pandemic prevention strategies and used "Number 1" as its article title:

Reuters also noted in a special report today that CPBL and Taiwan Football Premier League are kicking off as scheduled, which is an invaluable moment for fans […] Taiwan has successfully contained the spread of the virus […] The Taiwan Football Premier League will start on the 12th […] The opening game of CPBL, which was originally scheduled to start on April 11, was postponed due to the rain. The match between CTBC Brothers and Uni-Lions on the 12th will become the first game of all professional baseball leagues around the world.

(Liberty Times, 2020a)

The local media's description of "world number one" also includes other details in the game, such as the CPBL's first home run in the world's professional baseball in 2020, describing the pitcher in the opposing team as a "top player of the world" who used to play in the MLB:

Kai-Wen Cheng, an outfielder with the Uni-Lions, hit the world's first meaningful home run of the year. The pitcher who served up was Ariel Miranda, who spent parts of three seasons in the MLB with the Seattle Mariners and Baltimore Orioles.

(Wu, C., 2020; see Anderson, 2020)

As the world's number one, CPBL has become the hope of baseball fans worldwide. For example, a commentator of the MLB's Baltimore Orioles remarked in a Twitter post that they must "rely on CPBL to get through the COVID-19 period" (Liberty Times, 2020e), quoting the US media's commentary on Taiwan's professional baseball as a "new hope for baseball fans":

A news article in *Time* magazine wrote, […] "there's new hope for fans sorely missing America's past-time. They merely need to look across the world to Taiwan, where the island's Chinese Professional Baseball League played the first Opening Day ballgame of the 2020 season on April 11."

(Su, 2020; see Zennie, 2020)

When South Korea's professional baseball, the KBO, resumed without live spectators in May, Taiwan's professional baseball is once again the first in the world to kick off its games with live spectators. News reports highlighted how this "world's first" achievement attracted the attention of foreign media:

> Taiwan announced that it will allow live spectators to watch CPBL matches again from the 8th, a feat that is the first in the world, attracting approximately 200 domestic and foreign journalists to apply for interviews. This will become the focus of world-class sports events.
>
> (Wong, 2020)

There are even reports that listed the news coverages from foreign media at the time, referring to them as Taiwan's "micro-propaganda":

> The Boston Globe interviewed English anchors, Richard Wang and Chien-Ming Wang, about the pride and glory of Taiwan. ESPN published an interview with Josh Roenicke of Uni-Lion; Japan's *Nikkan Sports* published a series of stories with 12 CPBL cheerleaders yesterday, and *The Sankei Sports* published the news story of Xinzhuang Baseball Stadium's support for the Koshien History Museum. Recently, there will also be reports on CPBL in *The New York Times* and *Sports Illustrated*. Zhao-Ru Chen, the deputy leader of Fubon Guardians, said, "This is CPBL's micro-propaganda for Taiwan."
>
> (Hsieh, 2020)

Conflicting Identities and Renaming the CPBL

Due to the rare international attention that CPBL gained, its English name (Chinese Professional Baseball League) has repeatedly confused foreign fans and players who mistake CPBL for a professional baseball league in China. Thus, political leaders, sports fans, and the media began debating the issue of renaming CPBL. During the pandemic, the debate reflected the conflict between different national identities in Taiwan, as well as the confrontation between the pro-China and anti-China political camps.

The anti-independence/pro-unification/pan-Blue (which is called 統派 or 泛藍) and pro-independence/anti-China/pan-Green (which is called 獨派 or 泛綠) media, subsequently, respectively, promoted their political perspectives in news reports about this controversy. Despite their considerably different positions, both factions adopted similar discourse strategies. These nationalist discourses drew the boundary of "others" and "us" and distinguished "enemies" from "companions." The anti-independence/pro-China media saw both the Taiwanese government and those who support the renaming campaign as "others" and portrayed them as "irrational" and "far-politicized" fanatics. Conversely, the anti-China/pro-independence discourse emphasized that "our" Taiwanese baseball and public health system are "for all people" and "civilized" and, therefore, differ from "others" such as the Chinese "uncivilized" regime and society.

After the CPBL kicked off on April 12, it attracted the attention of US baseball critics, leading to many reports that "mistook" it for originating from China. For example, Jeffrey Bellone, a columnist for the sports website FanSided, mistook the "Chinese Professional Baseball League" for the "China Professional Baseball League" (Liberty Times, 2020d). Even the agent of the retired MLB star Manny Ramirez, who played for the CPBL for six months in 2013, mistook the CPBL for a league in China (Chen, 2020a). These misunderstandings led to corrections from various sources, including the Taiwanese president, on social media:

> Despite the international attention gained by the CPBL, some foreign media mistakenly presented that the game was held in China. The US baseball writer Jared Carrabis retweeted a video of CPBL on Twitter and wrote "We are playing Baseball in China," and was immediately corrected that the actual location was in Taiwan. President Ing-Wen Tsai also posted on Facebook: "The CPBL is Taiwan's Baseball League."
>
> (Wu, C., 2020)

Even naming "China" in the news coverage is significantly different among the different political camps. Most pro-China or Pan-Blue (泛藍) newspapers referred to China as Mainland China (中國大陸) or Mainland (大陸) in their headlines (Lan, 2020), whereas most anti-China or Pan-Green (泛綠) newspapers directly used China in their headlines and referred to our country as Taiwan instead of Republic of China (Liberty Times, 2020k).

The political differences in the use of words by the media with different political positions can also be seen in naming the disease. As the earliest case and large-scale pandemic involving COVID-19 were first reported in Wuhan, China, in early 2020, the Chinese-language media in China, Taiwan, and other regions referred to it as "Wuhan pneumonia." However, to avoid discrimination, the World Health Organization requested that pandemics not be named with geographical or country names. Therefore, after March 2020, Chinese media began to refer to COVID-19 as "corona pneumonia" (新冠肺炎) or "coronavirus" (新冠病毒). However, the Taiwanese government and anti-China media still referred to COVID-19 as "Wuhan pneumonia" or "*wufei*"(武肺) for short by 2022 (Lin, 2020).

In addition to the differences in word usage, most reports by the anti-independence media described the proposal of renaming CPBL as "unnecessary" and "irrational." On the second day of the CPBL's opening, *The United Daily News*, an anti-independence newspaper, reported that

> CPBL's Secretary-General Sheng-Hsien Feng stressed that [...] the US media mistook CPBL for a mainland baseball league. He said that as long as everyone is watching CPBL and the league is doing a good job in its publicity, people will know that the CPBL is in Taiwan."
>
> (Lin, 2020)

When the government clearly suggested that CPBL should consider adopting a different name, Chih-Yang Wu, the commissioner of CPBL who was a former KMT politician, firmly responded with his refusal to do so, and *The United Daily News* also emphasized in its headlines that "(the league) is a nongovernmental unit" and "the government should not interfere" (Wu, M., 2020a). The American Institute in Taiwan (AIT) issued an article calling for the CPBL to be renamed TPBL (Taiwan Professional Baseball League) in May, and *The United Daily News* also quoted in its headline the KMT politicians' adoption of Chinese diplomatic vocabularies—"Don't interfere in other country's internal affairs" (Gao, 2020).

On the other hand, when reporting the responses of the CPBL commissioner, the pro-independence *Liberty Time* emphasized in its headline that "China took advantage of the confusing name of CPBL" (Lo, 2020a). In addition to distinguishing the difference between Taiwan and China, *The Liberty Times* also emphasized that the renaming of CPBL is a matter of sovereignty and national interest, which has also won support from the US:

> Playing baseball is an internal affair in that no country has the right to interfere and using the name of Taiwan is justifiable. Although the professional baseball league is a nongovernmental organization, it involves national interests, and the government should not stand idly by and watch. Even AIT suggested that the CPBL should rename as Taiwan Professional Baseball League. The government can no longer refuse to rectify this name for excuses. He further emphasized that CPBL was the first to kick off its season in the world, but because of its name "Chinese Professional Baseball League," it was mistaken for the China Professional Baseball League.
>
> (Wang, 2020)

After live spectators were allowed back to the game in May, *The Apple Daily*, which similarly took an anti-China stance, also emphasized in the report:

> Taiwan's professional baseball [...] today, will be the only one in the world to allow attendance of up to 1,000 for each game. Media from other countries, including the world's three major news agencies, have published special reports on this event. However, the "C" of CPBL, the English abbreviation of the Chinese Professional Baseball League, is often misunderstood as related to "China" while live games were streamed online to world fans in the past month.
>
> (Hsieh et al., 2020)

Imagined Global Communities: The Hierarchy of the Global Baseball System

The nationalist discourse of baseball in Taiwan during the pandemic is an ideology under globalization. While exalting Taiwan's achievements in professional baseball and pandemic prevention, the discourse of coronationalism still regards capitalist centers—such as the US and Japan—as the standard for self-identity. In short, the nationalist narration replicates the hierarchy in baseball's "world system."

Local media emphasized that fans in the US and Japan often use the well-known MLB or Japanese baseball as a metaphor for understanding or introducing CPBL that they were unfamiliar with in the past. For example, a story reported that the US baseball columnist used "Taiwan's Yankees" to introduce the CTBC Brothers or Rakuten Monkeys, or that they referred to the Rakuten Monkeys' game against the Fubon Guardians as the "the New York Yankees versus the Boston Red Sox" (Liberty Times, 2020b; 2020c; 2020q).

Local media also translate how the US and Japan fans understand Taiwanese baseball by "transforming" CPBL players into MLB or NPB figures, such as An-Ke Lin (林安可) of the Uni-Lions as "Taiwan's Ohtani Shohei/大谷翔平" in the eyes of Japanese fans, Jing-Kai Lin (林靖凱) of the Uni-Lions as the Taiwanese Roberto Alomar, or Yu-Hsien Chu (朱育賢) of the Rakuten Monkeys as Aaron Judge (Apple Daily, 2020b; 2020c; Liberty Times, 2020j).

The vision of taking the US as the center of the baseball world system is even more prominent in the controversy over the report that "CPBL's competence or skill level is between the 1A and Advanced A of the Minor League Baseball." Since the era of globalization in the 2000s, Taiwanese media and fans usually employed the MLB system to define the competency of individual countries' baseball. For example, CPBL is positioned at 1A and thus inferior to Japan (better than AAA) and South Korea (roughly at AAA level). However, such perspectives and comparisons are usually limited to Taiwanese baseball commentators and fans. During the pandemic, the major league-centric viewpoints were mentioned again when American journalists introduced CPBL to MLB fans, which was subsequently reported by Taiwanese media. For example, at the end of April, Taiwanese media reprinted a Canadian media report:

> Radio-Canada, the French division of the Canadian Broadcasting Corporation, interviewed [...] Rob Ducey, the Canadian coach for Fubon Guardians [...] (He) said, "Taiwan's skill level is probably equivalent to the AA of the Minor League Baseball. CPBL has many good batters, but the rest are probably at 1A level [...]" This article also mentioned that there are some former MLB pitchers in CPBL [...] Ducey was a previous MLB player with 13 years of experience.
>
> (Liberty Times, 2020g)

Subsequently, in early May, following the opening of the South Korean professional baseball tournament, the US media compared the baseball leagues in South Korea and Taiwan in their reports, leading to more comparisons and discussions about the competency of CPBL. Because the comparisons and comments were from the US, the center of the baseball world system, they garnered attention in Taiwanese media and among baseball fans. The dispute was started by Kyle Glaser, a journalist from the sports magazine *Baseball America*, who noted the MLB's following evaluation of Asian countries such as Japan, South Korea, and Taiwan: "the Japanese professional baseball (NPB) falls between the level of the MLB and AAA, South Korean professional baseball (KBO) is between AA and AAA, and CPBL ranges between 1A and Advanced A" (Liberty Times, 2020l). As KBO began the new season, CPBL gradually lost overseas fans and audiences. Taiwanese media quoted a Twitter post by Clinton Yates, a US baseball commentator, saying, "The opening of KBO… snatched the spotlight from CPBL [...] This is very much like a guy friend I know who looks back and peeks at other pretty girls" to describe the bitter national sentiment (Liberty Times, 2020m; see Yates, 2020).

An outcry of injustice proliferated among the Taiwanese media's nationalist discourse regarding the evaluation of Taiwan's baseball performance being inferior to that of South Korea. Some critics emphasized that a few CPBL batters exceeded the average standard and were equivalent to AAA hitters (Ni, 2020; Liberty Times 2020l). However, it is better to provide a good explanation through "authorities" from the US:

> Glaser wrote, "MLB teams usually signed Taiwanese players when they were amateur athletes, just like those in Dominica and Venezuela. Thus, most of Taiwan's top young players left Taiwan instead of joining CPBL."
>
> (Chen, 2020b)

Furthermore, despite the inferiority of Taiwan's CPBL to South Korea's KBO, Taiwan's baseball still occupies a place in global baseball through the viewing and affirmation of American fans. Through the positioning of the baseball world system, it shows that Taiwan is "accepted" and "recognized" by the global baseball village:

> There are many American fans on Twitter who are still supporting CPBL. ESPN reporter Marly Rivera watched yesterday's game between CTBC Brothers and Uni-Lions on time: "It's the 3rd inning, and the score is 6:4, this is going to be a long game!" A Philadelphia teacher responded, "It's 8:4 in the 4th inning, I think I'll stick with Taiwan's baseball."
>
> (Liberty Times, 2020p)

Despite its inability to surpass South Korea's KBO in its skill evaluation, the viewership and affirmation of US fans is still evidence that Taiwan's CPBL is recognized by the world. For example,

> (a fan in the US) he said the lower quality of the Taiwan league didn't bother him … "I'm not opposed to watching a bad team. I found the sound of the bat to be almost therapeutic" [...] (another fan in the US) [...] said he tuned in, especially because … it was also interesting to see a familiar name in the Guardians' pitcher, Henry Sosa, a former MLB player.
>
> (Liberty Times, 2020f; see Steger, 2020)

Conclusion

As many important sports events were canceled or postponed due to the COVID-19 pandemic at the beginning of 2020, Taiwanese professional sports—the Chinese Professional Baseball League (CPBL)—started in April and became the first and the "only" professional baseball season in the world at that time. Taiwan's success in containing the COVID-19 pandemic provided local baseball a rare opportunity for international exposure. As CPBL launched English-language online streaming via Twitter, Taiwan's baseball suddenly became popular worldwide—the broadcasting of each game attracted more than one million viewers worldwide. Taiwanese baseball, therefore, has become a national glory that represents the achievement of preventing the pandemic.

Through discourse analysis of a total of 285 news articles in three mainstream newspapers between April 12 and May 12, this study illustrates how the nationalist discourse of baseball during the pandemic was characterized. First, by associating professional baseball with the nation's success and international reputation in containing the COVID-19 pandemic, the nationalist discourses during the pandemic have formed the CPBL games as "a national glory" and Taiwan as "a community/country against the viral threat." Local media tended to connect the success of virus prevention with the achievement of being "the first nation to kick off professional baseball season amid global lockdowns." Furthermore, local news reports are inclined to emphasize that "the whole world is watching our games" by translating and reediting foreign media's reports and tweets of sportswriters and fans about CPBL, including those from the US, Japan, Korea, and European countries.

Second, the nationalist discourses during the pandemic reflected the conflict of national identities in Taiwan, as well as different attitudes toward political and military oppressions from China. In news reports about the controversy around "renaming the CPBL"—replacing "Chinese" with "Taiwanese," the results suggest that rival national identities, which are represented by different media, employed similar discursive strategies to distinguish "they/the others" from "we/the selves." The pro-unification/pro-China media regarded the Taiwanese government and supporters of the renaming movement as "the others," who are "irrational" and "far-politicalized." On the contrary, the pro-independence/anti-China discourse regards "our" sporting and medical system as "popular" and "advanced," which should be distinguished from "others," especially from China.

Third, the nationalist discourse during the pandemic also duplicated the global hierarchy, which represents the "world system" of globalization. In order to introduce the CPBL to international baseball fans, news reports usually depicted Taiwanese baseball clubs and players as those famous MLB or Japanese teams and athletes. Moreover, media reports usually defined Taiwanese baseball by the MLB system—positioning the CPBL as "1A" level and inferior to Japan (better than AAA) and Korea (equivalent to AAA). By doing so, Taiwan has been "accepted" and "recognized" by global baseball fans and institutions through integration into the baseball world system—or being incorporated into the MLB global empire.

While racism and xenophobia dominated many societies during the era of the pandemic, which was called "coronationalism," "Covid nationalism," "viral/vaccine nationalism" by critics and scholars, the nationalist discourses about the CPBL games during the outbreak of coronavirus in Taiwan have presented a set of different sentiments and identities. CoroNationalism as a discursive struggle has reinforced the conflicts of contesting national identities in Taiwan, as well as in Taiwanese baseball. These emerging nationalist sentiments during the global risk of the public health crisis, moreover, replicate and represent the anxiety of Taiwanese nationalism that an "isolated" country has expected to be recognized. The nationalist responses to COVID-19 in Taiwan interweave with the global, regional, and local contexts of politics, economy, and culture.

References

Anderson, B. (1983). *Imagined Communities: Reflections on the Origin and Spread of Nationalism*. Verso.

Anderson, R. (2020, April 13). Professional baseball League becomes first to play ball in 2020. CBS. https://www.cbssports.com/mlb/news/actual-baseball-highlights-chinese-professional-baseball-league-becomes-first-to-play-ball-in-2020/

Bairner, A. (2001). *Sport, Nationalism, and Globalization: European and North American Perspectives*. SUNY.

BBC News Chinese. (2020, Feb 11). Coronavirus: Racism widespread over the world. https://www.bbc.com/zhongwen/trad/world-51454984 [In Chinese].

Beck, U. (1996). World risk society as cosmopolitan society? Ecological questions in a framework of manufactured uncertainties. *Theory, Culture & Society, 13*(4), 1–32.

Beck, U., Giddens, A., & Lash, S. (1994) *Reflexive Modernization: Politics, Tradition and Aesthetics in the Modern Social Order*. Polity.

Bieber, F. (2020). Global nationalism in times of the COVID-19 pandemic. *Nationalities Papers, 2020*, 1–13.

Bloomberg. (2020, December 22). World's longest virus-free streak ends with new Taiwan case. https://www.bloomberg.com/news/articles/2020-12-22/world-s-longest-virus-free-streak-ends-as-taiwan-case-emerges

Brookes, R. (1999). Newspapers and national identity: The BSE/CJD crisis and the British Press. *Media, Culture and Society, 21*, 247–263.

Brooks, R. (2020, October 5). Why African Americans Were More Likely to Die During the 1918 Flu Pandemic. *History TV*. Available at: https://www.history.com/news/1918-flu-pandemic-african-americans-healthcare-black-nurses

Chang, Y. (2020, May 9). Taiwan baseball league reopens stadiums to fans. https://www.scmp.com/video/coronavirus/3083616/taiwan-baseball-league-reopens-stadiums-fans

Cho, Y. (2008). The national crisis and de/reconstructing nationalism in South Korea during the IMF intervention. *Inter-Asia Cultural Studies, 9*(1), 82–96.

Chung, A., Jo, H., Lee, J., & Yang, F. (2021). COVID-19 and the political framing of China, nationalism, and borders in the U.S. and South Korean news media. *Sociological Perspectives, 64*(5), 747–764.

Colijn, K. (2020, March 18). Coronationalisme. Available at: https://spectator.clingendael.org/nl/publicatie/coronationalisme

Ellis, S. (2020, May 9). Post on twitter. https://twitter.com/samsonellis/status/1258931691361427456

Fitzgerald, D. (2021). Normal Island: COVID-19, border control, and viral nationalism in UK public health discourse. *Sociological Research Online*. https://doi.org/10.1177/13607804211049464

Gamble, V. N. (2010). "There wasn't a lot of comforts in those days:" African Americans, public health, and the 1918 influenza epidemic. *Public Health Report*, *125*(Suppl 3), 114–122.

Gottweis, H., & Kim, B. (2010) Explaining Hwang-gate: South Korean identity politics between bionationalism and globalization. *Science, Technology, & Human Values*, *35*(4), 501–524.

Hardt, M., & Negri, A. (2000). *Empire*. Harvard University.

Hobsbawm, E. (1983). Mass-producing traditions: Europe, 1870–1914. In Hobsbawm, E. & Ranger, T. (Eds.). *The Invention of Tradition* (pp. 263–307). Cambridge University Press.

John, A., & Jackson, S. (2010). Call me loyal: Globalization, corporate nationalism and the America's Cup. *International Review for the Sociology of Sport*, *46*(4), 399–417.

Juergensmeyer, M. (2020, September 6). Covid nationalism. Available at: https://www.e-ir.info/2020/09/06/covid-nationalism/

Kobayashi, K. (2011). Globalization, corporate nationalism and Japanese cultural intermediaries: Representation of bukatsu through Nike advertising at the global-local nexus. *International Review for the Sociology of Sport*, *47*(6), 724–742.

Lee, J. (2012). Commodifying colonial histories: Korea versus Japan and the re/productions of colonial violence in the World Baseball Classic. *Journal of Sport and Social Issues*, *36*(3), 231–244.

Liu, C. (2008). The development of baseball's international division of labor and the transformation of sporting nationalism in Taiwan. *Taiwan: A Radical Quarterly in Social Studies*, *70*, 33–77. [In Chinese]

Maguire, J., Jarvie, G., Bradley, J., & Mansfield, L. (2002). *Sport Worlds: A Sociological Perspective*. Human Kinetics.

Miller, T., Rowe, D., McKay, J., & Lawrence, G. (2003). The over-production of US sports and the new international division of cultural labor. *International Review for the Sociology of Sport*, *38*(4), 427–440.

Mittelman, J. (2021). Global transitioning: beyond the Covid-19 pandemic. *Globalizations*, *19*(3), 439–449. DOI: 10.1080/14747731.2021.1963201

Ong, A., & Chen, N. N. (Eds.). (2010). *Asian Biotech Ethics and Communities of Fate*. Duke University Press.

Oxfam. (2021, December 24). Rich countries have received more vaccines in run-up to Christmas than African countries have all year. https://reliefweb.int/report/world/rich-countries-have-received-more-vaccines-run-christmas-african-countries-have-all

Ozkirimli, U. (2020, April 14). Coronationalism?. *OpenDemocracy*, 2020. https://www.opendemocracy.net/en/caneurope-make-it/coronationalism.

Rogers, K., Jakes, L., & Swanson, A. (2020, March 18). Trump defends using 'Chinese virus' label, ignoring growing criticism. *New York Times*. https://www.nytimes.com/2020/03/18/us/politics/china-virus.html?_ga=2.160095540.849900311.1642494506-2061640437.1633943144

Silk, M., Andrews, D., & Cole, C. (2005). *Sport and Corporate Nationalisms*. Berg.

Steger, I. (2020, April 23). The world's baseball fans are being kept entertained by just four pro teams in Taiwan. *Quartz*. https://qz.com/1842138/baseball-fans-turn-to-taiwan-pro-league-for-entertainment/

Tsai, W., Lai, H., Chang, J., & Hsieh, J. (2020, April 13). Mask donation is wasted. *Liberty Times*. https://news.ltn.com.tw/news/politics/paper/1365493. [In Chinese]

Tsai, Y. (2020, May 14). Imagined viral communities: The global/local bionationalist war. *Reporter*. https://www.twreporter.org/a/opinion-covid-19-imagined-communities [in Chinese]

WHO. (2020, March 11). WHO Director-General's opening remarks at the media briefing on COVID-19. https://www.who.int/director-general/speeches/detail/who-director-general-s-opening-remarks-at-the-media-briefing-on-covid-19---11-march-2020

Yates, C. (2020, May 4). Thank you. https://twitter.com/clintonyates/status/1257437908614754310?ref_src=twsrc%5Etfw

Zennie, M. (2020, April 16). Missing baseball? Taiwanese games are now broadcasting in english. Here's how to watch live. https://time.com/5822240/watch-taiwan-baseball-live-free/

Zhou, Y. (2021). Vaccine nationalism: Contested relationships between COVID-19 and globalization. *Globalizations, 19*(3), 450–465. DOI: 10.1080/14747731.2021.1963202

News articles for analysis (In Chinese)

Apple Daily. (2020a, April 12). Foreign media pile in as the world watches CPBL. https://tw.appledaily.com/sports/20200412/3K3N5VPYW7CGODKBU6L5GKJ2AQ/

Apple Daily. (2020b, May 7). Yu Hsien Chu's superb skills earns comparison by US media to yankees' AARON JUDGE. *Apple Daily*. https://tw.appledaily.com/sports/20200507/ATJVLNQ2WB43SV5UPHLGEHSGX4/

Apple Daily. (2020c, May 12). Japanese media names An-Ke Lin: Taiwan's Ohtani hits home run. *Apple Daily*. https://tw.appledaily.com/sports/20200512/ONVGU7UWKGKWIWDHHMAXRCLCGM/

Central News Agency. (2020, May 9) Taiwan's national flag makes headlines in international media: Foreign media exmedia envy as Taiwan opens stadium to live audience. *United Daily News*.

Chen, W. (2020a, April 30). Manny Ramirez's manager mistaken CPBL for China professional baseball league. *United Daily News*.

Chen, W. (2020b, May 7). CPBL's 1A Ranking Sparks Debate — US Baseball: Exodus of Top Amateur Players. *United Daily News*.

Gao, Y. (2020, May 9). W. Brent Christensen Urges CPBL to be Renamed as Taiwan Professional Baseball League: Pan-Blue Politicians: Don't interfere in other Country's Internal Affairs. *United Daily News*.

Hsieh, D. (2020, May 4). Micro-propaganda moves US and Japan: Foreign media frenzy on CPBL. *Apple Daily*. https://www.appledaily.com.tw/sports/20200504/BEMWANS4H4FNYLPXR4RVWFYA2E/

Hsieh, D., Lai, D., & Wang, Y. (2020, May 8). The fans are back: Thousands enter the stadium today as CPBL urged to be renamed as TPBL. *Apple Daily*. https://tw.appledaily.com/sports/20200508/OUY3JIICI33XJPJPWUPPWHHJME/

Lan, Z. (2020, April 13). CPBL mistaken for China professional baseball league: Sheng-Hsien Feng: People will know CPBL is in Taiwan if publicity is done right. *United Daily News.*

Liberty Times. (2020a, April 14). Taiwan's exceptional success in pandemic prevention: Reuters marvels at the start of baseball and football season as scheduled. https://sports.ltn.com.tw/news/breakingnews/3133360

Liberty Times. (2020b, April 17). "Rakuten Monkeys is Taiwan's Yankees" US Correspondent's Frivolous Analogy Corrected. *Liberty Times.* https://sports.ltn.com.tw/news/breakingnews/3136848

Liberty Times. (2020c, April 19). Foreign correspondent watch CPBL: Rakuten monkeys vs fubon guardians "similar to yankees vs red sox." *Liberty Times.* https://sports.ltn.com.tw/news/breakingnews/3138261

Liberty Times. (2020d, April 19). Jin-Lung Hu achieved fastest 1000 hits but mistaken by US media for playing in China. *Liberty Times.* https://sports.ltn.com.tw/news/breakingnews/3138430

Liberty Times. (2020e, April 20). How does one survive the Wuhan Pneumonia? Orioles writer: By relying on CPBL. *Liberty Times.* https://sports.ltn.com.tw/news/breakingnews/3139017

Liberty Times. (2020f, April 24). Not objected to watching matches involving weaker teams: US fans keen on Taiwan's professional baseball. *Liberty Times.* https://sports.ltn.com.tw/news/breakingnews/3144029

Liberty Times. (2020g, April 24). What is the level of baseball in Taiwan? 30-year MLB Veteran coach comments. *Liberty Times.* https://sports.ltn.com.tw/news/breakingnews/3144030

Liberty Times. (2020h, April 26). "I'm really lucky." Feierabend Applauds Taiwan's achievement in pandemic prevention on Canadian media. *Liberty Times.* https://sports.ltn.com.tw/news/breakingnews/3145918

Liberty Times. (2020i, May 1). "Taiwan is a great country" Former Dodgers general manager happy that the world witnesses CPBL. *Liberty Times.* https://sports.ltn.com.tw/news/breakingnews/3151548

Liberty Times. (2020j, May 2). Famous even in the Caribbeans: Jing-Kai Lin's amazing skills earned him the name of "Taiwan's Aloma" *Liberty Times.* https://sports.ltn.com.tw/news/breakingnews/3152573

Liberty Times. (2020k, May 2). Taiwan professional baseball blooms: British media: A symbol of resistance to China's isolation. *Liberty Times.* https://sports.ltn.com.tw/news/breakingnews/3152541

Liberty Times. (2020l, May 5). "CPBL ranked between low-level and high-level 1A," US reporter disclosed internal evaluation of MLB. *Liberty Times.* https://sports.ltn.com.tw/news/breakingnews/3155127

Liberty Times. (2020m, May 5). KBO steals limelight from CPBL: US correspondent's apt description through meme. https://sports.ltn.com.tw/news/breakingnews/3155050

Liberty Times. (2020n, May 6). Taiwan's CPBL featured in the New York Times as "symbol of success in fighting the pandemic." *Liberty Times,* https://sports.ltn.com.tw/news/breakingnews/31559662020.5.6

Liberty Times. (2020o, May 7). CPBL introduced in AFP Article: The secret alliance that attracts foreign audiences. *Liberty Times.* https://sports.ltn.com.tw/news/breakingnews/315807320200507

Libety Times. (2020p, May 7). Taiwan's CPBL not outshined by South Korea's KBO: The reason why US fans support CPBL. *Liberty Times.* https://sports.ltn.com.tw/news/breakingnews/3157648

Liberty Times. (2020q, May 11). CTBC brothers is Taiwan's Yankees: Foreign media provides analogy for US fans to get started in CPBL. *Liberty Times.* https://sports.ltn.com.tw/news/breakingnews/3162027

Lin, Y. (2020, April 16). Wuhan Pneumonia presents opportunity: Kai-Wen Cheng's home run gives Taiwan more exposure. *Liberty Times.* https://sports.ltn.com.tw/news/paper/1366108

Lo, Z. (2020a, April 16). CPBL misunderstanding taken advantage of by China: Chih-Yang Wu: There's no problem calling it Chinese professional baseball league. *Liberty Times,* https://sports.ltn.com.tw/news/paper/1366110

Lo, Z. (2020b, April 19). Benches cleared following Sosa's hit-by-pitch as fans worldwide watch. *Liberty Times.* https://sports.ltn.com.tw/news/breakingnews/3138932

Ni, W. (2020, May 6). CPBL rated as equivalent to MiLB's level 1A: Sheng-Hsien Feng: This is unfair to the players. *Liberty Times.* https://sports.ltn.com.tw/news/paper/1370821

Su, Z. (2020, April 17). CPBL kicks off during pandemic: Times magazine: New hope for baseball fans. *United Daily News.*

Wang, Y., & Wang, J. (2020, April 16). CPBL kicks off and makes headlines on Yahoo Japan. *Apple Daily.* https://tw.appledaily.com/sports/20200416/4PWYHR6WOQI5W736RTJ7MIAV5Q/20200416

Wang, Z. (2020, May 12). Foreign media mistook CPBL as "China": Tainan councilor calls for immediate renaming for CPBL. *Liberty Times.* https://sports.ltn.com.tw/news/breakingnews/3162934

Wong, Y. (2020, May 7). World's first professional baseball with live spectator: The whole world is watching. *Liberty Times.* https://sports.ltn.com.tw/news/breakingnews/3158332

Wu, C. (2020, April 14). World's first home run this year hit in Taiwan. *Liberty Times.* https://sports.ltn.com.tw/news/paper/1365822

Wu, M. (2020a, April 15). Tseng-Chang Su calls for CPBL renaming: Chih-Yang Wu shot back: CPBL is a nongovernmental organization. *United Daily News.*

Wu, M. (2020b, April 18). The only world-class baseball tournament live broadcast with CNN also reporting. *United Daily News.*

10 Troubled Togetherness in the Pandemic

The Analysis of "Special Social Cluster" in Taiwan

Nien Hsuan Fang

Introduction

For the past two years, the World Health Organization (WHO) and governments worldwide have been urging vigilance against the spread of the coronavirus. At the same time, news media and social media act as COVID vigilantes; these actors keep calling out people and groups who behave against the new norms while a global pandemic rages. To hold people accountable to get through the pandemic together and supervise any possible outlaws are the agenda held by the media. However, as labels are attached by local government and news media, those few who seemed to defy coronavirus safety measures are prejudiced in the news. The association between certain groups and the pandemic is built, and stereotypes are thus fixed.

Taiwan has kept the pandemic well under control because of the adoption of early and effective prevention measures. Most cases of infection have been ones coming from abroad, yet the island did see an outbreak of domestic infections in the middle of 2021. On July 20, the local English news outlet only reported the latest local cases including 13 males and five females between the ages of 20 and 80, and as for the distribution of these cases, seven were in Taipei City, six were in New Taipei City, three were in Keelung City, and two were in Taoyuan City. However, most of the local news media in Chinese highlighted the fact that the two newly found in Taoyuan City were also part of the "special social cluster" (「特殊交友圈」), and there were already 16 cases found within 10 days who are involved in the same cluster. In fact, the newly coined term "special social cluster" refers to the COVID-infected gay people who interacted with each other and were found infected. The investigation of COVID infection and the daily press release on the development of infection resulting from a "special social cluster" brought the issue to the general public's attention. Precarious social gathering is warned in news headlines and the report, and the public either learned what the term conveyed, or they checked with others online about what "special social cluster" really means. For the next few months, the term "special social cluster" and its variants (such as "X men party") were used repeatedly in most news outlets. From 2020 till the end of 2021, the cases found due to the same link of COVID transmission in Taiwan may also be labeled by the government and news

DOI: 10.4324/9781003286684-10

media to identify the path of transmission as addressed in press conferences and reports. The occupation of some spreaders is revealed, and the occupation may be used to label the cluster (such as "a growing cluster of pilots"), but never has the word "special" been used before. Advocating to cut the links in the developing coronavirus transmission chain since mid-2021, the news media and the local government at the same time have fostered gaying the pandemic by using the term "special social cluster." Purportedly "factual" questions about virus transmission or epidemiology are treated as inextricably related to questions of prejudice and discrimination against homosexuals. The terms that at first adopted and used in the press conference were not the common phrases that government officials, authorities of public health, and journalists would use in their expressions in the past. The professional stocks of interactional knowledge in addressing LGBT communities in public pave the way for the modification of word use. However, the new usage still conveys a certain degree of prejudice and sensationalization in terms of social education.

Taiwan is the first country in Asia to legalize same-sex marriage as two-thirds of the legislators voted in favor of four key articles guaranteeing same-sex couples the right to marry in 2019. The movement for marriage equality is considered a conjuncture achievement rather than a necessary result of social evolution. Ho's (2019) analysis shows that a historical conjuncture takes place when different causal factors intersect at a particular moment, which gives rise to an unexpected trajectory. Favorable cultural endowments, supportive public opinion, international linkages, the certain changes in a political context, such as the electoral reform in 2008, the eruption of the Sunflower Movement in 2014, and the electoral victory of the Democratic Progressive Party (DPP) in 2016 all helped to stimulate Taiwan's lesbian and gay mobilization and fueled the legalization of same-sex marriage (Ho, 2019). A government survey released in May 2021 shows that Taiwanese people's acceptance of same-sex marriage has significantly increased to 60.4% in 2021 from 37.4% in 2018 before the country legalized same-sex marriage. A total of 5,871 couples have registered for marriage two years after the legalization of same-sex marriage. However, COVID did shadow the situation which some transnational lesbian and gay couples experienced since the Taiwanese cannot legally marry a same-sex partner in a country where same-sex marriage is not officially recognized. The challenge has been exacerbated by the COVID-19 pandemic due to travel restrictions in the past two years. For those couples whose marriages are transnational and the partner is from a country where same-sex marriage is forbidden, they experienced long periods of separation since the status cannot be warranted by marriage, and partners were not allowed to stay in Taiwan for good. The regular hosting of the largest annual pride parade in Asia and the legalization of same-sex marriage seem to paint Taiwan as a highly gay-friendly country worldwide. However, at the Taipei City Government's press conference, Taipei Mayor Wen-je Ko made controversial claims about gay people as the ones who carry responsibility for the outbreak of coronavirus among non-family members at that time. He was chastised by LGBT groups; then, leaders of the groups refuted the mayor's claims by saying that being gay does not result in transmission, high-risk interaction does. How the association of the gay community and the pandemic influenced the public's perceptions remains to be studied after the media and public figures' continual homophobic insinuation.

The research reported here analyzes the news report containing the term "special social cluster" related to the outbreak of the infection taking place in the mid-2021 in Taiwan. The scope of the use of the term and how the usage was received by the gay community are analyzed in this exploratory study. The study aims to analyze how COVID is gayed in the news report as the related cases emerged and how the association influenced social perception.

Literature Review

Visibility of Gay and Lesbian People in News Media

While the efforts instilled to "de-gay" AIDS were visible and claims such as AIDS is an "equal opportunity" virus to all were heard since the last century, the news media are the target of analyses. As a key apparatus for the dissemination of ideology and a major site of contestation over meaning buildings, the news is constantly singled out as the analysis target. In Meyers' research (1994), extensive news coverage in *The Washington Post* was generated regarding the life of ban on gay and lesbian people serving in the military proposed by the then-presidential candidate Bill Clinton. The examination of news coverage surrounding the proposed repeal showed the representation of homosexuals and the social construction of homophobia in the US then. The research findings indicate that the coverage presented a male, heterosexist discourse that reinforced homophobic myths and stereotypes. The analysis shows that in the argument, the integration of lesbians and gay men in the military is framed as a possible precursor to violence and a breakdown in morale, efficiency, and effectiveness, rather than a gesture of justice. Repeal of the ban is constructed as jeopardizing the readiness and morale of the American military in return for serving the political correctness demanded by certain interest groups. The stereotypes of gay men and lesbians being sexually deviant are activated discursively so as to convince the readers that the life of the ban would destroy the social and moral fiber of the nation. Meyer highlighted in the analyses that the lack of quoted lesbians and gay men in dispelling the myths and assumptions of the right-winged religious group raised served to sustain their doubtful images as qualified military people. The non-discriminatory social policy is thus challenged and the homophobia narrative is legitimized as the argument is buttressed by the discourse of militarism. The study conducted by Jacobs and Meeusen (2021) documents the results of a longitudinal content analysis of televised news about LGBT people with regard to representation and framing in Flanders from 1986 to 2017. The results show that although deviance and abnormality frames have decreased in favor of a rise in equal rights and victim frames, news remains negatively biased. The authors highlighted that it is imperative to have the image and voice of LGBT people in the news. Lack of subjective narratives risks reducing individuals to their group membership as the within-group diversity is disregarded. By giving LGBTs the floor to express themselves to elaborate on issues, TV audiences would get to see individuals instead of cat-egorized and stereotyped informants. To reduce prejudice and reveal the diverse nature of the LGBT community, news no longer depicted LGBT as a large and anonymous group (p. 7).

The Stress Gay and Lesbian People Experience during COVID

The prejudice against lesbians and gay men was first studied systematically by psychologists in the early 1970s. MacDonald (1976) defined the term "homo-phobia" as "an irrational persistent fear of dread of homosexuals." Kitzinger and Peel (2005) state that one of the challenges confronting the researchers studying prejudices like this has been "to define which attitudes, beliefs and/or behaviors are appropriately characterized as 'homophobic'" (p. 174). Scales to measure individual levels of prejudice are developed since then and the liberal-humanist conceptions of gay and lesbians are critiqued by Kitzinger as the shift from under-standing lesbian and gay sexuality as a sickness to the one as a lifestyle, which is no different from heterosexual men and women. Instead of targeting social and institutional structures, the liberal-humanist approach pinpoints the problem of homophobia to always lie with the individual and not the social structures through which the individual learns to legitimize the meanings they ascribed to the abnormality as Kitzinger criticized. MacBride-Stewart (2004) highlights Kitzinger's argument as Kitzinger noted that

> the attention to lesbian "health" may simply be a reversal of the historical discourse of lesbian "sickness" in which notions of the bad and sick les-bian have been merely replaced by conceptualizations of the good (happy) healthy lesbian. In this way, the production of a discourse about the healthy lesbian does not challenge the structures, apparatuses, institutions and binary relations that support the view of the "sick" lesbian. A dominant ideology in lesbian health research that remains largely unexamined is that health is a stable and achievable outcome for lesbians. For example, an understanding of lesbians "as healthier" overall than heterosexuals appears to be grounded in the belief that lesbian health is a personal achievement for overcoming the societal oppression of lesbians (MacBride-Stewart, 2001). This psychological state of achievement is regarded as producing both phys-ical and mental health.
>
> (p. 524)

As MacBride-Stewart (2004) mentions in her piece, Kitzinger talks about her re-assessing of the scientific research that health professionals and academics have done in theorizing lesbian experience, the intriguing relationship between indi-vidual psychology and social construction of gay and lesbian sexuality situated in the discourse of pandemic cannot be analyzed through the individual-biased lens. How is the concept "social" constructed as it comes to the experiences of gay and lesbian during the pandemic times as opposed to their heterosexual counterparts' experiences? Hafford-Letchfield, Toze, and Westwood (2021) analyze health inequalities and structural disadvantages faced by marginalized communities. Their paper explores the experiences of LGBT+ older people in several LGBT+ community organizations working in England, Scotland, and Wales from July to August 2020. As the result of the interviews show, some participants provided a positive narrative of social inclusion: "we are all in this together." But negative experiences also emerged as tensions, intolerance, and inequalities towards stigmatized groups. For the older LGBT+ people, rather than passive receipt of care and support, their narratives are full of strong self-agency. The participants of the study expressed highlighted intersecting discrimination based on gender and sexual identities during the lockdown. They shared their experiences of lack of trust and the findings emphasize the outreach from organizations with grassroots knowledge.

McKay et al. (2021) conducted a study collecting data from 728 gay and bisexual men from April to May 2020 to examine changes in their sexual behaviors during the first wave of the pandemic in the US. The result shows that dramatic voluntary and mandated behavioral responses among sexual minority men. Those who are most at risk (the ones with HIV) respond dynamically to new threats by adapting new coping strategies to reduce risks to themselves and others. Suen et al. (2020) study the effects of COVID-19-related stressors on the mental health of lesbian, gay, and bisexual people in Hong Kong. They pointed out that fear of getting infected with COVID-19, stay-at-home order, unstable work and unstable income, disorders of daily routines, loneliness and distress, and insufficient mental and physical healthcare services are found to be contributed to deteriorating mental health uniquely in the COVID-19 pandemic. For LGB people, family conflict related to their sexual orientation may be worsened since the lockdown confines them to stay in a not-so-friendly environment all the time and they may not come out of the closet yet. At the same time, LGBT people experience reduced connection to their communities and they thus lost the resilience resource they need most. The findings of the survey in Hong Kong showed that the depressive and anxiety symptoms of LGB people were "even more pronounced during the COVID-19 pandemic'"(p. 5). The reduced social contact with friends was a vital factor affecting their mental health. The enforced social distancing guidelines inhibit sexual minority people from socializing in LGBT+ spaces. In the findings, the LGB who were younger and with a lower socioeconomic status were found to have a higher degree of disruption in daily routine and a greater level of financial difficulty. Social and financial support to LGB people in Hong Kong is advised in the paper

Reinventing Intimacy

On March 11, 2020, the WHO declared the coronavirus disease (COVID-19) a pandemic. Severe disciplinary policies were adopted by most authorities and regulatory agencies worldwide since then in order to reduce the spread of the disease. The Centers for Disease Control and Prevention (CDC) in the US and the WHO guidance all have it that there are three main ways through which COVID-19 can spread. First, by breathing in the air carrying droplets or aerosol particles that contain the SARS-CoV-2 virus when close to an infected person or in poorly ventilated spaces with infected persons, the disease will be transmitted to the ones situated in that context; second, by having droplets and particles that contain the SARS-CoV-2 virus land on the eyes, nose, or mouth, the person will be the target of the virus. Last but not least, one will also be infected by touching the eyes, nose, or mouth with hands that have the SARS-CoV-2 virus particles on them. Science studies also have the result that infection may happen through contact with the blood, feces, and semen of a contaminated person (Cheung et al., 2020). Social/physical distancing and stay-at-home requests are issued by governments as a strategy to prevent the dissemination of SARS-CoV-2. Lopes et al. (2020) stated that as a consequence, sexual contact is thus discouraged, as it might increase the risk of transmission of SARS-CoV-2, mainly for those who do not live together. As for those who do live together, the effects of social isolation can impose variable impacts on sex life (Turban, Keuroghlian, & Mayer, 2020). Researchers highlighted the fact that studies on sexual health during the pandemic are limited and while the regulation of social distance is still enforced, the provision of counseling on sexual behavior during the pandemic is urged by the science community.

As Lopes et al. (2020) have stated in their paper entitled "COVID-19 and Sexuality: Reinventing Intimacy" for people living apart from their steady partners, they are advised to "reinvent intimacy with each other" since physical separation is the fact due to social distancing, and therefore they're advised to, except getting physically together, awaken other sources of pleasure and create new habits. Those who do not have steady intimate partners—the group that tends to be viewed as the main risk group for COVID-19—are suggested to meet new people online instead of meeting people in person. In the analysis of Lopes et al. (2020), it seems that physical intimacy is only reserved for partners' isolation together even though being confined at home with the partner may pose some unprecedented challenges to intimacy. In facing COVID, it is necessary to reinvent oneself in relating to others, as Lopes et al. (2020) have put near the end of their analysis. Since social distancing is still the best measure regulators can come up with, people have to reinvent intimacy. For the past two years, physical proximity and touch are seen with great discomfort following the advice given by the authorities of public health and physical contact has never been more discouraged. At the same time, new forms of intimacy are encouraged during uncertain times, even though the essence of the new intimacy has not been thoroughly studied yet.

Cultural anthropologist Thomas Strong may be one of the few researchers who delve into the concept of intimacy during the pandemic time. The word "intimacy" presupposes the embodied spatial imagery of closeness as indicated by Strong (2021). However, after the outbreak of COVID-19, closeness "suggests an emergent ethical rival of intimacy" since closeness suggests proximity and the nearness conveys the high risk of infection. The new ethics of proximity rewrite the conventional idea of being intimate, everyone constantly polices the social distance between himself and others so as to elicit a grid of separation. Strong (2021) in his article addressed the arguments taking place during the holiday season of 2020 in North America and Europe. The gay community was torn apart as they argued about the social media shaming of gay men partaking in parties characterized as potential "superspreader" events. The antipathy toward "irresponsible gays" has emerged even though in the broader world, other than gay people, family gatherings are visible in Europe and the States during holiday seasons. The ethics of proximity seem to discriminate against LGBT people as they are the only ones who do not move away from each other and an unfriendly gesture of breaching the solidarity in the pandemic is thus shown.

Method

The data of the analysis are twofold. One set of the data comes from news online, mainly from *The Liberty Times* (*LT*). *The Liberty Times* is founded in 1980. According to Nielsen data, the LT "had an average daily readership of 2.55 million in 2014, followed by Apple Daily with 2.45 million, the United Daily News with 993,000, and the China Times with 692,000" (Rickards, 2016, in Lynch & Yau, 2022). Therefore, the *LT* might be considered Taiwan's most popular newspaper. *LT* is aligned with the Pan-Green political parties led by the Democratic Progressive Party (DPP), the ruling party in Taiwan since 2016. The press emphasizes the local values of Taiwan and supports Taiwan's independence (cf. Curran & Park 2000). In the current study, *LT* online is the major site the news is sampled. A corpus was constructed using text from web pages. Web pages were queried and identified manually using the Google search engine with search terms related to the special social cluster. The URLs for each page were collected and the text from the associated webpages was extracted and the corpus was thus formed. Among the linguistic devices available for the analysis of *LT* News discourse, collocation analysis that identifies collocates and phrases around significant words is considered useful as the presence of recurring patterns can identify specific indicators established around words immediately adjacent to each other (Baker et al., 2013; Potts et al., 2015).

The second set of data comes from an interview study conducted at the end of 2021 in Taiwan. The researcher herself carried out eight interviews in one month and transcribed all the recorded interviews on her own due to the extremely private nature of the talks. In line with the rules of confidentiality, the analysis uses pseudonyms for all the interviewees. The interviewees consisted of eight gay men with college education, aged 25 to 35 years, born and/or brought up in Taiwan. The method of snowballing is adopted in this search for recruiting interviewees who self-identified as gay. Six out of the eight interviewees are active in gay-related non-government organizations. None of the interviewees was married at the time of the interview; half of the interviewees had a steady relationship with their partners, and the other two interviewees just broke up with their partners and were into hook-up arrangements before COVID started to spread. Two of the eight interviewees remained single. Widest possible diversity among the interviewees is not the researcher's major concern since the nature of the study is not the analysis of the reception of the news. The perceptions of how gay communities and different age groups cope with COVID and restrictions are the research concern. The governmental and media representations of the infections of gay men serve as the framework within which gay men were situated. Interviews began with a general open question: "Please tell me about your experience of personal life during COVID in the past year." The interview proceeded from there, guided flexibly by an interview protocol aimed at covering various aspects of the interviewee's experience in abiding by the rules the government set to prevent virus transmission. All the interviews were conducted in person at locations that allowed for private conversation, such as coffee shops or a university office where the interviewers felt secure. The interviews lasted from an hour to two were audio-recorded and subsequently transcribed (Table 10.1).

Analysis

News Analysis

The corpus is composed of *LT* News content with the use of the phrase "special social cluster" (Table 10.2).

Table 10.1 Characteristics of Interview's Sample

Code Band	Age	Gender	Sexuality	Living Along/with Others
SAM1	30–35	Male	Gay	Alone
SAM2	30–35	Male	Gay	With partner
SAM3	25–30	Male	Gay	With partner
SAM4	25–30	Male	Gay	With partner
SAM5	25–30	Male	Gay	With partner
SAM6	30–35	Male	Gay	Alone
SAM7	30–35	Male	Gay	With parents
SAM8	30–35	Male	Gay	With mother

Table 10.2 The Basic Statistics of the News Corpus

Number of news stories	78
Total words	32,163
Total words (without stop words)	19,076

In this study, I examined collocates, words that co-occur more frequently than normal distribution with the search term "special," in order to capture its most frequent lexical associations. The list of collocates was obtained by using the t-score statistic (which calculates the co-occurrence frequencies expected from corpus frequencies and compares this with the actual number of co-occurrences) and sorted by frequency. The procedure yielded the following results (Table 10.3).

I then categorized the collocations into groups. Clusters, infection/transmission, and cities are identified. The word "gay" was never used in the news stories, but the words such as male, member, aggregation, cluster, and social all were collocated with the word "special" throughout the news.

The search for the phrase Special Social Cluster in the *LT* corpus yielded 544 occurrences (the size of the corpus: 32,163 words, 78 pieces of news stories). There are a few other words that are interchangeably used with "special social cluster" such as Xmen, Party-Thrower (kāi pā), and Gang of men. With concordance analysis, the words before or after the keyword in the concordance line are

Table 10.3 The 25 Most Frequent Collocates of the Word "Special" within a −5 to +5 Span

	Word	Z_score	t_score
1	Social	9.32	19.964
2	Cluster	9.085	18.639
3	Confirmed	4.118	5.439
4	Reported	3.794	6.118
5	Taoyuan (county)	3.706	5.621
6	Journalist	3.664	5.7
7	Cases	3.608	4.81
8	Member	3.457	6.976
9	Aggregation	3.45	5.08
10	Chain of transmission	3.335	5.573
11	One case	3.303	4.524
12	Pandemic	3.268	4.497
13	Increase	3.082	5.386
14	Taoyuan City	3.045	4.569
15	Expansion	2.941	4.915
16	Infect	2.662	3.939
17	Local	2.618	3.837
18	Kaohsiung	2.53	3.639
19	Family	2.414	4.198
20	Outbreak	2.414	4.198
21	Today	2.376	3.345
22	Intercept	2.345	4.332
23	Male	2.338	3.433
24	Team	2.285	3.918
25	Related	2.262	3.217

"the expansion of the chain of transmission" and "youth (special social cluster)." If we check to see what words sit adjacent to the word "special" in the concordance line, other than the words "social cluster," the word "male" and city names such as Taoyuan and Kaohsiung preceded our keyword several times in the corpus. As for the words that showed up after the keyword "special," the words "gathering," "type," and "case" are the ones and these expressions the newsroom adopted accentuated the nature of the infection and transmission. Without uttering the word "gay," the newsroom still gayed the infected group by framing the groups composed of men as "special." Instead of focusing on the way that the general public may interact with each other, the newsroom focused on the people as if by nature the community carries more risks.

Among the 78 news stories by *The Liberty Times* that adopted the expression "special social cluster," the very first news story that showed up online on July 20 has the headline read as such, "Special Social Cluster" 16 Infected Tracked in 10 days! Department of Health in Taoyuan Calls for Safety Precautions on Risky Social Gatherings (「特殊交友圈」10天16確診！桃園衛生局：嚴防危險社交環境). The phrase "special social cluster" became a common expression since. On August 3, the news report used the term "alternative special social cluster" to denote an infected drug addict who passed COVID-19 to a group of people. The news did not dwell upon the sexual orientation of the infected but the negative connotation carried by the expression "special social cluster" is conveyed in the news. The news story containing the term "special social cluster" on August 5 reported on police raiding a gay spa in Kaohsiung for allegedly operating an illegal adult business and supplying prostitutes. The news was pandemic-irrelevant, but the journalist used the term "special social cluster" to indicate how the words about the newly-opened store went viral in gay communities. The newly coined expression "special social cluster" replaced the representation of all the interactions among gay people in the news and the seemingly vague expression in fact functions to demean the gay community repeatedly.

Interview Analysis

Most of the interviewees have unanimous responses to the question regarding the implications of the expression "special social cluster." As the word "special" implies that gay men's promiscuous conducts are the major cause of the spread and transmission of COVID, and then in Taiwan, interviewees responded by saying that the gay community is in fact far more resilient to illness,

> I think people in the community are more prepared for something like COVID, you know, that our sexuality has been stigmatized for almost 30 years, whether we like it or not, we as gay people are more or less weary of being HIV positive, so I think people in the community here in Taiwan has a certain immunity to COVID-19, at least more than other people because we're more aware of personal hygiene and public health, we know how to protect ourselves from viruses, like HIV, or COVID.
>
> (SAM2)

Indeed, the gay community has been stigmatized and suppressed since I can remember. Obviously, some are better informed about viruses, how it gets transmitted, and so on. For these people, COVID is just like AIDS, it's just another virus, so these people are less worried than most. But obviously, some gay people could care less about their lives. I know people who, during semi-lockdown, were still out and about finding sexual partners; but I've got nothing to comment on that.

(SAM8)

More resilient to illness as the interviewees explain, they revealed they are being anxious as the interpersonal contacts during COVID-19 are considered risky and the habit of self-monitor they acquired seems to increase their anxiety level.

Personally, I am. I work at the hospital and people tend to think hospitals are dreadful places to stay during a pandemic time. It worries me to get close to others.

(SAM 7)

I asked my ex to come over. It is risky to date someone you don't know before. But even for someone I am familiar with, I checked on him, and tried to make sure that he did not fool around before he came to my place. Variety is good, but during the pandemic time, I control myself. I don't ask for trouble.

My college friends who know my sexual orientation would ask me directly, 'do you go for hook-ups lately? Do not join our get-together this time if you do have.' I don't mind them saying that. We have known each other for quite some time, I know they're worried, and I am ok with the reminder.

(SAM 3)

And maybe it's because I work at a place where people constantly visit and seek help, they are stressed out. As for my gay friends, their anxiety level is high because, first, they can no longer have regular gym workouts. This freaks them out. They are body-conscious, and they talk about the alternative workout one can adopt at home all the time. Secondly, gay people have HIV screening tests checked regularly. But the services came to a stop during the pandemic time, it's not resumed yet. And some people cannot get the prescriptions they need then. The anxiety level is high for the ones who used to have all the support and now most of the support comes to a full stop temporarily.

(SAM 7)

I do not moralize the thing, the sex, when we have COVID-19 around. Gay people would message me privately, not in public, as they have sex-related questions. We at the mental health center provide all the needed information with the hope that you can make up your mind and have informed decisions. Now the screening information one provides at some online dating apps includes 'vaxed or not'. People get to know the partner's status, for better or for worse.

(SAM 7)

All of the interviewees are aware of the expression that gained its popularity after mid-July 2021 since the local government and media used it on daily basis. Contrary to the public's stereotypes, they talked about how LGBT communities are always keeping alert to viruses so as to rid of worries about being labeled as the black sheep. The more relaxed attitudes toward viruses are said to acquire in the past. As SAM8 puts it, the infection has little to do with ones' sexual orientation; it has more to do with the understanding of it and how one reacts to it.

I've always been a more "traditional" person, if you will, when it comes to relationships, love, and sex. Basically, I'm for monogamy. Then this NGO called "HotLine" widened my perspective on hook-ups and non-monogamous relationships. It was there that I also realized, "Oh, HIV and such viruses aren't all that scary." It's just like any type of virus. If you understand it and take the time to do so, it becomes just another part of this world we live in.

(SAM8)

However, gay people became more visible during the pandemic. Most gay people felt more self-conscious about the possibility of hostility,

If you are straight, and you got COVID, it's a personal issue. But if you are gay, you got COVID, then it becomes a gay issue and suddenly being gay becomes morally incorrect again.

(SAM2)

I personally don't mind the use of the phrase "special social clusters," because I believe those CDC officials who coined this term used it for the very purpose of not insinuating anything. This is obviously based on the fact that, from what I have gathered, they are heterosexuals who aren't as sensitive or aware of certain phrases. I mean, I think the point of using such a phrase was to hopefully dissipate the amount of public reproach. But, yes, I also get how this phrase is problematic. I mean, it's that classic misuse of the word "abnormal" or "special," whenever describing homosexuals. Like, what's so special about us gay people, and what's so "normal" about heterosexuals? In this case, it's "what's so special about our friend groups or hookups?" "What's so normal about the promiscuous sex heterosexual people are having?"

(SAM8)

The expression obscured the deeds that led to infection. The news report ascribed the practice to gay people only as if heterosexual people do not have hook-ups.

The interviewee SAM4 first learned the expression online. He described the flaming taking place at the gay-related bulletin board then, and the reposted news report on a special social cluster caught all the participants' eyes and fueled the flaming ever since. Contrary to all other interviewees, interviewee SAM4 considered the expression not malicious; it was meant to be creative and divert readers' attention to the expansion of the pandemic instead of stigmatizing gay people,

> Personally, I consider it to be a sign of progress. Government officials and media began to ponder an alternative way to report the gay-involved social issue. As opposed to the nasty terms people came up with online, such as 'venomous faggot'(毒甲), the 'special social cluster' is rather implicit, and also, the man who transmitted the virus is said to be the one who used to upload his sexual images onto Twitter before the pandemic. And as the pandemic broke out, he did not stop doing what he used to do. The word 'special' may refer to his own deeds and cluster, not his sexual identity.
>
> (SAM4)

The interviewees were not harsh towards the government and media for using the expression since the implicit expression revealed the intention to cover up the identity. And yet, gay men are not treated equally after all,

> Back in 2019, Taiwan was the first country in Asia to legalize gay marriage, at the time we were so proud that we are one of the first to value equality and love being equal. And then you have COVID, not long after the passing of the law, and suddenly we are not so equal anymore. Our actions are deemed 'special' and the clusters are […] may not convey, may not be a negative adjective (bad connotations) but still.
>
> The officials know that it's not right to finger-point gay men as they address infected people, but to use the word 'special,' the public knows who are the ones the news media implied.
>
> (SAM2)

Much was revealed about LGBT+ via mass media. Some interviewees described how people other than LGBT+ acquired stereotyped impressions about gay people and believed that gay people are promiscuous and drug-addicted,

> But straight people only know about us from TV shows, and movies, can't help to have these stereotypes about us.
>
> (SAM7)

> Obviously, it's different for everyone, I was born in 1986, and I still remember learning that homosexuals are more prone to AIDs, promiscuous people are more prone to AIDs, and things like that from watching TV. It wasn't

until college (as a bio major too) that I learned how viruses spread; It wasn't until then that I felt more at ease about viruses.

(SAM8)

And the heated debates online help to fuel the fight also,

Although homosexuals have been stigmatized since I can remember, and although the public knew about these gay sex workers through daily news; I personally think that anonymous users on the internet are more at fault. I believe they're also to blame for making the connection between "hook-ups," "COVID," and "being gay." It's not like every homosexual being has promiscuous sex.

(SAM8)

When asked how to name the infected cases as news media need to address the new cases in reporting the chain of transmission, interviewees reminded me the practices media took in the past were sufficient,

I don't think there's a need to put any kind of label. Just state the facts, the numbers. That's all you need. You don't need to make any comments or add any fancy titles. We had media naming the case by his occupation, like the pilot. Pilot as he is, the label works well for the public to know the differences among cases.

(SAM1)

Socially active or hotel-hopping? I don't think it's necessary to give labels to all the chains of transmission. The public should focus on the places where the infected cases had been to. That's all. No need to label the persons.

(SAM 7)

A study of LGBTQ people's experience during the pandemic conducted by University College London (UCL) and Sussex University found that 69% of respondents suffered depressive symptoms. The interviewees offered their observations on how the gay youth who did not come out of the closet experienced,

They are forced to stay at home, which means they are forced to be someone they are not without having a chance to take a breather. You live with people who either didn't know your sexual orientation or gender identity, or they were not supportive of it. They experience a high level of depression, but they cannot offer the use of the resources schools since all the counseling centers are shut down at that time also.

(SAM 1)

Interviewees shared their thoughts on the most vulnerable groups during the pandemic time,

Gay men, transgender communities, and the youth.

(SAM 7)

Besides gay people and the youth who did not come out of the closet, the disabled people, especially the young ones, they have a hard time socializing with others before COVID-19 hits, now it is extremely difficult for them to interact with others. For those who seek the service of sexual surrogates we provide before the pandemic prevails, now they cannot have the service anymore. Their family members would not allow strangers to come into their house and the disabled people have a hard time going to hotels.

(SAM 2)

Meeting up with others online serves as a way to reinvent intimacy. However, as an alternative to meeting up in person, a get-together online may help to change the norm of isolation, but it cannot bring the needed intimacy to lives.

I think the biggest difference between going there in person and meeting everyone online is, that you cannot just sit around and chat, take your time online. Being online always has a purpose. For example, if I go there in person to have meetings, I can see people walk by I can take my time. But I can't do any of that online. And it's not as intimate online as in person.

(SAM 6)

It's very purposeful, it's for meetings. It's not the place for hanging out. You don't stay there for chit-chat.

(SAM 7)

Almost all the interviewees mentioned the flaming taking place on the gay-related bulletin boards since the pandemic erupted. The flaming was not the exchanges among people who really know each other. Participants constantly monitored gay-related news and the posts netizens uploaded elsewhere. The constant reposting was used to evoke accusations against indiscreet gay people. The deeds and words were scrutinized to make sure people abide by certain norms of behavior, especially when sexual contact is involved.

People within our circle were very high strung about anyone in the community who might breach the regulation. Almost no one posted photos of his having sex with others. If someone did, the photos will have the captions saying something like 'it is taken at the time before 2020.' They would get told off for something they were so used to doing, something they used to get extremely positive feedback. Now everyone is on high alert.

And for the LGBT-related NGOs, the pandemic and the public opinions pose challenges to their active promotion of the prevention measures for LGBT people,

NGOs faced great challenges in reminding LGBT communities of the importance of sexual safety and the prevention of infection. The central government has high hopes for our being the ones to constantly remind community members, but the general public finger-points at us when the promotion is out there. People are harsh to our promotion, and they tend to look at it as pieces of evidence that gay people are an infection control breach.

(SAM 2)

Conclusion

Gay men are subject to a concealable social stigma. Although same-sex marriage has been legalized in Taiwan in 2019 and it is believed that Taiwan is more gay-friendly as compared with other Asian countries, the social stigma and discrimination against gay people are still obstacles to be overcome. The adoption of the term "special social cluster" by the government and news media in Taiwan in 2021 is a delicate linguistic move for some since the term helped to alert the public regarding the development of the transmission without explicitly pinpointing the sexual orientation of the infected ones. However, for most of the interviewees, the term "special social cluster" is problematic in that the use of "special" replicates the stereotypes of being abnormal. The newly coined term "special social cluster" soon becomes the expression that news media employed to convey the implication of "gay-involved" while the news even has nothing to do with COVID-19.

Throughout the COVID-19 pandemic, advocates worldwide have argued for the inclusion of LGBT people in the design of infection prevention measures. How sexual orientation and gender identity impact gay people's experiences of crisis is not static and greatly varies depending on an individual's status, such as their having a stable relationship or not. It is similar to heterosexual people's experiences; the level of complexity of interpersonal networks varies and to use identity-based categories as an analytical lens is problematic. The totalizing focus on sexual identity and ignoring the different factors that contribute to the diverse LGBT populations are how we depoliticized the category and fixed gay people in one fixed, stable, and yet unrealistic position.

References

Baker, P., Gabrielatos, C., & McEnery, T. (2013). Sketching Muslims: A corpus driven analysis of representations around the word 'Muslim' in the British Press 1998–2009. *Applied Linguistics, 34*(3), 255–278. https://doi.org/10.1093/applin/ams048

Cheung, K. S., Hung, I. F., Chan, P. P., Lung, K. C., Tso, E., Liu, R., Ng, Y. Y., Chu, M. Y., Chung, T. W., Tam, A. R., & Yip, C. C. (2020). Gastrointestinal manifestations of SARS-CoV-2 infection and virus load in fecal samples from a Hong Kong cohort: Systematic review and meta-analysis. *Gastroenterology, 159*(1), 81–95. doi: 10.1053/j.gastro.2020.03.065.

Curran, J., & Park, M.-J. (Eds.). (2000). *De-westernizing Media Studies*. Routledge.

Gailey, J. A., & Prohaska, A. (2011). Power and gender negotiations during interviews with men about sex and sexually degrading practices. *Qualitative Research, 11*(4), 365–380. doi.org/10.1177/1468794111404315

Hafford-Letchfield, T., Toze, M., & Westwood, S. (2021). Unheard voices: A qualitative study of LGBT+ older people experiences during the first wave of the COVID-19 pandemic in the UK. *Health & Social Care in the Community*. First published: 06 August 2021. doi.org/10.1111/hsc.13531

Ho, M. (2019). Taiwan's road to marriage equality: Politics of legalizing same-sex marriage. *The China Quarterly*, *238*, 482–503. doi:10.1017/S0305741018001765

Jacobs, L., & Meeusen, C., (2021). Coming out of the closet, also on the news? A longitudinal content analysis of patterns in visibility, tone and framing of LGBTs on television news (1986–2017). *Journal of Homosexuality*, *68*(13), 2144–2168. DOI: 10.1080/00918369.2020.1733352

Kitzinger, C., & Peel, E. (2005). The de-gaying and re-gaying of AIDS: Contested homophobias in lesbian and gay awareness training. *Discourse & Society*, *16*(2), 173–197.

Lynch, D. C., & Yau, C. W. (2022). What Exactly is it that the Taiwan Greens Want?: Extracting "Taiwan Subjectivity" from the Liberty Times Newspaper. *Journal of East Asian Studies*. doi.org/10.1017/jea.2021.37

Lopes, G. P., Vale, F., Vieira, I., da Silva Filho, A. L., Abuhid, C., & Geber, S. (2020). COVID-19 and Sexuality: Reinventing intimacy. *Archives of Sexual Behavior*, *49*(8), 2735–2738. doi.org/10.1007/s10508-020-01796-7

MacBride-Stewart, S. (2001) Health "in queer street": Constituting sickness, sexualities and bodies in the spaces of lesbian health [Unpublished doctoral dissertation]. University of Waikato, Hamilton, New Zealand.

MacBride-Stewart, S. (2004). VI. Kitzinger's pivotal text on the social construction of lesbianism. *Feminist & Psychology*, *14*(4), 522–526.

MacDonald, A. P. (1976). Homophobia: Its roots and meanings. *Homosexual Counseling Journal*, *3*(1), 23–33.

McKay, T., Henne, J., Gonzales, G., Gavulic, K. A., Quarles, R., & Gallegos, S. G. (2021). Sexual behavior change among gay and bisexual men during the first COVID-19 pandemic wave in the United States. *Sexuality Research & Social Policy*, (Aug 20, 2021), 1–15. doi.org/10.1007/s13178-021-00625-3[Epub ahead of print]

Meyers, M. (1994). Defining homosexuality: News coverage of the 'Repeal the Ban' Controversy. *Discourse & Society*, 5(3), 321–344. https://doi.org/10.1177/0957926594005003004

Potts, A., Bednarek, M., & Caple, H. (2015). How can computer-based methods help researchers to investigate news values in large datasets? A corpus linguistic study of the construction of newsworthiness in the reporting on Hurricane Katrina. *Discourse and Communication*, *9*(2), 149–172. https://doi.org/10.1177/1750481314568548

Rickards, J. (2016). Taiwan's changing media landscape. *Taiwan Business Topics*, March 25. https:// topics.amcham.com.tw/2016/03/taiwans-changing-media-landscape/.

Strong, T. (2021). The end of intimacy. *Cultural Anthropology*, *36*(3):381–390.

Suen, Y. T., Chan, R., & Wong, E. (2020). Effects of general and sexual minority-specific COVID-19-related stressors on the mental health of lesbian, gay, and bisexual people in Hong Kong. *Psychiatry Research*, *292*, 113365. https://doi.org/10.1016/j.psychres.2020.113365

Turban, J. L., Keuroghlian, A. S., & Mayer, K. H. (2020). Sexual health in the SARS-CoV-2 era. *Annals of Internal Medicine*, *173*, 387–389. doi: 10.7326/M20-2004

11 The Digital Divide among Women Slum Dwellers during the Pandemic

Violet B. Valdez and Samantha P. Javier

We are witnessing the first great pandemic of the digital age, set against the backdrop of a worsening digital divide. In normal circumstances, the digital divide already puts individuals and groups who are located on the deficit side of the divide at a disadvantage. It is reasonable to expect that the pandemic would pose an aggravation. In this chapter, we present the results of a study that examined the consequences of digital inequalities to women in a low-socioeconomic urban setting in Metro Manila and looked into how they appropriated the internet into their everyday life during the COVID-19 pandemic.

Literature Review

The digital divide refers to the disparities and inequalities in access, skills, and knowledge of information and communication technologies (ICTs) which lead to differentials in use, opportunities, and benefits or consequences. Dominant conceptions view the digital divide as a binary (Valdez & Javier, 2020) consisting of those who have and those who do not have ICTs. However, it is argued that this model may not adequately reflect the complexity of the technosocial dynamics of rapidly industrializing societies like China and the ICT-related development experience of much of the Global South (Qiu, 2009) where an array of low-end ICT devices, uses, applications, and practices has emerged particularly in low socio-economic settings such as slum areas and other informal settlements. Qiu (2009) views the divide more as information stratification where there are degrees of information deprivation or privilege that give rise to other categories of deprivation or privilege, notably the "information have-less," which is a broad category of low-income consumers and providers of low-end digital media products and services while Uy-Tioco (2017) has proposed the concept of "good enough" access that is characterized by limited, unequal, and constrained access to digital technologies.

The consequences of the digital divide are manifested in differentials in the quality and quantity of participation and performance in educational, political, social, and economic activities (Helsper, 2016; Quan-Haase et al., 2018; Underwood, 2009; Van Dijk & van Deursen, 2014; ITU, 2018). Limited access to digital technologies generally implies limited access to services, resources, and

DOI: 10.4324/9781003286684-11

information, and their potential benefits. Digital inequalities were starkly evident during the COVID-19 pandemic when ICTs became the dominant tool for communication, interactions, business, education, interpersonal relations, and participation in social life (Guitton, 2020). Especially during periods of forced isolation, there was hardly any alternative to the use of ICTs to deal with even the most mundane tasks. Hence, lack of access to ICT worsened the material and social deprivation of the poor during the COVID-19 pandemic. Being digitally disadvantaged, they were more at risk of contracting the virus itself and to suffer from negative outcomes related to the crisis, in general.

Digital inequalities during the COVID-19 pandemic are exacerbated, according to Beaunoyer et al. (2020), along a number of factors including physical and material access (speed of connections is dependent on the features of the digital gadget and speed of the internet connection, number of persons connecting to the internet), and social support networks (isolation requirements complicate access to support in technology use, for instance, of the elderly). Moreover, digital inequalities are bound to deepen vulnerability to COVID-19 and its consequences, first, through vulnerability to the virus itself due, for example, to the lack of access to telemedicine and low level of e-health literacy, and second, through vulnerability to the repercussions of the crisis such as unemployment, mental health issues, and access to online education.

Studies of individual and household digital divides show that the digital divide occurs along socio-demographic lines such as gender, age or generation, education, income, employment status, and ethnicity. Gender is one of the most important individual-level determinants of ICT inequalities. In 2018, the proportion of women using the internet globally was 48% compared to 58% of men, a differentiation that is evident in all regions of the world although the gap is small in developed countries, and large in developing countries, especially among the least developed countries or LDCs (ITU, 2019). This gender gap is consistent globally, varying between 11% and 19% in Nigeria, Tanzania, India, Pakistan, and Japan, with differences as high as 31% in the least developed settings (Singh, 2017). Research also shows gender differentials in internet use and skills. Women tend to use the internet for communication while men use it for entertainment, commerce, and online gaming (Hargittai & Shafer, 2006). A survey done in Ghana that examined the digital literacy of lay consumers of online COVID-19-related information found high overall digital literacy among the respondents, but men were more likely than women to have high digital literacy related to internet-based information (Abdulai, Tiffere, Adam, & Kabanunye, 2021).

Gender-based digital inequalities in low socio-economic settings have been attributed to various factors including unequal access to education among young women leading to their low literacy levels, limited institutional opportunities to access ICTs, personal safety issues in regard to access, and the leaky pipeline phenomenon, i.e., the gender difference in individuals' personal aspirations where women tend to rank work–life balance, parenthood related-issues and their family's welfare as more important than men do (Joshi et al., 2020; United Nations, 2019). These obstacles are perpetuated by structural factors such as extreme poverty and highly patriarchal societies and psychological barriers, for example, limited confidence among women in their capacity to learn ICT skills, and the belief that technology is reserved for men (Singh, 2017).

In general, research on digital inequalities especially its occurrence among poor populations is infrequent in countries of the Global South. In the Philippines, a handful of studies on this population exist. Among these is a study that shows that the mobile phone provided women a tool for performing their roles as mothers, and wives, i.e., the exercise of parental authority over their children and caring and nurturing functions vis-à-vis the children and husbands (Portus, 2008). In a study of the *Pisonet* (one peso-net), a public access ICT that is in wide use in low-income communities in the Philippines, Soriano (2019) found that users were mostly young people who used it for social networking, watching YouTube, gaming, exploring employment opportunities, and engaging in digital labor.

Research on underprivileged communities and their internet practices would present data that could challenge dominant assumptions and conceptualizations in particular those developed within affluent contexts and the context of the Global North.

Research Objectives and Conceptual Framework

In this chapter, we present the results of a study that sought to examine the digital inequalities experienced by women dwellers in a slum area in Metro Manila, the Philippines, during the COVID-19 pandemic. We examined, first, the women's profile along the dimensions of access, skills, and use. Second, we looked into the ways in which women slum dwellers appropriated the internet and integrated it into the routines of everyday life.

To examine digital inequalities, we employed the conceptualization of the digital divide as a phenomenon that involves differentials in physical and material access, digital skills, and usage. To look into how the internet was appropriated for everyday life by this unique user population, we used the conceptualization of ICTs as meaningful tools bearing social value and as a meaningful phenomenon that exists only in a particular place (Miller & Slater 2000). The social value of ICT is brought about through conscious acts of configuration, mediation, and active interpretation by social actors (Zwick & Dholakia 2004; Rangaswamy & Cutrell, 2013).

Method of Data-Gathering

This exploratory study sought to uncover broad trends and patterns of ICT-related behaviors through a focused engagement with a small sample of women within the context of the lockdowns and social distancing measures that were in place in Metro Manila in the course of the pandemic.

The study area is Ronas Garden, one of five slum communities in Barangay Loyola Heights in Quezon City. Typically, this slum community exists side-by-side with affluence. Its boundaries are defined by the peripheries of upscale-gated communities (referred to in local usage as "villages"). It can be reached from the main street through a narrow passageway about 1.8 m wide and 25 m in length. The land belongs to the Manila Electric Company (Meralco), the major electric power distribution company in the country. More information about life in the community is discussed in the findings below.

We conducted in-depth interviews, with follow-ups, of 10 women who met the following criteria: residents of a selected slum area; with a family of their own; and with access to a smartphone. As the study took place at the height of the pandemic, we refrained from conducting a face-to-face interview and instead held synchronous video interviews using the instant messaging app and platform Messenger. All the interviewees knew how to operate Messenger. Follow-ups were done through instant messaging.

Three of the interviewees also acted as key informants who provided baseline information and other data which were needed to achieve a "thick description" (Geertz 1973) of the contexts of internet use by the women such as a description of community life in the slum area. They were selected on the basis of the informal leadership positions they held in their slum community. They helped identify potential respondents who met the selection criteria and provided data, including those on living conditions, infrastructure, and available facilities, which would have been collected from observations of community life if the study took place at a time when social movement was not restricted. The semi-structured interviews took about 40 minutes to one hour, depending on the quality of the Wi-Fi connection.

The conversations with the women took place in Filipino, the national language. Filipino and English, the country's two official languages are associated with different social classes with the latter being a sign of elite status (Reyes, 2017).

Poverty and Living Conditions in a Slum

The Philippines is among the countries in Asia with a large number of urban slum dwellers. In 2010, an estimated 37% of the population of Metro Manila, or over 4.0 million people, lived in slums. The slum population was increasing at an annual rate of over 3.5%. About 32% of the slum population are poor, i.e., had household incomes below the national poverty threshold and 12% lived in extreme poverty (Ballesteros, 2010). Ballesteros (2010) describes the slum environment as follows:

> Slums are characterized by poor sanitation, overcrowded and crude habitation, inadequate water supply, hazardous location and insecurity of tenure. The people living in slums are highly vulnerable to different forms of risks — both natural and man-made. Their living conditions depict poverty in terms of both inadequate incomes and environmental deprivation. Studies show that slum poverty puts major stress on people's lives through pollution, congestion, noise, stagnant water and flooding. Households living in these poor

environs pay more for basic services (i.e., water and electricity), have poorer health status, have poorer school performance, have lower productivity and are vulnerable to crimes and violence.

In Quezon City, one of the cities comprising Metropolitan Manila, 20.6% of the city's 634,436 households lived in slum areas (*Demographic Profile and Social Development by Government of Quezon City*, 2018).

On the eve of the pandemic, in the first semester of 2018, the proportion of poor Filipinos, or those whose per capita income was not sufficient to meet their basic food and non-food needs, was estimated at 21.1% of the population. At that time, the poverty threshold was placed at an average of PHP 10,532 per month for a family of five. During the same period in 2021, the proportion of poor Filipinos had risen to 23.7%, which translates to 26.14 million Filipinos living below the poverty threshold estimated at an average of PHP 12,082 per month for a family of five. The deprivation is reflected in the housing situation.

Findings

Living Conditions

Ronas Garden has been described as the area with the worst condition among the slum areas in Barangay[1] Loyola Heights (Zakir, 2013). In a telephone interview, barangay officials said the community housed approximately 300 families with an average of three to four members. Community facilities included a chapel and a "plaza" with a half basketball court and a stage. A number of small retail stores ("sari-sari" stores) dotted the area, and there were three stations for *Pisonet* computer devices and one spot for a *Piso Wi-Fi* device. About a kilometer away is the Santa Clara Monastery, which draws a large number of Catholic pilgrims, spawning income-generating opportunities for many residents of Ronas Garden, including women and children who typically sell Sampaguita flowers and food-stuff, and men and boys who act as parking assistants.

The 10 women study participants, aged from 22 to 42 years, were living in extended families consisting of the husband, children, and other relatives, usually siblings and parents. The women had from one to four children residing with them. The majority of the women had a high school diploma; one was a college graduate. Using an income group typology devised by Albert et al. (2018), the women could be classified into poor (four women), low income but not poor (four women), and lower-middle-income (two women) households. The two women in the lower-middle-income households had husbands who earned about PHP 25,000 per month from regular formal employment and did not engage in paid work outside the house. The eight women in the low-income and poor groups were engaged in at least two types of casual work[1] to augment the family income. They typically worked as household help, as vendors at the Santa Clara Monastery, as gatherers of "kalakal," i.e., scraps, trash, and recyclable materials that are sold to junkyards, and as producers of "eco-bricks," i.e., building blocks made of solid non-recyclables. The daily household income of the low-income and poor groups ranged from PHP 100 to 600 (USD 1.9–11.5 per day). With a daily household income of USD 1.90 per day, the families of two of the women fell in the category of the extremely poor (ILO, 2021). For these women, additional support, mostly in kind, came from the government's social amelioration program and from private persons and organizations engaged in charity work in the area. Some of the women said they "owned" their houses, having bought them for a sum ranging from PHP 10,000 to PHP 20,000 while the others rented their houses or were living with their parents. Most of the houses did not have a toilet and bath and no running water. Water was bought from neighboring households that had a piped water supply in quantities defined by units of time, for instance, PHP 20 pesos for 15 minutes of use, or other units of measure such as a pail.

The pandemic brought greater hardship in particular to the families of the eight women who were engaged in casual work as they lost their sources of income due to the economic lockdown.[2] Establishments such as restaurants and offices which were the sources of the scraps and recyclable materials had shut down. Santa Clara Monastery stopped holding religious services and closed its premises to the pilgrims who bought flower and other goods. Affluent families confined themselves in their bubbles and dreaded employing casual household help. Schools and universities shifted to online learning, thus stopping the flow of clients of services such as transport via tricycle, laundry, hawker food, and the like. All the women received funds from the government's social amelioration program (SAP) emergency subsidy meant for low-income families most affected by the community quarantine measures. Occasionally they received assistance in kind such as rice and canned goods from the local government.

Some women were beneficiaries of the 4Ps, a program of the national government that provided conditional cash grants to the poorest of the poor.[3] Under 4Ps, a household with three children could receive PHP 1,400 every month, or a total of PHP 15,000 every year for five years, from two types of cash grants— health and education grants.

The women's struggle for subsistence is mirrored in the way they managed their ICT needs. In the following sections, we present the ICT profile of the women in the context of the concept of the digital divide, i.e., inequalities in access to the physical-digital tool and to the means to purchase the services and requirements of internet connectivity and their sustained use over time (van Deursen & van Dijk, 2019).

Acquiring ICT

ICT as an expense item had the least priority in the women's limited budget. Four of the women did not have a digital device when the health crisis broke out; they acquired one only in 2021, which was the second year of the pandemic. At the time of data-gathering in early 2022, nine women had a mobile phone and one had a tablet, all of which had internet capability. All the phones were smartphones of a low- to mid-range level, i.e., capable of storing apps for messaging, gaming, and social networking. No one had a desktop or laptop computer.

Since buying a phone would cut a significant chunk from the women's incomes, the women's phones were either bought on installment or were lent to them by relatives or friends. The cost of the phones ranged from USD 60 to 150. For the poorest among the women, the cheapest phone meant a full month's household income. So the cost would not eat into their usual budgets, some women used the sum obtained from the government's pandemic subsidy program called SAP or obtained a loan from an employer or a relative.

Borrowed gadgets were obtained from a relative or neighbor who specifically lent these to enable the women's children to attend online learning classes. Indeed a strong motivation to acquire an internet-ready gadget arose from the women's desire to see their children continue their schooling as all Philippine schools shifted to online learning starting the school year of 2020. As one participant remarked:

> Inutang po ng asawa ko sa trabaho po niya kasi kailangan mag-online ng anak ko. Ito po ang ginagamit namin. November 2020. Dati po nanghihiram lang po ako sa kapatid ko. Nandito lang po sa Ronas. Katabi ng bahay namin.
>
> [My husband borrowed money from his job because my child had to go online. This is what we have been using since November 2020. (Up until then) I used to just borrow (a gadget) from my sibling who's just here in Ronas. Next to our house.]

Shared Access

Shared ownership of an ICT device within the household was the norm as most of the women lived in single-ICT-unit households. They shared with their husbands and children the one gadget available for the household. A participant described her situation as follows:

> Kaming dalawa at mga anak ko ang gumagamit. Wala akong sariling cell phone. Shared phone po sa buong pamilya. Sa ngayon, ako ang madalas humawak kasi may online ako. Walang cell phone ang asawa ko. Nakiki-text siya sa iba.
>
> [Both of us, and the children are the users. I don't have my own cell phone. (What I have is) Shared phone with the whole family. Right now, I'm the one who has it most of the time because I have online-related tasks. My husband doesn't have a cell phone. He just borrows the device of others to send text messages.]

The women had priority claim for use of the mobile phone because they had to supervise and assist their children who were learning from home. They helped the children in their online classes and occasionally they communicated online with the teachers. But even if she had priority claim to the mobile phone, one of the women would leave the phone at home whenever she went out on errands or for work so the husband and children could use it.

Connectivity

Among the women it was one thing to have access to a digital device and quite another to have uninterrupted access to internet services. Intermittent and limited access characterized the women's internet access because they did not have sufficient means to purchase prepaid, much less postpaid, services that would give unlimited access for a long period of time. To obtain internet services, the women either bought prepaid mobile data services at the best bargain available, for instance, PHP 50 that lasts for about three days, shared the Wi-Fi connection of a neighbor, or switched between Wi-Fi and prepaid services depending on the speed of the shared Wi-Fi services (usually shared with an entire household and many others and hence has slow connectivity) and on whether they had the money to buy prepaid services. Another option was to use public access ICT devices such as *Pisonet* and *Piso Wi-Fi* which sell internet services in retail.

The women spent from PHP 100 to PHP 1,500 (USD 2 to 30) or an average of PHP 565 (USD 11.30) per month to buy prepaid services for their mobile phones. The cost of sharing a neighbor's Wi-Fi access ranged from PHP 150 pesos to PHP 500 per month. They usually bought prepaid cards costing PHP 50 for three days of access. Once the card was used up, they would buy a new prepaid subscription right away if they had the money. If they did not, they abstained from the internet for as long as it took for them to afford a new card, even if being offline meant that their children would not attend online classes. As one woman matter-of-factly explained:

> 'pag wala pong pang-load, hindi po sila nakakapasok.
> [If there are no funds to buy load, they are not able to attend classes.]

If the budget was too tight, what would make the women decide to place priority on the purchase of prepaid data services? One woman said:

> Nag-lo-load lang po ako pag importante lang po. Ano ang importante? Para sa school. Pag may FDS (Family Development Sessions) and 4Ps.
> [I only buy load when it's important. What is important? For school. For the FDS (Family Development Sessions) and 4Ps.]

Or, with much less money, they could continue accessing the internet through two more affordable means: the public access ICTs - *Pisonet* and *Piso Wi-Fi*. Both devices are vending machines that provide internet connectivity in retail for at least a peso for a specific amount of time. The two differ in that the *Pisonet* is a computer station that is activated by a peso coin while the *Piso Wi-Fi* gives internet access via Wi-Fi in exchange for a peso coin. In the *Piso Wi-Fi*, a peso coin is fed into the machine which then provides an access code that connects the user's smartphone to Wi-Fi. A peso gets the user about five min of Wi-Fi which may be enough to check one's Messenger and send a message. As one woman explained:

> Depende kung may pera, saka nagpapa-load. Meron namang *Pisonet o PisoWi-Fi*. Piso kada minuto. Meron isang piso Wi-Fi sa Plaza sa loob ng Ronas Garden. Dati kahit magdamag mag-Wi-Fi dahil wala pang curfew. Ngayon, patay na 'pag 10 pm. Malapit lang sa bahay namin.
>
> [It depends. If there is money, then I buy load. But there is *Pisonet and PisoWi-Fi*. A peso for a minute. There is a *Piso Wi-Fi* in the plaza inside Ronas Garden. I even used to use Wi-Fi overnight because there was no curfew. These days they shut down at 10 p.m. It's just near our house.]

There were two *Piso Wi-Fi* units and three *Pisonet* centers in the community. The *Piso Wi-Fi* units could provide internet access to as many as 30 gadgets at one time. Each of the three *Pisonet* centers was equipped with multiple workstations which added up to a total of 19 stations serving the community. Among the interviewees, three women used the *Pisonet* regularly whenever they run out of prepaid data load and needed internet access. But their use of it was restricted during the pandemic when social distancing rules and curfew were imposed forcing the Pisonet centers to close early. Moreover, the opportunities provided by *Pisonet* computers were limited because these usually were not installed with work-oriented software. Game apps were the typical software in the computers, luring children who asked a few pesos from their parents purportedly to buy food but would spend the money to use the *Pisonet*. Similar findings were obtained by Soriano (2019) (Figures 11.1 and 11.2).

A participant explained that she turned to *Pisonet* during the pandemic whenever her prepaid service ran out when she had to reply to a client of her buy-and-sell business. Another said she used it to comply with the requirements of the government social welfare agency that provided her with much-needed medicines. She had to submit the video recording that provided proof that she was taking her medication regularly.

Other Sources of ICT and Connectivity

In addition to the smartphones and the tablet for personal use, some women reported that there was at least one tablet in their households that was loaned to their children in the third quarter of 2021 by the Quezon City local government so their children could follow online lessons. To obtain connectivity, the children received a data load of PHP 150 per month which, the women said, was insufficient for the children's needs. Hence, the women were keen to obtain support for internet services. Other sources of funds for internet access were charitable organizations. For instance, the women who attended a series of talks and discussions called "Tahanan ng Panginoon" (Filipino version of "Life in the Spirit Seminar") received data subsidies on the day of the activity. Moreover, the child of one of the women received a monthly internet subsidy of about PHP 400 from a religious organization while the monthly Wi-Fi fee of one of the women was paid for by her grandfather.

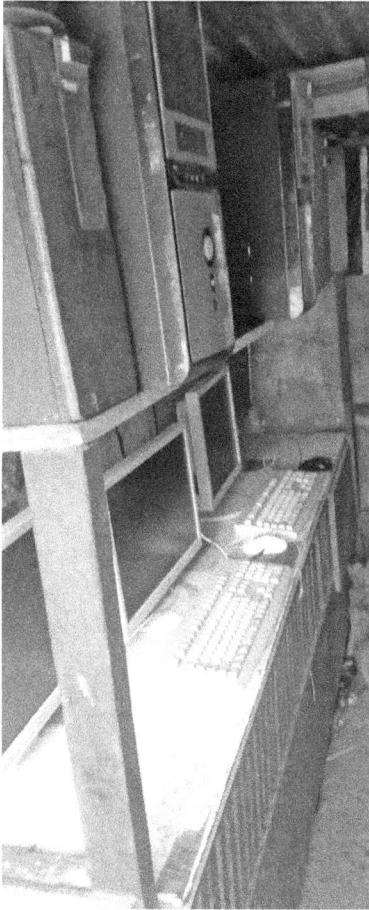

Figure 11.1 Pisonet. This *Pisonet* device, measuring about 132 × 48 cm, sits on top of a ledge, with the monitor and keyboard on the desk underneath. Eight *Pisonet* devices were operating in this alternative form of an internet café at Ronas Garden.

In general, the data suggest that contextual experiences such as income levels and living arrangements are important to understanding the methods the women of Ronas Garden used to obtain internet access during periods of isolation and social distancing.

Insufficient Monetary Resources and Access

Of paramount importance is income. Access to ICT presupposes purchasing power; the quantity and quality of access to ICT are directly related to the

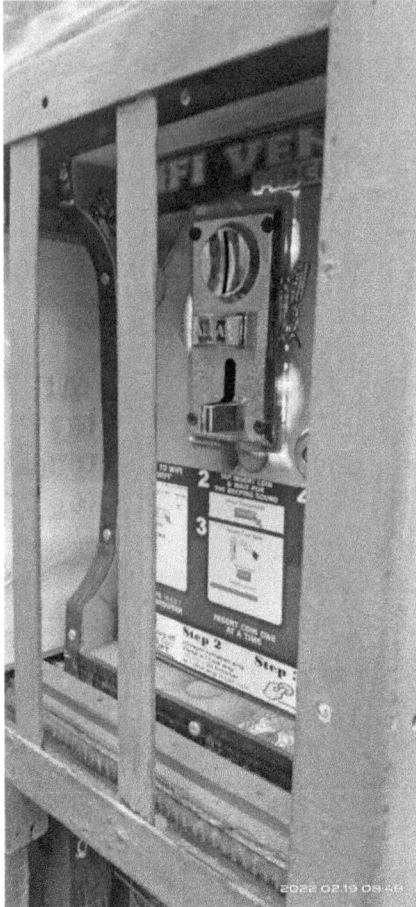

Figure 11.2 Piso Wifi. This *Piso-WiFi* vending machine operating in Ronas Garden
can provide internet access to a maximum of 100 clients simultaneously.
It is a relatively small box-like structure (approx. 28 × 20 cm) secured
in a metal casing with bars. A coin slot and instructions are displayed
prominently on the front.

strength of a user's purchasing power. One way in which the negative consequences of the pandemic impact disproportionately on the already underprivileged is through their relative inability to replace in-person communication
with digital communication (Robinson et al., 2020). We see this in the way the
women of Ronas Garden managed their ICT. Their gadgets had marginal capa-
bilities, and their access to the internet was likewise marginal—reduced to the
bare minimum, barely enough to fulfill day-to-day communication needs, much

less the in-person needs that have been replaced by digital communication such as classroom learning. Research suggests that low-income households suffer from the immediate and long-term economic consequences of the pandemic more severely so that expenses for ICT devices will unlikely rank high in their priority expenditures. The consequences of low-end ICT are explained by Bergman & Iyengar (2020):

> [...] using outdated equipment generates longer delays in accessing online resources, if accessible at all, which can create a less satisfying experience, resulting in fewer opportunities to use Internet technologies and consequently fewer opportunities to develop digital literacy skills. In contrast, more economically favored households will have a high incentive to upgrade their equipment—whether for telework, learning or entertainment. This will result in a worsening of pre-existing equipment-based digital inequalities. COVID-19-triggered home confinement creates an unprecedented Internet traffic load, which results in slower connections for multiple Internet users.

Beaunoyer et al (2020) elaborates that

> households with low incomes might not be able to afford the best connection both in terms of speed and data usage, without sacrificing essential spending. In opposition, those with the greatest Internet packages subscription will likely not experience the slower connections at the same scale. Furthermore, households with more members will have to share Internet devices, downloading data and entertainment modules (such as Netflix accounts or television decoder).

Using ICT

The user's skills level likewise influences internet use during a pandemic. The use of ICT is premised on a person's possession of a specific set of skills to achieve one's purposes. The digital skills divide refers to the gap that separates those individuals and groups who possess the set of skills needed to use ICT in beneficial ways from those who do not possess those skills.

The study participants had the technical skills to operate their mobile phones to use a number of apps, notably Facebook and Messenger, and the apps their children needed for their online classes such as Zoom and Google Meet. They used the apps to produce content for "My Day"; help their children look for materials for research projects; assist their children during online classes; communicate with their children's teachers; locate recipes and medical advice; chat with their children who were living elsewhere, and with, relatives, and friends; post news, photos, and videos of themselves and their children in Facebook and Messenger; access children's programs; watch shows (e.g., "Mukbang") and videos in Facebook and TikTok; attend meetings organized by authorities such as the Department of Social Welfare and Development (DSWD), attend religious services, discussions and training programs, and deal with customers and benefactors.

Above all, the women accessed the internet for the education of their children. A popular tool is Zoom which they used for their children's classes, and to attend a reflection and sharing activity organized by a charismatic Christian group, and chat with family members, especially those who lived out of town.

The women hardly used the internet for entertainment and medical purposes and did not use it at all for shopping, food delivery, banking, or payment of services. The two women who reported using the apps for leisure purposes said they watched news and variety shows. Those who had game apps on their phones, for instance, *Snake* and *Tom and Jerry,* said these were for their children.

The youngest among the women, a mother of two, was the only one who used the internet to access health services. She used it to set the appointment for her prenatal check-up and to consult a doctor about her husband's illness. The others were not aware of telehealth services. They did not find the need to see a doctor during the pandemic and preferred to shrug away their health complaints or self-medicate. Some said they searched the internet for treatments for minor complaints. According to them no one contracted COVID-19 in their community during the first two years of the pandemic. They attributed this to the strict entry and exit rules enforced in their community by volunteer guards.

The internet activities of the women give evidence that they were equipped with important digital skills such as the ability to communicate and interact online and find solutions to everyday problems through web-based information sources. However, the women's intermittent and restricted access to the internet prevented them from using these skills to the utmost to help them cope with the challenges posed by the pandemic. Often they had to give up on certain important activities due to lack of access as in those times when their children could not attend online classes because their prepaid data services had run out. Moreover, income-earning opportunities were missed because they were unable to sustain communication with potential employers or clients. Or, these were not explored at all.

As the women scrimped on their prepaid data services, they restricted their online activities to those which they considered most valuable—the education of their children. Online alternatives to public services such as health care, and information on work opportunities, were rarely explored. This finding shows how digital inequalities can put already disadvantaged groups at greater risk as a result of diminished social contact during a pandemic. On one hand, the women's vulnerability to the economic and health consequences of the pandemic was heightened by their restricted access to the internet. On the other hand, the internet reinforced the women's ability to cope with day-to-day life struggles brought about by restrictions in social movement, especially during the lengthy lockdown periods as they harnessed personal benefits by using it as a tool for maintaining meaningful relationships with friends and family, for accessing services that provide moral and psychological support for their daily struggles, and for leisure.

ICT in Everyday Life

With the data at hand what could be inferred about the ways in which the women slum dwellers appropriated the internet in their everyday life? We examined the ways in which the women used and integrated the internet into the routines of everyday life.

Most of the women were uprooted from their families. Some were local migrants who originated from the provinces, settling in Ronas Garden after marriage. Others were born and raised in Ronas Garden but had family members such as parents, children, and siblings who were living in other parts of the city. For all of them, the internet provided the space in which they could connect with families and so live with them in a "natural" way and enact their roles as parent, child, or sibling, and be involved in mutual support. For instance, they regularly chatted via Messenger with children or siblings who were living in youth shelters, or with parents and siblings who lived in different provinces. For one study participant, the regular chats with family members were the most important use of *Messenger*:

> Kinakausap ko ang mga magulang ko na taga-Romblon. Regular na chi-na-chat. Mga kapatid ko din, kasi malayo sila sa akin"
> [I talk to my parents who live in Romblon. I chat regularly with them. My brothers and sisters too, because they are far from me]

Similarly, the ICT provided the women a space for family bonding during the enforced isolation periods:

> Na-mi-miss ko po ang kapatid ko na nasa Cainta. Kasi minsan gusto ko silang tulungan kasi kapos sila talaga. Tapos yung mga pamangkin kong yun, miss na miss ko talaga. Minsan nag-video chat kami. Malaking tulong ang cell phone kasi kahit malayo sila nakakausap ko sila. At naiibsan ang lungkot ko [...] Kasi dati kahit saan pwede kang pumunta sa mga mahal mo sa buhay. E ngayon, bawal mag-biyahe. E sa cellphone, pwedeng magkumustahan.
> [I miss my sibling who lives in Cainta. Because sometimes I want to help them as they are really needy. And I miss my nephews and nieces. Sometimes we video-chat. The cell phone is a big help because I am able to talk to them even if they are far away. That way my sadness is relieved. One used to be able to go anywhere to visit loved ones. But now, traveling is not allowed. But on the cell phone, you can chat and find out how everyone is doing.]

Indeed for the women, the internet had a strong impact on the extended family during the pandemic as it allowed the continuation of family bonds during periods of enforced spatial separation.

Moreover, the internet provided the women a space to enact their aspirations. None of them had a profession to speak of although one had a college degree and was employed before marriage. The youngest among the participants was a Grade

11 pupil who used mobile phone apps to attend classes. She and many of the other women were enrolled in an online non-formal course in housekeeping that was run by the barangay. Invariably they aspired for better life circumstances and were convinced that this was possible only through education.

> Pinipilit ko pong makatapos. High school graduate po ako. Para hindi naman po habang-buhay nangangalakal.
> [I am doing my utmost to finish the course. I am just a high school graduate. I do not want to be gathering scraps and recyclables all my life.]

> Lahat kailangang mag-aral. Sana lahat makapag-college. Yun ang pangarap ko na gusto kong matupad.
> [Everyone has to study. I hope all of them will be able to finish college. That's my dream that I want to come true.]

Furthermore, with the churches shuttered during the pandemic, the women found on the internet the space where they could continue to give expression to their faith and enact their spirituality. As one woman who attended daily mass online said:

> Dasal lang din po ang pinanghahawakan ko sa buhay. Para din po sa mga anak ko. Sa awa ng Diyos, nakakaraos naman. Mas mahirap ngayon kasi pandemic nga.
> [In life I just hold on to prayer. That's also for my children. By God's mercy, we are able to cope. Although it's harder now because of the pandemic.]

In the structure of the Catholic church to which the women belonged, Ronas Garden was part of the Our Lady of Pentecost Parish. The parish church is about half a kilometer away from the community. While not all the women attended mass online, almost all of them attended a weekend activity called "Tahanan ng Panginoon," a program run by a Catholic charismatic movement called Ligaya ng Panginoon, described on its website as: "The Ministry of Compassion [...] focused not merely on evangelizing the faithful, but even more, on the evangelization of the poor, the needy and those in the fringes of society." The group describes its mission, thus: "We want to love God by loving and caring for the poor He has given us" (Tahanan ng Panginoon, n.d.).

Through talks, reflections, and sharing in small groups, the online gathering provided the women a space to express their frustrations in life, unburden themselves of the challenges of daily living, for instance, with husbands who were perennially unemployed or underemployed, with perennial scarcity in material goods, find support for their struggles, articulate a sense of community and neighborly compassion, and express their gratitude to God. The activity literally brought the women together whenever they would use only one device to attend it. This device-sharing happened when some of them did not have prepaid data service at the time of the activity or whenever they wanted to scrimp on the use of their data. They would gather in an open space to attend the activity and sit themselves apart from each other following social distancing guidelines.

Indeed ICT has become essential to the women's lives during the pandemic.

Ending Thoughts

The consequences of the digital divide to underprivileged communities during the pandemic are evident in the situation of the women of Ronas Garden. While the motivation to want and obtain access to the internet was strong, the women did not have the physical and material resources for reliable and efficient access that opens up to the wide range of possibilities found on the internet.

At best the women of Ronas Garden had marginal access to the internet, akin to "good enough access" (Uy Tioco, 2019) or the benefits enjoyed by the "information have less" (Qiu, 2009). The economic consequences of the pandemic are likely to have worsened the social inequalities and the disparities in internet access and skills arising from marginal access that existed even before the pandemic.

A relatively new manifestation of the digital divide was also evident among the women of Ronas Garden. All the women had access to the internet either through a smartphone or a tablet although access was intermittent and unstable due to low internet speeds. No one had access to a computer. Indeed, the smartphone, in particular, with its relatively low price, ease of operation and multiple functions, narrows the digital divide that runs along the lines of income, education, and occupation. There are, however, differences in the technical capacities of smartphones and tablets, on the one hand, and desktops and laptop computers on the other hand. While their functionalities have increased in recent years to include video streaming, mobile conferencing, and word processing, smartphones are not a substitute for desktop or laptop computers as they offer lower memory, storage capacity, and speed, and are unable to support advanced applications (Mossberger, Tolbert, & Hamilton, 2012). Hence, smartphones lend themselves more to social networking and leisure while computers are best suited for tasks or work purposes (Murphy et al., 2016). Thus, the women were missing out on important benefits that could be derived from the internet, which could be useful for the betterment of their life circumstances.

Nevertheless, the low-end ICTs that were accessible to the women—whether shared with family members or not—were of tremendous value in the time of the pandemic. Most importantly for the women, through ICT their children were able to attend online classes. The women also used the devices to communicate with their extended families and social network, to find solutions to everyday problems such as doing business and seeking medical help, and to take part in life-support activities like sharing and reflection sessions and church services.

As such the women appropriated the ICTs for everyday life in many meaningful ways during the pandemic. The internet afforded them a space for familial connectivity and for the enactment of their aspirations and their core values. Not least it afforded them a crutch for their daily struggles as they found there a space for sharing experiences of uplifting, optimism, community building, and suffering from persistent structural inequality. Ultimately in spite of access limitations, the internet provided the women of Ronas Garden with a meaningful tool for coping and survival during the pandemic.

Acknowledgment

We are grateful to Dr. Jozon A. Lorenzana for valuable critical comments at various stages of this project.

Notes

1 Barangay is the smallest political unit in the Philippines.
2 Casual work is defined by the ILO as "the engagement of workers on a very short term or on an occasional and intermittent basis, often for a specific number of hours, days or weeks, in return for a wage set by the terms of the daily or periodic work agreement. Casual work is a prominent feature of informal wage employment in low-income developing countries, but it has also emerged more recently in industrialized economies, particularly in jobs associated with the 'on-demand' or 'gig economy'" (https://www.ilo.org/global/topics/non-standard-employment/WCMS_534826/lang--en/index.htm).
3 The implementation of 4Ps or *Pantawid Pamilyang Pilipino Program*, which is based on similar modes of conditional cash transfer in Latin American and African Countries, is led by the Department of Social Welfare and Development. It "is a human development measure of the national government that provides conditional cash grants to the poorest of the poor, to improve the health, nutrition, and the education of children aged 0-18" (https://www.officialgazette.gov.ph/programs/conditional-cash-transfer/).

References

Abdulai, A., Tiffere, A., Adam, F. & Kabanunye, M. (2021). COVID-19 information-related digital literacy among online health consumers in a low-income country. *International Journal of Medical Informatics*, *145*, 104322. https://doi.org/10.1016/j.ijmedinf.2020.104322

Albert, J., Santos, A. & Vizmanos, F. (2018). Profile and determinants of the middle income class in the Philippines. Quezon City: Philippine Institute for Development Studies.

Ballesteros, M. (2010). *Linking Poverty and the Environment: Evidence from Slums in Philippine Cities*. Discussion Paper Series no. 2010-33. Philippine Institute for Development Studies.

Beaunoyer, E., Dupéré, S. & Guitton, M. J. (2020). COVID-19 and digital inequalities: Reciprocal impacts and mitigation strategies. *Computers in Human Behavior*, *111*, 106424. https://doi.org/10.1016/j.chb.2020.106424

Bergman, A. & Iyengar, J. (2020 April 8). How COVID-19 is affecting internet performance. *Fastly*, https://www.fastly.com/blog/how-covid-19-is-affecting-internet-performance. Accessed 19 February 2021.

Demographic Profile and Social Development. (2018). https://quezoncity.gov.ph/wp-content/uploads/2021/01/Eco_Profile_2018_Chapter-3.pdf

Dholakia, N. & Zwick, D. (2004). Cultural contradictions of the anytime, anywhere economy: Reframing communication technology. *Telematics and Informatics*, 2(2), 123–141. https://doi.org/10.1016/S0736-5853(03)00052-2

Geertz, C. (1973). *Thick Description: Toward an Interpretive Theory of Culture*. Basic Books.

Guitton, M. J. (2020). Cyberpsychology research and COVID-19. *Computers in Human Behavior, 2020*, 106357. https://doi.org/10.1016/j.chb.2020.106357

Hargittai, E. & Shafer, S. (2006). Differences in actual and perceived online skills: The role of gender. *Social Science Quarterly*, 87(2), 432–448.

Helsper, E. J. (2016). *Slipping Through the Net Report: Are Disadvantaged Young People Being Further Left Behind in the Digital Era?* Prince's Trust. https://www.princes -trust.org.uk/about-the-trust/research-policies-reports/slipping-through-the-net

International Labour Organization. (2021). *Statistics on the Working Poor*. https:// ilostat.ilo.org/topics/working-poor/

International Telecommunication Union. (2018) *Measuring the Information Society Version 1.01*. ITU.

International Telecommunication Union. (2019). *The ICT Development Index (IDI): Conceptual Framework and Methodology*. ITU. https://www.itu.int/en/ITU-D/ Statistics/Pages/publications/mis/methodology.aspx

Joshi, A. Malhotra, B., Amadi, C., Loomba, M., Misra, A., Sharma, S., Arora, A. & Amatya, J. (2020). Gender and the digital divide across urban slums of New Delhi, India: Cross-sectional study. *Journal of Medical Internet Research*, 22(6), e14714. https://www.jmir.org/2020/6/e14714/

MB Technews. (2021). GCash doubles user base to 40 million in one year. In *Manila Bulletin* Online. https://mb.com.ph/2021/05/28/gcash-doubles-user-base-to -40-million-in-one-year/

Miller, D. & Slater, D. (2000). *The Internet: An Ethnographic Approach*. Berg.

Mossberger, K., Tolbert, C. J. & Hamilton, A. (2012). Measuring Digital Citizenship: Mobile Access and Broadband. *International Journal of Communication*, 6, 2492–2528. https://ijoc.org/index.php/ijoc/article/download/1777/808

Murphy, H. C. et al. (2016) An investigation of multiple devices and information sources used in the hotel booking process. *Tourism Management*, 52, 44–51.

Portus, L. (2008). How the urban poor acquire, negotiate, resist and give meanings to the mobile phone. In Katz, J. E. (Ed.). *Handbook of Mobile Communication Studies*. MIT Press.

Qiu, J. L. (2009). *Working-Class Network Society: Communication Technology and the Information Have-Less in Urban China*. MIT Press.

Quan-Haase, A., Williams C., Kicevski, M., Elueze, I. & Wellman, B. (2018). Dividing the grey divide. *American Behavioral Scientist*, 62(1207). https://doi .org/10.1177/000276 4218777572

Rangaswamy, N. & Cutrell, E. (2013). Anthropology, development, and ICTs: Slums, youth, and the mobile internet in urban India. *Information Technologies & International Development*, 9(2), 51–63. https://itidjournal.org/index.php/itid /article/download/1052/1052-2949-1-PB.pdf

Reyes, A. (2017). Inventing postcolonial elites: Race, language, mix, excess. *Journal of Linguistic Anthropology*, 27(2), 210–231.

Robinson, L. et al. (2020). Digital inequalities in time of pandemic: COVID-19 exposure risk profiles and new forms of vulnerability. First Monday. https:// firstmonday.org/ojs/index.php/fm/article/view/10845/9563

Singh, S. (2017). Bridging the gender digital divide in developing countries. *Journal of Children and Media*, *11*(2), 245–247. https://doi.org/10.1080/17482798 .2017.1305604

Soriano, C. R. R. (2019). Communicative assemblages of the pisonet and the translocal context of ICT for the "Have-less": Innovation, inclusion, stratification. *International Journal of Communication*, *13*, 4682–4701. https://doi.org/ https://ijoc.org/index.php/ijoc/article/view/10931/2806

Tahanan ng Panginoon. (n.d.). *Brief History*. http://www.tahananngpanginoon.org /aboutus.html

Underwood, J. D. M. (2009). *The Impact of Digital Technology: A Review of the Evidence of the Impact of Digital Technologies on Formal Education*. Becta. http:// dera.ioe.ac.uk/10491/3/A9RF934_Redacted.pdf

United Nations. (2019). *Goal 5: Achieve Gender Equality and Empower All Women and Girls*. Sustainable Development Goals. https://www.un.org/sustainabledeve lopment/gender-equality/

Uy-Tioco, C. (2017). Transnational ties: Elite Filipino migrants and polymedia environments. In Lopez, L. K. & Pham, V. (Eds.). *The Routledge Companion to Asian American Media* (pp. 249–260). Routledge.

Uy-Tioco, C. (2019). 'Good enough' access: Digital inclusion, social stratification, and the reinforcement of class in the Philippines. *Communication Research and Practice*, *5*, 156–171. https://doi.org/10.1080/22041451.2019.1601492

Valdez, V. B. & Javier, S. P. (2020). Digital divide: From a peripheral to a core issue for all SDGs. In Leal Filho, W., Azul, A. M., Brandli, L., Özuyar, P. G., Lange Salvia, A. & Wall, T. (Eds). *Reduced Inequalities (Encyclopedia of the UN Sustainable Development Goals)*. Springer. https://doi.org/10.1007/978-3-319 -71060-0_107-1

van Deursen, A. & van Dijk, J. A. G. M. (2014). The digital divide shifts to differences in usage. *New Media Society*, *16*(3), 507–526. https://doi.org/10 .1177/1461444813 487959

van Deursen, A. & van Dijk, J. A. G. M. (2019). The first-level digital divide shifts from inequalities in physical access to inequalities in material access. *New Media Society*, *21*(2), 354–375. https://doi.org/10.1177/14614448 18797082

Zakir, S. (2013). The slum community and street vendor in Quezon City, Metro Manila: Lesson for Palembang City. *Demography Journal of Sriwijaya*, *1*(1), 4–13. http://ejournal-pps.unsri.ac.id/index.php/dejos/article/view/1

Index

For Product Safety Concerns and Information please contact our EU
representative GPSR@taylorandfrancis.com
Taylor & Francis Verlag GmbH, Kaufingerstraße 24, 80331 München, Germany

www.ingramcontent.com/pod-product-compliance
Lightning Source LLC
Chambersburg PA
CBHW060253220326
41598CB00027B/4085

9 781032 261386